SPEECH-LANGUAGE PROGRAMMING
IN THE SCHOOLS

SPEECH-LANGUAGE PROGRAMMING IN THE SCHOOLS

Second Edition

By

ROLLAND J. VAN HATTUM, Ph.D.

*Professor, Communication Disorders
Exceptional Children Education Department
State University of New York College at Buffalo*

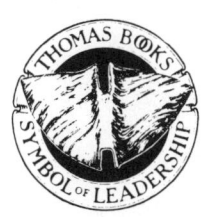

CHARLES C THOMAS • PUBLISHER
Springfield • Illinois • U.S.A.

Published and Distributed Throughout the World by
CHARLES C THOMAS • PUBLISHER
2600 South First Street
Springfield, Illinois 62712 • U.S.A.

This book is protected by copyright. No part of it may be reproduced in any manner without written permission from the publisher.

© *1969, 1982, by* CHARLES C THOMAS • PUBLISHER
ISBN 0-398-04542-9
Library of Congress Catalog Card Number: 81-8990

First Printing, 1969
Second Printing, 1970
Third Printing, 1971
Fourth Printing, 1972
Fifth Printing, 1973
Sixth Printing, 1974
Seventh Printing, 1976
Eighth Printing, 1978
Second Edition, 1982

With THOMAS BOOKS careful attention is given to all details of manufacturing and design. It is the Publisher's desire to present books that are satisfactory as to their physical qualities and artistic possibilities and appropriate for their particular use. THOMAS BOOKS will be true to those laws of quality that assure a good name and good will.

Library of Congress Cataloging in Publication Data
Main entry under title:

Speech-language programming in the schools.

Previously published as: Clinical speech in the schools. 1969.
Bibliography: p.
Includes index.
1. Speech therapy.   2. Speech, Disorders of.
I. Van Hattum, Rolland James, 1924–
II. Clinical speech in the school.   [DNLM:
1. Education, Special.   2. Speech therapy—In infancy and childhood.   3. Organization and administration.   WM 475 S7413]
LB3454.S66   1981   371.91′4   81-8990
ISBN 0-398-04542-9   AACR2

Printed in the United States of America
SC-OK-1

ABOUT THE AUTHORS

Editor

Rolland J. Van Hattum received his B.S. at Western Michigan University and his M.S. and Ph.D. at the Pennsylvania State University. He has previously held administrative posts in the schools of Rochester, New York, and Kent County, Michigan, before assuming his present position as Professor of Communication Disorders at the State University of New York College at Buffalo. Dr. Van Hattum is past president of the American Speech-Language-Hearing Association, the Division for Children with Communication Disorders of the Council for Exceptional Children, and the New York State Speech and Hearing Association. He has been a major contributor to the literature of his profession, including *Developmental Language Programming for the Retarded* and *Communication Disorders: An Introduction* among his book credits. He has received the Honors of the New York State Speech and Hearing Association and has been elected a Fellow of the American Speech-Language-Hearing Association.

Other Contributors

Thelma P. Albritton was awarded her A.B. from Greensboro College and her M. Ed. from the University of Oregon. She has previously been Associate Secretary for School Affairs for the American Speech-Language-Hearing Association and is currently Associate Professor, Speech Pathology, at Eastern Michigan University. Professor Albritton is a former Vice President for Planning for the American Speech-Language-Hearing Association and has been elected a Fellow by that group. She is a past president of the Michigan Speech and Hearing Association. Among her contributions to the literature has been her service as first editor of *Language Speech and Hearing Services in Schools.*

Delores E. Battle is currently Associate Professor, Communication Disorders, State University of New York College at Buffalo. She received her M.A. at the University of Massachusetts and her M.Sc. and Ph.D. at the State University of New York at Buffalo. She served as a Speech-Language Pathologist at the Children's Rehabilitation Center in Buffalo and was in charge of speech-language-hearing services for the Campus Learning Laboratory at the State University of New York College at Buffalo. Dr. Battle has served on many local, state and national committees as well as publishing in various journals, including *Seminars in Speech, Language, Hearing*.

Lee I. Fisher is currently Hearing Consultant for the United States Public Health Service, Indian Health Services, in Bemidji, Minnesota, after having served as Supervisor, Hearing Conservation and Education, Grant Wood Area Education Agency, Cedar Rapids, Iowa. He received his B.A. and M.A. from the University of Iowa. Mr. Fisher is past president of the Iowa Speech and Hearing Association as well as having served on numerous local, state and national committees, notably the American Speech-Language-Hearing Association's Committee on Speech, Language, and Hearing Services in Schools. He was a contributor to *Clinical Speech in the Schools* as well as authoring many other articles and presentations dealing with aspects of speech-language-hearing services in schools.

Gerald G. Freeman is Director of Special Education for the Oakland Schools, Pontiac, Michigan. He has previously served as consultant to speech-language programs in twenty-eight school districts in Oakland County, Michigan, and functioned as a visiting faculty member at eight universities. Dr. Freeman received his Ph.D. at the University of Michigan. He is a past Vice President for Clinical Affairs for the American Speech-Language-Hearing Association and has been elected a Fellow of that organization. He has served as editor of *Language, Speech and Hearing Services in Schools* as well as being a contributor to that journal, *Asha* and the *Journal of Speech and Hearing Disorders*. He was an author for *Clinical Speech in the Schools*.

About the Authors

Frederick E. Garbee is currently Consultant, Communicatively Handicapped, Language, Speech and Hearing, for the Department of Education, State of California. He was previously Coordinator, Communicatively Handicapped, Orange County, California, Department of Education. Dr. Garbee received his B.A. and M.Ed. from the University of Virginia and his Ph.D. from Claremont Graduate School. He is a former Vice President for Standards and Ethics of the American Speech-Language-Hearing Association and has received their election as Fellow. He has received the Honors of the California Speech and Hearing Association. Dr. Garbee has made numerous presentations regarding speech-language-hearing services in schools as well as serving as a panelist for the Bureau of Education for the Handicapped, the United States Office of Education. He has authored articles in the *Journal of Speech and Hearing Disorders, Asha* and *The Voice* as well as contributing to *Clinical Speech in the Schools.*

Margaret E. Hatton is Assistant Professor of Speech and is Coordinator of Clinical Practicum in the Schools for Kent State University. She received her M.A. from Case-Western Reserve University. Professor Hatton is a past president of the Michigan Speech and Hearing Association and of the National Council of University Supervisors of Practicum in Speech Pathology and Audiology.

William C. Healey is Acting Assistant Dean for Research and Graduate Studies; Professor, Department of Special Education; and Adjunct Professor, Department of Speech and Hearing Sciences, University of Arizona. He was previously Director of School Service Programs for the American Speech-Language-Hearing Association and has been elected a Fellow by that group. He also formerly was Assistant Superintendent and Director of Research for the St. Louis County, Missouri, Special School District, and previous to that he was Director of Special Education for the Missouri Department of Education. He is a former president of the Missouri Speech and Hearing Association and has served at numerous times as a consultant to the federal government. Dr. Healey has published extensively and has been a significant participant in the preparation of many publications and policies of the American Speech-Language-Hearing Association.

Oliver M. Nikoloff is Professor and Chairman, Special Education Committee, Department of Educational Psychology and Statistics, State University of New York at Albany. He received his B.A. and B.S. at the University of Cincinnati, his M.S. at Xavier University and his Ph.D. at Syracuse University. He is a former classroom teacher and school psychologist. He authored a chapter in *Clinical Speech in the Schools* and has published regarding educational psychology and special education.

Ronald K. Sommers is Professor, Speech Pathology/Audiology at Kent State University. He received his B.A. at Kent State University, his M.A. at Northwestern University and his D.Ed. at the University of Pittsburgh. He previously has been a speech and hearing clinician in the public schools and was the Supervisor of Speech and Hearing Services for the Montgomery County, Pennsylvania, schools. Dr. Sommers is a Fellow of the American Speech-Language-Hearing Association and has served that association in numerous capacities. He has contributed to the *Journal of Speech and Hearing Disorders, Journal of Speech and Hearing Research, Journal of Special Education* and several textbooks, including *Clinical Speech in the Schools.*

Rhonda S. Work is Consultant, Speech and Language Impaired, Bureau of Education for Exceptional Students, Florida Department of Education. She previously was a clinician in schools and a supervisor of speech-language-hearing programs in schools. Miss Work received her B.S. from Northwestern University and her M.A. from the University of Florida. She has been president of the Florida Language, Speech and Hearing Association and has received the Honors of that organization. She has been Vice President for Professional and Governmental Affairs for the American Speech-Language-Hearing Association and has been elected a Fellow of that organization. She has participated extensively in research in the schools and has numerous presentations regarding programming in schools to her credit.

PREFACE TO THE SECOND EDITION

The acceptance of *Clinical Speech in the Schools* as a reference for professionals functioning in school environments and as a textbook for students preparing for careers in schools justifies the efforts and the views of the authors of that book. This current revision is an effort to retain the values that book possessed but update and expand on the initial efforts. As was true with the earlier text, this book is not intended to duplicate material included in books dealing with description, diagnosis, and remediation of speech-language-hearing disorders. Information is not provided regarding the "what," "why," or "how" of remediation. Rather, the content of this offering is intended to be a practical rather than theoretical presentation of the varied roles of the specialist assigned responsibility for assisting children with communication disorders in the schools and the organizational/management responsibilities of this expert.

Some of the material may seem too basic for veteran clinicians, and some material may initially seem to have little meaning for beginning students. It is intended that each individual will draw out the level of information that is helpful for her or him. In addition to students and professionals in communication disorders, the content can serve as valuable information for board of education members, administrators, other special service personnel, classroom teachers, and interested community members in developing better understanding of the significant roles the specialist fills in the educational program and the complexities of program organization/management.

The focus in this presentation is on the concept of "program." More than "speech therapy" is needed. Well-planned, integrated, coordinated programming is essential. I have often used the example of a late fall meeting I attended in Michigan. On departure day it suddenly snowed approximately 8 inches, and a colleague remarked that he was concerned that he would have difficulty driving home. In response to my query, he indicated that he did have snow tires. I commented that he should have no difficulty then, to which he replied, "But they are bald." When is a snow tire not a snow tire? Merely labelling a clinician's activities a "program" does not make it so. Knowledge of the many factors involved, comprehensive planning, and efficient implementation are needed. This is what this book attempts to provide.

The current book includes suggestions offered by many persons in our profession. It also includes several new contributors, all well-known experts in school programming. Their willingness to take time from their busy schedules is greatly appreciated. I feel that this has significantly strengthened the content.

Acknowledgment is due Dale Bingham and Ronald Sommers for their assistance in planning the first book many years ago. Their interest and encouragement are well remembered. Also, the efforts of Charles Mange in the first text and his generosity in allowing use of his material in this one is appreciated. Christina Kane's and Sandra McDonnell's efforts also deserve thanks.

This book is dedicated to the late Myfanwy Chapman and the other pioneers who gave so much of themselves in establishing our profession in school environments. Since our profession is a relatively young one, we are fortunate that many of them still live. Hopefully all of them derive satisfaction from the recognition that their efforts have meant so much to so many.

ROLLAND J. VAN HATTUM

PREFACE TO THE FIRST EDITION

Many fine textbooks are available in the area of therapeutic handling of speech problems. This book is not intended to duplicate the material included in these books. It does not provide information regarding the anatomy of the speech mechanism, the etiology of speech problems, the descriptions of speech problems, or the remedial techniques for speech problems. In other words, it does not seek to provide the "what" or the "why" of speech problems or the "how" of therapeutic handling. Rather, it seeks to fill a gap which has existed for some time in the professional literature in the areas of program organization and management. Persons working in supervisory capacities in schools have noted, and recent graduates entering the schools as speech clinicians have reported, a deficiency in training in these areas. In recognition of this situation, many states have added a course to their certification requirements which covers this subject area. Even in states where such a course is not required for certification, it has been added to the curricula of many training institutions. This addition has created a problem in that no textbook has existed which adequately covers the information essential for such a course. True, much of the material is available, in part, in various articles and books but not in a compiled and complete manner.

The content of this text is intended to be practical rather than theoretical. To accomplish this, persons with extensive experience in the schools have been selected as authors. In fact, every author was employed in the school environment at the inception of this book. Although the finished product contains the weaknesses of multi-authored books, in that writing styles are not consistent and some of the information is restated, the book does have the strengths of one jointly authored by persons who represent over a hundred years experience in the schools, who represent a wide variety of training and experience backgrounds, and who represent a wide area geographically.

A companion benefit of this book is the opportunity for school administrators and other professional workers in schools to better acquaint themselves with the organizational and management aspects of clinical speech programs in schools.

Special mention is due Dale Bingham for his original interest in such a text and for the contributions he has made to speech and hearing programs during his many years of association with school programs. It was Mr. Bingham who, with Dr. Rolland Van Hattum and Dr. Ronald Sommers, originally conceived this book and planned the content. Although other commitments made it impossible for Mr. Bingham to participate in the final production of the book, his contribution is acknowledged and appreciated.

Several other persons made important contributions of labor and deserve mention. These include Mrs. Joyce H. Van Hattum, Mrs. Thelma Kingsley, Mrs. Judith Janus, Miss Caroline Will, Mrs. Juanita Garner, Mrs. Ruth Smith.

In this joint endeavor an attempt has been made to combine the traditional and proven with the new and promising in an effort to carry on the relatively new but wise traditions established by the pioneers in speech and hearing services in schools, many of whom still live and many of whom are still active professionally.

It is to these pioneers, with affection and admiration, and to those speech and hearing handicapped individuals we have all chosen to serve that the authors dedicate this book.

ROLLAND J. VAN HATTUM

CONTENTS

Preface to the Second Edition ix
Preface to the First Edition xi

Chapter

1. INTRODUCTION
   Rolland J. Van Hattum 3

2. THE SPEECH–LANGUAGE PATHOLOGIST AS A PROFESSIONAL
   Rolland J. Van Hattum and Oliver M. Nikoloff 38

3. THE SPEECH–LANGUAGE PATHOLOGIST AS A MEMBER OF THE EDUCATIONAL TEAM
   Frederick E. Garbee 72

4. CONSULTATION
   Gerald G. Freeman 144

5. SUPERVISION
   Lee I. Fisher 176

6. SYSTEMS FOR PROGRAM PLANNING, MANAGEMENT, AND EVALUATION
   William C. Healey 245

7. COMMUNICATION: IN THE SCHOOLS, TO THE COMMUNITY
   Thelma P. Albritton 323

8. ESTABLISHING THE THERAPY PROGRAM: CASE FINDING, CASE SELECTION, AND CASE LOAD
   Ronald K. Sommers and Margaret E. Hatton 354

9. SCHEDULING
   Dolores E. Battle and Rolland J. Van Hattum 448

10. THE THERAPY PROGRAM
    Rhonda S. Work 510

11. LEARNING DISABILITIES
    Lee I. Fisher 561

Author Index 625
Subject Index 631

ILLUSTRATIONS

Figure		Page
1-1.	Activities included in speech-language-hearing programming.	12
1-2.	Possible sources of assistance for the communicatively handicapped.	31
2-1.	Violations of professional conduct can injure public relations.	40
3-1.	Organization of the United States Department of Education.	79
3-2.	The continuum of language, speech, and hearing services for children and youth.	94
3-3.	A broad view of communication development, an alternative placement model, and an education team approach demand a fusion of educational services.	95
5-1.	Processes and activities involved in supervision.	204
5-2.	Suggested parameters for school practicum experience.	238
6-1.	Program planning, development, management, and evaluation model.	247
6-2.	Continuum of communication needs.	264
6-3.	Conceptualization of administrative arrangements for serving handicapped children.	264
6-4.	Prevalence of handicapping conditions.	265
6-5.	Continuum of services.	266
6-6.	Per pupil cost indices.	271
6-7.	Assessment and placement.	272
6-8.	Hearing process.	273
6-9.	Management-by-objectives cycle.	278
6-10.	Possible format for a Delphi Probe.	280
6-11.	Implementation steps for PPBS.	282
6-12.	Program request.	283
6-13.	Implementation calendar.	286
6-14.	Plotting personnel activities.	286
6-15.	Information needs.	290
6-16.	MIS as system coordination.	293
6-17.	Management cycle.	294

6-18.	CSRS audit cycle.	301
6-19.	The evaluation cycle.	309
7-1.	Speech-Language-Hearing Referral Form.	328
7-2.	A form for notifying parents.	329
7-3.	Progress report.	332
7-4.	Statistical summary.	341
7-5.	End of Year Disposition Report.	342
8-1.	Speech-Language-Hearing Evaluation Roster.	359
8-2.	Hypothetical schedule of high school English classes.	363
8-3.	Functional areas of language.	388
8-4.	Broward County Phoneme Development Chart.	395
8-5.	Recommended guide for providing indirect or direct speech and language services.	398
8-6.	States randomly selected to represent regions of the country and respondents.	413
8-7.	Levels of training and accreditation of respondents.	415
8-8.	Number of years practicing per region.	416
8-9.	School districts having the services of educational audiologists by region.	417
8-10.	Numbers, types, and percentages of communication disorders in school case loads.	419
8-11.	Mean and range of children having language and articulation disorders, nationally and by region.	421
8-12.	Mean and range of children having language but no articulation disorders, nationally and regionally in case loads.	422
8-13.	Mean and range of children having articulation with language disorders in case loads, nationally and regionally.	423
8-14.	Mean and range of children having articulation but no language disorders in case loads, nationally and regionally.	424
8-15.	Mean and range of children with fluency disorders found in national and regional case loads by grade levels.	425
8-16.	Average number of individual sessions per week, per region.	430
8-17.	Average length of group sessions in minutes.	431
8-18.	Average number of children seen in speech improvement classes per region.	433

Illustrations

8-19.	Percentage of usage of operant versus traditional therapy by grade level, regions, and for regions combined.	434
8-20.	A comparison of the results from the 1961 Purdue Survey, the 1976 Survey by Neal and the 1979 Sommers and Hatton Investigation.	437
10-1.	Suggested materials, equipment, and supplies.	539
10-2.	Recommendations for facilities.	543
11-1.	Two articulation curves for a single list of words.	583
11-2.	Fisher's Auditory Problems Checklist.	594
11-3.	Normative data for Fisher's Auditory Problems Checklist.	595

SPEECH-LANGUAGE PROGRAMMING
IN THE SCHOOLS

CHAPTER 1

INTRODUCTION*

ROLLAND J. VAN HATTUM

The conspicuous growth of the speech-language-hearing profession attests to the constantly increasing recognition of the importance of disorders of communication. The ability to use appropriate communication behaviors is exceeded in importance only by the ability to breathe in the life of each individual (Van Hattum, 1980). Emotional and social adjustment and educational achievement are intimately related to each individual's communication behavior. Persons with communication skills commensurate with their total abilities are better adjusted, possess better social skills, and are more likely to perform to their potentials in school environments and in later occupational pursuits then those who do not develop these skills to their ultimate potential.

Those specialists responsible for helping individuals to develop communication skills to their capacities, particularly those who aid persons with defective communication, accept awesome responsibilities. It is a credit to members of the profession serving the communication handicapped that they have accepted this challenge with an admirable degree of commitment and, in slightly over half a century, have forged a profession with efficient methodology, ever improving instrumentation and materials, professional integrity, and scientific orientation. That some much older professions have altered their courses and new professions have developed that impinge on speech-language-hearing areas is a noteworthy tribute to the truth of these assertions.

Speech-language pathologists (SLPs), audiologists, and scien-

---

*Some of the material in this chapter is based on Rolland J. Van Hattum. Speech and Language Services in the Schools, *Audio Journal*, 4, 1977. Courtesy of Grune and Stratton, Inc.

tists who function in these areas apply their skills in a wide variety of professional environments such as schools, community clinics, hospitals, universities, laboratories, rehabilitation centers, and, in growing numbers, private practice. The information in this book is primarily intended for those persons who function in school environments and seeks to present information pertaining to the organizational and management aspects of speech-language-hearing programs.

A basic premise of this presentation is that it is not only clinical skills but the *manner* in which these skills are used and the *environment* in which the skills are used that leads to the degree of success each specialist experiences. An attempt has been made to avoid proposing *the* way of functioning in recognition that too many varying situations exist to be able to apply one solution. From the information provided, each individual must provide his or her own application.

In 1969, *Clinical Speech in the Schools* (Van Hattum) attempted to provide recommendations for structuring programs in the schools. It is tempting to claim credit for the outstanding growth of programs in schools, not only in numbers, but in the level of professional competence, innovation, and commitment to scientific ideals that can now be observed. In truth, the credit is due the professionals who labor in the schools and those who have shared their experiences as teachers in colleges and universities. No other area of the profession has advanced further more rapidly than the services provided in the schools. Not only has the number and size of programs increased and the level of professional function improved, but there have been significant changes in the character of programs. As Garrard (1979) points out, the advent of Public Law 94–142, described in Chapter 3, has resulted in a significantly greater number of language disorders being included in case loads and more mentally retarded, learning disabled, emotionally disturbed, visually impaired, and physically disabled being served. Additionally, more attention is being given to earlier identification of communication disorders, learning disabilities, the effects of problems associated with auditory processing disorders, interaction with special and regular education personnel, and a wider variety of alternatives in program presentation.

Ten years ago it would not have been possible to predict the current status of speech-language-hearing services in schools. The next decade will surely bring additional changes and challenge. To be part of this rapidly developing and constantly changing profession is indeed an exciting experience! Regardless of the direction of growth, our goals should include a commitment to a "Bill of Rights for Children and their Communication Skills," briefly stated as follows:

- Every school-aged child should have her or his communication evaluated early in the educational experience.
- Each child with a speech-language-hearing difference should have that difference evaluated further to determine the potential impact on the child's social, emotional, and educational future. In this process, the importance of differentiating between the severity of symptoms and the potential effect of the problem must be recognized. It is likely that there is no such thing as a mild communication disorder.
- Each child with a speech-language-hearing difference should have a plan developed for the handling of that difference. The least action appropriate for each child should be recommendations to classroom teachers and parents and an evaluation scheduled for a specific later time to note the childs' progress and for additional recommendations.
- Each child in need of speech-language-hearing therapy should have such therapy. The exact type and amount of therapy must be left to the professional discretion of the appropriate specialist, speech-language pathologist (SLP), or audiologist, as should all decisions regarding the child's communication abilities.
- Efforts should be made to extend downward to at least three years of age the evaluation of speech-language-hearing so that preventative measures can be initiated at the earliest possible time, rather than allowing the ravishes of communication disorders to take their toll.

If we could accomplish what this "Bill of Rights" suggests in the next ten years, our society would be much the better for it, and the lives of millions of women and men would be greatly enriched.

Placing our future in perspective can be greatly enhanced by examining our past and examining our present status. Although all aspects of communication are important, the primary emphasis will be speech-language pathologists and their areas of responsibility.

A LOOK BACKWARD

Although descriptions of persons with speech problems can be found dating centuries back and, similarly, assistance for them is reported in documents preceding the Bible by some 3,000 years, the speech-language-hearing profession as an organized, scientific group is extremely young. In fact, it is only within the last sixty years that assistance has been provided the speech-language-hearing handicapped by persons specifically trained for this purpose.

Just before the turn of the present century, changing educational philosophy brought about an awareness of the needs of exceptional children. This led to assistance for the speech-language-hearing handicapped by classroom teachers and speech arts teachers who particularly recognized the debilitating effects of speech differences. No special training was required for these persons, although, at a later time, courses were offered at training centers. Originally these persons were certified only as teachers. In educational settings, the methods tended to be curricular in nature, to use instructional methods and materials, and to be best suited for large groups of children. The techniques employed frequently included breathing exercises, poetry reading, and choral speaking. These techniques were aimed at goals of general speech improvement. Because of the backgrounds of these individuals and the settings in which they worked, it is understandable that they often became known as "speech teachers." Probably this is where the idea originated that such a person should also hold certification for classroom teaching, a requirement that still persists in some localities. While knowledge of the educational process and educational environment is very important, excessive educational requirements can reduce the amount of time available for preparation in the specialized areas.

The role of the "speech teacher" was easily misinterpreted. There was confusion regarding the responsibilities of a person in such a position. The speech-language pathologist had her concept; administrators and others had theirs. The frequent remark upon introduction to the SLP was "Oh, I'll have to watch my English!" The difference in function of the newly emerging profession from that of curriculum-oriented personnel—teachers of general speech, drama, debate, and English and other instructional personnel—often had to be interpreted.

Since speech services were offered within the organizational framework of a school where the primary objective of the majority of staff personnel was classroom teaching largely involved with subject matter, it was difficult for educational personnel to understand the status of the SLP and the need for flexibility. Often, since she was a "speech teacher" she was expected to work in speech improvement in the classroom in addition to carrying a heavy case load. There was little understanding as to why the individual should be privileged to work with individuals and small groups, why her schedule was flexible, and why she did not have certain responsibilities assigned classroom teachers.

While all this was occuring, a second type of help was being provided persons with communication disorders by specialists such as psychologists and physicians. Their activities tended more towards adult patients and were characterized by the application of clinical skills relating to diagnosis, prognosis, and prescription of therapeutic needs. They functioned in hospital settings, universities, and private offices, applied their ethical codes, and dealt with total habilitation based on individual need. Many of them viewed speech and hearing as an extension of their basic professional affiliation rather than a new profession. Finally, and unfortunately, many of these persons did not view the school setting as an environment capable of supporting competent professional activity.

Between these major groups existed many variations and even other types, all providing contributions to the emerging profession. It is little wonder that from these many and diverse backgrounds came persons sharing common interests and goals for speech-language-hearing handicapped persons and yet differing markedly in ideas pertaining to causation, diagnostic techniques, methods, and program organization. In fact, to this day some of these differences exist. Fortunately, the differences are diminishing; the chasm is narrowing. Much of the credit for this is due to those individuals who had the foresight to create a national organization, the American Speech-Language-Hearing Association, the courage to discuss their viewpoints in open forum, and the flexibility to alter their views and practices based on discussion, research, and clinical experience. These activities continue to weld professional agreement, which is resulting in better understanding of role, qualifications, and function. In many respects, the speech-language-hearing profession has accomplished in several decades what other professions required centuries to attain.

A LOOK AT THE PRESENT

Although the profession is displaying remarkable progress, there is no reason for complacency. Many problems remain. Perhaps it is because of the profession's interest in accuracy of communication that the problem of a title for one of the specialists remains unresolved. The title "audiologist" for the specialist interested in hearing, its functions, its disorders, and remediation of the resulting problems has been well established. However, the person who detects, prevents, diagnoses, prescribes for, and remediates speech-language disorders still is known by many labels. Rather than attempting to establish one unified title, many persons pursue their own special interests, and these variations have led to continuing confusion in establishing a consistent title. The previous text (Van Hattum, 1969) used the title "speech clinician." The purpose at that time was to attempt to promote the school environment as a place capable of providing a clinical setting where "a highly professional manner of conduct" could occur and "whereby the speech clinician in appearance, demeanor and action, utilizes ethical conduct, enlightened judgment and skilled methods and techniques" (Van Hattum, 1969). At the present time, the need for the title is to describe the professional in the broadest sense, to use one title for all professionals, regardless of employment environment. To accomplish this it is first of all important to add the word "language" to the title. The specialist now possesses the skills to diagnose and remediate disordered language. In fact, he or she has primary responsibility for the communication skills of individuals with language disorders (phonology, morphology, syntax, prosody, semantics, and pragmatics) as well as speech (articulation, voice, rhythm). This includes children with specific learning disabilities.

Healey (1981) conducted a survey of specialists in schools regarding the title to be used. The results noted that "speech-language pathologist" was ranked first, followed, in order, by "speech-language specialist," "communication disorder specialist," and "speech and hearing clinician." Subsequent to this, the American Speech-Language-Hearing Association officially adopted the title of speech-language pathologist (SLP) to be used in all employment environments. Other terms, such as "speech-language specialist" (SLS), are acceptable and might offer advantages in various school environments. For example, some school personnel believe that "speech-language specialist" suggests interests and skills not only in the pathologies of communication but also in aspects such as development and prevention. I view this as an acceptable additional title.

In deciding on a preferred title we must be aware of the full impact. If we members of the profession are to fulfill our total mission, we must make the world aware that we have the expertise and desire to provide a full range of services to those with communication deficits. In particular, we must convince those persons who control our professional actions in some way that we are independently functioning experts, without need of prescription or outside supervision. In some instances, this may be school boards who must also understand that children cannot profit totally from their educational experiences if they do not have intact speech and language systems; in other instances, it may be taxpayers who must be aware that children cannot achieve their potentials emotionally, socially or economically, as well as educationally if they have disordered communication systems; in still other instances, it is the lawmakers and other persons responsible for planning legislation and funding.

The commonly used and often harmful label of "speech therapist" fails us with all of the aforementioned individuals because it does not adequately denote the wide range of services we provide; because it does not suggest our commitment to language and the total communication systems of the child; and because it has been considered parallel to those practitioners who depend on other specialists, usually physicians, to diagnose and prescribe for persons with disordered structure or function. The speech-language pathologist is capable of detecting, preventing, diagnosing, prognosing, prescribing for, and remediating disordered communication. This is a simple message, but it has important ramifications. There is no doubt that some few persons *are* functioning as "speech therapists." These persons engage only in limited diagnosis, work almost exclusively with articulation disordered children, and follow a relatively similar routine with all children regardless of the specific problem, the severity, the etiology, the age level of the child, interest, motivation, and other variables that should influence planning. Such persons are running the risk of having programming eliminated because of low priorities currently attached to such activities. Most professionals perform many more services than these individuals, and not only must we demonstrate this, but we must also make the decision makers clearly aware of this.

Another example of a title that leads to confusion is the New York State Education Department term "Teacher of the Speech and Hearing Handicapped." In the school district in which I reside, Grand Island, New York, the recommendations for speech and hearing handicapped are reportedly interpreted by the Committee on the Handicapped, which includes no speech-language pathologists. School psychologists, I am told, are considered to have the necessary expertise to interpret the recommendations of the SLPs. SLPs are considered teachers whose major role is direct therapy to children, not consulting, diagnosing, and planning. The official title is clearly misleading, leading to problems such as this.

The term "speech-language pathologist" (SLP) is the one that will be used as the official designation in this book. One problem with this title is that it does not reveal that the specialist has knowledge and skills in the area of hearing impairments. The SLP does assist children with hearing impairments by aiding in their detection through screening measures and by remediating deficits in their speech and language behaviors. The more complete assessment and management of the hearing-impaired child is the responsibility of the audiologist.

The road ahead is not an easy one. We have failed to sell ourselves adequately. We must inform the public of our function and our worth. A logical first step is by clearly delineating our roles and functions and describing them through an appropriate title. Of those choices available, Speech-Language Pathologist better suggests who we are and what we do. Experience suggest that continuation of terms such as "Speech Therapist" and "Teacher of the Speech and Hearing Handicapped" may lead to unfortunate consequences.

Acceptance of any title would not in itself clarify roles. The SLP must still be the interpreter of the profession. A clear understanding of the nature of the work continues to be necessary and is extremely important to the program and to those we seek to help. The SLP must have an awareness that, in any effective clinical work, insightful liaison with other disciplines becomes an integral phase. The SLP cannot afford to be in conflict with the working environment, so she must be constantly alert to the need for good public relations. She must also be cognizant of the responsibility for offering professional service that will demand the respect of the many people with whom she works—the classroom teacher, parents, administrators, nurses, psychologists, counselors, physicians, and dental specialists.

The SLP, in any school, is the one who contributes most to the acceptance, or rejection, of the local speech-language program. The school is a natural place for the SLP to function because it is here those who need not only speech-language help but also help in adjusting to the educational environment are located. The public accepts the idea that all children should be served by schools. Parents look to schools for services of many kinds, including help for children with speech-language-hearing disorders. The SLP must do her utmost to see that those in her professional environment understand her aims, methods, and qualifications.

Since the early days of speech-language-hearing programs in schools, states have continued to raise certification requirements periodically, which have resulted in increased training requirements. Specific courses have been designated as a required background for the professional person. Some states indicate maximum case loads. This has assisted the SLP in making more time available for children with speech-language-hearing problems. Some states designate the number of times an individual must be seen per week or other professional rules and regulations. However, the profession will never really come of age until professional decisions such as the aforementioned ones are left to the professional — the SLP — not to national, state, or local rules and regulations.

Working conditions have improved, and many school systems have provided working facilities specifically designed for the speech-language-hearing program. However, in many instances SLPs work in undesirable work space. If this is temporary, it can be tolerated. However, experience indicates that the success of the program is related to facilities, at least in part, and the SLP and school administration should work towards improved facilities.

In addition to the adequacy of the facilities, the efficiency in program organization and management is critical. The specialist has so many more responsibilities than providing direct services to children. Figure 1-1 presents a number of these activities that will be discussed in detail throughout the remainder of this book.

Whether the individual is a member of a large staff in a major city program or the only specialist in an isolated area, attention

CLINICAL ACTIVITIES	ADMINISTRATIVE ACTIVITIES
DIRECT SERVICES TO CHILDREN	**CLINICAL RELATED**
EARLY DETECTION AND PREVENTION	EQUIPMENT AND MATERIALS ACQUISITION
SCREENING	OFFICE/CLINIC SPACE LAYOUT
DIAGNOSIS	
PRESCRIPTION	SCHEDULING
REMEDIATION	RECORD KEEPING
RELATED SERVICES	REPORT WRITING
PARENT COUNSELING	AIDE SUPERVISION
TEACHER CONSULTATION	PRACTICA SUPERVISION
REFERRALS	**PROGRAM MAINTENANCE**
INTERACTION WITH OTHER EDUCATIONAL/HEALTH SPECIALISTS	BUDGETING AND COSTS
	PROFESSIONAL INVOLVEMENT
	PROFESSIONAL IMPROVEMENT PLANNING
RESEARCH	
PROGRAM IMPROVEMENT	POLICIES, RULES, REGULATIONS
PROFESSIONAL CONTRIBUTION	PERSONNEL ACTIVITIES
	STAFF MEETINGS
	PUBLIC RELATIONS
	LIAISON WITH OTHER AGENCIES

Figure 1-1. Activities included in speech-language-hearing programming in schools. From R. J. Van Hattum, Speech and Language Services in Schools, *Communicative Disorders, 2(4)*, 1977. Courtesy of Grune and Stratton.

should be given to these matters. Every program should have a philosophy and operational procedures. Since it is difficult to evaluate an unwritten idea or plan it is suggested that a program manual be developed. The manual should be developed by those individuals who will be affected by it. Understandably, supervisors or administrators of speech-language-hearing programs should have the final responsibility for the completed product. Federal, state, and local rules and regulations are initial determiners of policy, but the manual should contain much more than this.

Involvement of school educational personnel at the planning stages is a logical first step in the public relations program, which will be discussed later. Suggestion for specific sections should be solicited from teachers, administrators, and other special personnel. The manual should be reviewed yearly and updated as needed. It can serve as the basis for providing guidance for those using it, as a means for evaluating program effectiveness, as a vehicle in interpreting the program to administration, and as a document of understanding for persons applying for positions. In other words, each applicant should be aware of the philosophical style before accepting employment. That this is more idealistic than realistic has not escaped the author. Where possible, long-range planning is much more effective and should be used. Long-range planning enables the supervisory personnel to keep the administration informed regarding personnel, equipment, and facility needs that may best be met over time. One of the major deterrents to a successful program is the constant turnover of personnel. Those programs which appear to be most successful almost invariably have a record of continuity of personnel and planning.

A LOOK FORWARD

We live at a time when new developments occur with such frequency and so rapidly that they are a way of life. There is as much change in ten years as there used to be in a hundred years. Advancement is cumulative and rapidly proliferating. SLPs must have a zest and hunger for new things and a desire to remain current. There will continue to be new knowledge, new techniques, new equipment and materials, and new professional demands. Each individual has responsibility for insuring orderly and profitable growth, not just change.

In the schools there will be increasing recognition of the importance of communication skills and the necessity for integrating therapeutic and developmental measures into the classroom. Attempts will be made to detect deviance in communication development as early as possible and measures undertaken to prevent the development of aberrant communication patterns. While SLPs will work with fewer children, more children will be assisted through alternate means such as the use of supportive personnel or aides.

Use of Supportive Personnel

Although the practice is currently still somewhat limited, the use of supportive personnel or communication aides offers opportunity for extending the services of the speech-language pathologist. Many of the activities to this point are time-consuming. Clinicians relate many of the shortcomings in school programming to inadequate time. Thus, one important solution to improved programming would appear to be to find a way to make more time available, since the school day cannot be lengthened. The best solution would appear to be the elimination or reduction of some of the specialist's current responsibilities. In a 1976 article that appeared in *Asha*, this author (Van Hattum) advocated an alteration in the style of service delivery. It has been my concern that working year after year with primarily articulation problems led to boredom on the part of some highly skilled speech-language pathologists, which has contributed to the turnover of personnel. Further, working with large numbers of children has limited the opportunity for greater involvement in the educational environment, interacting with administration, teachers, and other professional personnel in the schools. Services to special groups, such as the mentally retarded or behaviorally different, have been restricted. It has also limited the time available for report writing, record keeping, and many other administrative responsibilities. Diagnosis, prevention, parent contacts, and interaction with professionals outside the school environment are also necessarily minimized.

Related to the need for time for administrative tasks is the need for a different look at maturation of articulation. In 1959 this author suggested "waiting for maturation" as a method of reducing the number of articulation cases. I now feel I was wrong. The importance of communication disorders and the severity of the consequences to children suggests that assistance be provided as early as possible if the child is being adversely affected by a communication difference. Thus, the need for more time and the presence of a larger population suggests a need for the availability of more clinical services.

There has been increased interest in methods for meeting this problem through the use of assisting personnel, or aides. Cofey in 1973 points out the opportunity for greater achievement by the specialist through the use of aides. Both Braunstein (1972) and Jelinek (1976) discuss the use of aides in language programming. Scalero and Eskenazi (1976) present the use of aides in a manner that appears most productive. They train aides and volunteers to work with articulation and language disorders. My personal preference is that aides be used with very specific guidance, preferably planned programs. Among the programs that have been described as successful in articulation remediation are the 1971 Neidermeyer and Helbert SWRL program for remediation of the /s/, /r/, /l/ and /th/, McKee's (1972) phonemic approximation program for correcting lateral sibilants and fricatives, the Weston and Irwin (1971) program using paired associates, the Mowrer, Baker, and Schutz program (1970), titled "Modification of the Frontal Lisp," the Stimulus-Shift Articulation Program (McClean, 1980), and the Taped Articulation Therapy (TAT) (Van Hattum, Page, Duguay, Baskerville, Davis, and Conway, 1982). The relative merits of each program will not be evaluated here. However, I will summarize the program in the preparation of which I participated.

The Taped Articulation Therapy (TAT) program is based on the experiences of the authors in developing "The Speech Improvement System (SIS)" (Van Hattum et al, 1969). The program consists of audiotaped therapy programs for remediation of the /s/ and /r/. It was developed to provide increased services more efficiently to more children by relieving the SLP of some active responsibility for children with /s/ and /r/ disorders. These programs can be administered by an untrained person referred to as a communication aide. TAT does not replace the SLP, since the clinician supervises the programs and makes all professional decisions regarding placement in, progression through, and dismissal from each program. The communication aide can be scheduled with as many as 200 children during a year, significantly reducing the cost of therapy per child.

The communication aide plays the tapes, maintains the equipment, furnishes supplies and materials, and is responsible for controlling behavior and providing reinforcement. The aide's responsibilities are limited to those described; training beyond these areas has been found to be detrimental in that confusions regarding role sometimes develop. Both Taped Articulation Therapy programs include a training program that offers practice in the skills needed to participate in one of the two sound programs. After this preparatory training, the SLP places each child in either the /s/ or /r/ program. Each program consists of three phases. Phase I, Auditory Identification and Discrimination, consists of listening exercises. The child listens to the tapes and marks a "response form" to indicate her or his answers. The response form consists of geometric designs, numbers, or pictures. Reinforcement is immediately provided on the tape by the announcer, who informs the child of the correct response. The program is planned so that most children succeed at least 80 percent in this Phase. In Phase I, each lesson consists of one specific goal and includes sixteen listening tasks. At the beginning the child judges whether his or her target sound (the sound the child is working to correct) is present or absent in contexts of increasing difficulty. The child then makes other increasingly difficult judgments in discriminating the target sound from other sounds in words, phrases, and connected speech.

If the child is judged by the SLP to have successfully completed Phase I, he or she enters Phase II, the Production Phase. This is a short series of lessons that use description of placement of the articulators and manner of correct articulation to assist the child in learning to produce the sound correctly and then produce it in the initial position in eight frequently used words. When the clinician determines that the child can produce the target sound in six of the eight words, Phase III, Stabilization, is begun. Phase III requires that the child respond orally to taped instructions and monitor his or her production. The eight words from Phase II are initially used, and these words are then inflected so that the child proceeds from the eight familiar words to an increasingly widening and more difficult series of words and contexts until conversational speech is approximated by requiring the child to respond orally to questions designed to elicit responses containing the target sound.

The Taped Articulation Therapy /s/ program consists of 101 lessons and can be presented in thirty-three sessions of approximately fifteen minutes of tape time. The /r/ program has ninety-seven lessons and can be presented in thirty-two sessions. Four sessions a week are recommended, but more or fewer can be used. Also, although the programs are designed to be administered by an aide, some SLPs report that they administer the program, or sections of it, themselves or use high school seniors.

Programs such as these that use aides provide opportunity for the speech-language pathologist to meet the needs of expanded programming. In some states use of aides is not permissible. An alternate course should be to allow each professional to make such judgments.

In addition to increased use of aides, the future will include a period of difficulty regarding professional roles, hopefully followed by a division of responsibility, which will find the speech-language pathologist with major responsibilities for all speech-language-hearing problems with increased interaction with reading specialists and with learning disabilities specialists, working cooperatively in classrooms.

New tests, materials, and equipment will be available. The SLP will have to be familiar with rapidly changing developments. Remedial articulation programs have been described. In addition, more types of equipment such as the "s" indicator* will be available. This instrument illuminates an indicator light when the /s/ is correctly produced.

---

*"s" indicator, Guinta Associates, South Hackensack, New Jersey 07606

Advances and changes are a part of any profession. They are welcomed as worthwhile signs of progress by competent individuals.

THE PROFESSIONAL AS AN INDIVIDUAL

The individual who accepts responsibility for becoming involved in altering aspects of another's behavior must develop a number of important skills. Additionally, my observation has been that many successful professionals often *bring to* the educational part of their preparation certain traits, namely, enjoyment of other persons, the ability to accept and relate to other persons, and a genuine desire to assist others. Other personal characteristics are important too, and the individual must be prepared to function in a variety of roles. The speech-language pathologist in the schools, as was noted in Figure 1-1, has an amazingly broad range of responsibilities and fills a wide variety of roles. These will be discussed later. In this chapter, attention will be given to the individual.

Perhaps the first important factor in alertness to the problems of others is the ability to look at oneself. Unless the SLP is able to find a relatively satisfactory adjustment within herself, she will be poorly equipped for helping others. She must also be constantly making new adjustments because she has to work with and through others. She will need to explore her own reaction to frustrations, her assets, her liabilities, making the most of assets and learning to lessen liabilities. She must learn to relax and face problems. Included in this self-examination must be a study of health habits and an analysis of the ability to minimize wasted time and effort.

Since the SLP's duties are largely concerned with individuals having problems, unless she can realistically examine herself and have an understanding of her own behavior, be sensitive to the feelings of those with whom she associates, and have command of techniques for handling these feelings, confidence in her will be lacking. So long as the SLP is successful, that is, manages her adaptation to a succession of situations, she will fulfill her personal needs and those of the individuals with whom she is working.

Understanding Others

The understanding of others is equally necessary. This ability aids the SLP in working effectively with those having speech-language problems. Children can seldom, if ever, be deceived about one's deeper feeling towards them. Genuineness reveals itself in warmth, kindness, and frankness and leads to rapport with children as well as with co-workers. If the child knows that his clinician is interested in him personally, respects his rights, and makes fair decisions, much can be accomplished. Such understanding and interest help the SLP realize that a speech-language difference may lead to problems of adjustment, feelings of insecurity, inferiority, frustration, or defensiveness. She will have to make every effort to help the individual overcome not only the communication disorder but also personality and adjustment problems that may be involved. Recognition of these factors enables the clinician to guide the child in a realistic examination of his needs and abilities.

Professional Relationships

Being part of an emerging profession, which is growing in recognition of its importance on the part of others and is receiving increasing respect commensurate with this expanded awareness, is not an easy task. It is a greater adjustment for some individuals than for others. Persons entering the speech-language-hearing profession appear to be dedicated, informal, and warm in their approach to others, including other professionals and the children and parents they serve. A first name basis is more comfortable for many of them. However, we would do well to observe the behavior of physicians. Opinion polls consistently show that the public rates physicians at or near the top of polls in the area of professionalism. Physicians are well aware that respect is enhanced when professional distance is maintained and when an air of slight formality prevails. Physicians seldom are observed in professional settings using first names with their colleagues, even close friends. It may seem awkward to use "Miss" or "Mister" with persons one knows well, but in appropriate situations it establishes a professional climate that may well increase the level of professional acceptance one receives. If we show respect of other professions, we should demonstrate the same level of respect for members of our profession.

If a member of our profession has a doctorate, I believe he or she should always be addressed professionally as "Doctor." It is one thing to demonstrate humility, but to me, it is more important to demand respect for one's profession. I personally use the title of "Doctor" consistently. I do so not based on my own needs but out of deep respect for my profession, recognition of its importance, and in my attempt to bolster it. If we do not respect and advance our profession, who will?

Personality and Character

Humility—Modesty

The attitude one assumes and the manner in which one conducts oneself make a considerable difference in the way what one has to offer is received. The quality of humility or modesty, defined as relative freedom from vanity, boastfulness, egotism, great pretension, or attitudes of superiority and the presence of regard for decency of behavior, in speech and dress, is an asset to any clinician. If the SLP holds herself aloof as a very special sort of person, she aids neither herself nor those she seeks to help. She should remember that no matter how brilliant and how capable she considers herself, no one will discover this if by an attitude of superiority she builds a fence around herself.

The qualities of humility and modesty help the SLP modify her assumption about her professional role to fit the image expected of her and yet remain true to her convictions. These aspects of character and personality are often shown in subtle ways; the friendly fraternizing with staff members during breaks and lunch periods, as well as at staff social gatherings, help good relationships. Consider the difference between the SLP who becomes acquainted with staff members at such times as mentioned and the one who always seeks a place by herself during such periods with the excuse, "I don't like coffee, so I don't join the group."

Schools may have fund-raising affairs (such as school carnivals) for equipment, books, and other school supplies. Classroom teachers are usually asked to participate in these activities. The SLP who graciously offers to help and cooperate in whatever capacity she can is usually well received. Co-workers in the schools appreciate the SLP's involvement in such causes.

In any school setting, it is important to abide by rules and regulations set up for other staff members, as far as an itinerant schedule will permit. Usually staff members are expected to arrive at work at designated hours. The SLP should observe such rules. Occasionally circumstances make it imperative for the SLP to be off schedule. At such times she should explain this to persons involved. Principals appreciate knowing when exceptions to regular schedules are necessary. School systems differ in what is expected of staff members, but behavior such as suggested helps the clinician's relationships in the schools that she serves.

SLPs have become increasingly interested in nonverbal communication. The myriad ways in which we communicate include our appearance, our demeanor, and our various behaviors. With our knowledge of nonverbal communication, no one should be more aware that "clothes makes the man" (and woman) than each member of our profession. The manner in which we clothe ourselves is a very specific form of communication. It tells those who observe us how we feel about who we are and how we feel about our profession. Commentators reporting on Olympic events, figure skating for example, will often note that the judges' evaluation of a figure skater is due, in part, to the figure skater's previous reputation. As a young profession we do not have an established reputation, and we do have to try harder than more established professions. Our professionalism must be beyond reproach. If we are to attain our correct position among the professions we must be aware that our appearance and our actions are important. Further, we not only represent ourselves, each of us represents the entire profession. While members of the general public may know several physicians or dentists, they often know only one SLP and judge the entire profession based on their views of that single individual. Each of us must endeavor to appear "professional" at all times, particularly during our working hours. It is difficult to describe specific appropriate dress, since it varies by custom, location, and climate. However, dress should be consistent with professional standards in each community. Some persons have suggested that advice on how to dress is a violation of personal liberties. However, the person who becomes a part of a profession has an obligation both to herself and to the profession. The messages we send must be consistent with our charge.

A well-modulated voice adds to one's attractiveness. Also, there are many correct ways of behaving in almost any situation, so there is little reason for neglecting small courtesies. It is often surprising how seemingly insignificant courteous acts are noted and commented upon. One SLP was well regarded because of her careful attention to rising when guests entered her office, and another was censured because he failed to remove his hat on entering the building. All the things mentioned, although considered trivial by some, may make a difference in the acceptance or rejection of a person in a position such as the SLP holds.

Honesty

A necessary aspect of character and personality expected in persons to whom one turns for help is honesty. It reveals itself in many ways. Frankness, tempered by tactfulness, may be one way; truthfulness and trustworthiness are others. Fairness in all dealings and loyalty to those with whom one works are still further indications of this trait.

Honesty demands that the SLP examine her prejudices. Persons working in schools do not deal with select populations. The SLP working in the schools is not in a position to give service to one at the exclusion of another without defending the choice made. She should always realistically deal with what she is going to have to face. When she chooses to work in schools, she needs to be aware that she will find children and youths who came from varying socioeconomic backgrounds, attractive as well as less attractive children, some with high intelligence as well as those with lower intelligence. She will be dealing with the needs of children of all races and creeds. Some will be multiply handicapped. Professionals who work in large urban areas may face a greater range of differences than those in smaller communities, and some will have to carry on work with children from less privileged areas than others. Adjustment will have to be made to differences in parental cooperation and understanding. In some homes there is a constant state of tension, troublesome economic circumstances, dissension, and in some cases, broken homes. It is the responsibility of the SLP to modify tension to the best of her ability. In situations where there are working parents, special arrangements to confer with these parents may have to be made outside of regular working hours.

There is a need for acceptance and fairness to all, as each is an individual in his own right. The effort put forth must be as great for one as for another. The SLP should realize that some children have poor self-images. Some are aware of parental rejection. Clinicians who are strong, firm, and accepting create a feeling of security in children and give them increased satisfaction. Children feel more adequate, secure and comfortable. No clinician can afford to display strong likes and dislikes. Children are particularly sensitive to attitude. As noted in Chapter 2, listening is one of the important things the SLP can do. She can give support in a variety of ways. She should acknowledge people's strong feelings, and she should credit all with possessing human dignity. A child cannot be helped until the clinician has observed him. The SLP should look for the positive things in the child and point them out. There is a difference between tolerating and accepting. Each child should be given reassurance. The way in which this is done is important. Providing an example of fairness, firmness, and friendliness is one of the best ways to attain this objective. Reality sets limits. The SLP is wise not to become overly attached or emotionally involved. Better clinical work can be done without excessive emotional involvement.

If the SLP deals honestly and realistically with problems, facing up to what is good for the child and what will help him get along better, she will occasionally have to admit, "I don't know the answer right now," recognizing that there are certain things she cannot do. She is a better clinician if she recognizes and honestly admits her limitations. She must realize that there are circumstances in the life of the individual with whom she works that, though she wants very much to do something to help, make her sometimes accept slow gains and occasional failures. The important thing is that she honestly tries to find answers and does not give up because the challenge seems too great.

While there are no hard and fast rules regarding dismissing a child from speech-language therapy, the SLP should give considerable thought for discontinuing the work with any given child. She must objectively weigh all aspects to determine whether personal reasons (such as inability to understand the child and cope with his behavior, a feeling of inadequacy in coping with the specific speech-language problem involved, or even an actual dislike for the child in question) are reasons, or whether it is truly for the welfare of the child. Consider the reaction of those concerned in the following: Tommy had caused considerable disturbance in the small speech group to which he belonged. He very much needed speech therapy, but without conference with the classroom teacher, principal, or parents, the clinician sent a note to the teacher saying, "Tommy creates too much trouble in the speech group. Don't send him anymore." One can easily imagine the results of this type of handling of a problem and no doubt agree that the element of honest evaluation by the SLP, as well as professional responsibility, was completely lacking.

This SLP might have asked herself these questions: What are my feelings about this child? Do I dislike this child? Is it a temporary dislike? What are my feelings about my inability to cope with this? Did I ever talk with the child, try to become acquainted when others were not present? Does my handling of this child relate to any prejudices I have? Do I object to working in this particular school district? Am I tolerating or really accepting? What did I do to encourage the self-reliance and initiative in this child? Did I try to draw him out and get his ideas? Was I inclined to scold too much? How did this child behave in other situations?

Sense of Humor

The ability to see humor in a situation will not only tide one over many rough spots but certainly will be a salvation to those with whom one associates. Each day one becomes more aware of the importance and value of humor. It will aid one in appreciating many things that happen during the course of a day and will create the good will necessary to successful therapy. Obviously, this does not mean that the SLP should be a buffoon. A clown may be loved, but his judgment is usually not respected. Producing a smile or a laugh at appropriate times and with appropriate frequency is a sign of a well-rounded personality.

Patience

The SLP frequently hears the comment, "I think it would take so much patience to do the work you are doing." Patience is an essential quality in a clinician. Many times it takes infinite patience and calmness. The SLP is often called upon to help those whose improvement is slow and laborious, or possibly one who is multiply handicapped, or who has become frustrated because of inability to communicate adequately. In clinical work one will experience times when she exerts every effort to help a particular individual, yet a feeling of success eludes her. Sometimes she is dealing with an individual who cannot allow the clinician to know she is succeeding. In such an event, the clinician needs to realize that emotional first aid and other therapy are often slow processes. She must not be easily discouraged. The SLP never knows how much of herself she leaves.

Imagination, Creativeness, and Originality

Imagination, creativeness, and originality are all traits of the SLP that contribute to more effective therapy. There are many books and other resource materials available to those doing speech-language therapy, but the SLP must be adept in applying these to particular cases. It is also important for her to be able to draw upon her own resources, for often the material available does not meet the particular needs of the child or youth with whom she is working. The separateness and uniqueness of each human being calls upon the clinician's resourcefulness. There are no stereotyped methods that will apply. Her curiosity and imagination should lead her into developing ideas and materials that will often far surpass those already available and force her to see what she can work out to meet the needs of her clients. She may feel that she does not have skill in creative work, but upon putting forth effort she may surprise herself. Interest in the needs of others should provide the incentive.

Guides that present various phases of the clinical speech-language program, brochures that deal with it, and bulletins offering suggestions for helping the speech-language handicapped individual in the home and in the classroom all appeal to the creative imagination of the clinician and may become very useful tools in phases of therapy.

Resourcefulness

Resourcefulness is another personality trait observed in the successful SLP. It is demonstrated in her ability to hold the interest of those in therapy and maintain an atmosphere of alertness, good humor, and pleasant give-and-take conducive to harmonious, friendly, and pleasing relations. She needs to study the cause-and-effect relationship between procedures and results. The SLP must allow opportunities for expression of a variety of feelings and release of the child's energy in constructive ways. She needs to become acquainted with resource materials, which often provide clues for therapy. A study of learning principles, concepts, and behavior theories that have been applied to communication behavior is one source. Understanding the application of these and experimenting with various methods will help her find ways of promoting and maintaining the child's interest and drive to achieve. It is helpful to be knowledgeable about the disciplines and theories of learning. The SLP will have to decide whether individual or group therapy is indicated in planning a program for each child.

Group therapy requires considerable resourcefulness on the part of the clinician, since the desire for group approval is so prevalent under these circumstances. It takes careful handling so that competition does not discourage those with lower ability. The SLP needs to find ways for self-competition, that is, helping the child learn to compete with his own performance and record and thus gain approval. Clever handling will allow the child to have a balance of success and failure. One cannot always succeed; neither can one always fail. He must be helped to accept realities of self—his strengths and his needs. Sometimes lack of success needs to be evaluated. Apropos here might be the comment made by Edison when confronted with the statement, "You have failed a thousand times." "No," he answered, "I've only found a thousand ways not to do a thing." Variation in therapy procedures, provision for new experiences, and the use of differing media to promote various aspects of treatment challenge the resourcefulness of the clinician. The SLP needs to recognize that the motivational force that exerts the greatest influence is not the same for all children, for all time, for all situations.

Dependability and Responsibility

Dependability and responsibility rank high among the assets of a good clinician. She must recognize that her first responsibility is to the child, the school, the parents, the community, and to the profession as a whole. This is shown in promptness in attending to schedules, reports, and records, by care of materials and equipment entrusted to her, by reliability in following through on suggestions, and by general thoughtfulness and cooperation. These traits result in purposeful activity of those involved. To achieve this, a minimum of one hour a day must be spent in reviewing and evaluating the day's activities and planning the therapy session for the following day. No successful clinician functions without evaluation and planning. It should be habitual. The SLP should also experience a sense of accomplishment and satisfaction as an outgrowth of reasonable effort.

Finally, she should make certain that each child with whom she works understands the aims and purposes of therapeutic activities and their relation to his particular problem. If the clinician is one who uses games as a part of therapy, she needs to check carefully to see that the game actually has therapeutic value and is not merely a busywork measure. Games and other devices of this nature can serve as motivational material but should be used judiciously. Therapy time is usually at a premium and must be used in ways that can be of greatest value.

Self-Improvement

Self-improvement has much to do with the attitude one assumes towards himself and his work. The difference between merely fulfilling attendance requirements and the demands of the moment and moving toward a goal of self-improvement must be recognized by every clinician. There are many ways of looking at this and many goals one may set for oneself.

The SLP may be located where classes for professional and self-improvement are available, such as college and university centers. This of course is not always true, but it would be difficult to imagine a situation where it would not be possible to gain knowledge through reading. Literature, journals and books, will prove helpful in promoting professional and personal maturity. Summer session courses are often especially designed for professional growth. In large urban areas one has the advantage of being with others who are in the same or related fields. Each can be of mutual assistance. In-service courses can be planned and visits to those doing speech therapy in clinics located in hospitals, universities, and rehabilitation centers can be arranged. The work that is required of SLPs in such centers is very closely related to school speech-language therapy.

The SLP must remember that good clinical work doesn't just happen. Wide knowledge and, above all, an acquisitive obsession beyond the call of duty are important attributes. Since assessment is a continuous process, one must be constantly on the alert. This is an increasingly scientific age. It is an age of intense competition, bringing with it strains upon human relations and demanding higher social and professional skills. It is an age that will tolerate less and less of anything that hinders smooth and efficient relations. Continuing education is almost certainly a part of our future. The competent, devoted professional need not wait for "requirements." Continued self-improvement is a responsibility for each of us.

Self-Rating

Since it is imperative that each of us strive for self-improvement, not only professionally but in understanding and improvement in personality and character, an exercise in self-analysis is suggested.

For each of the following the student or professional should rate "Excellent," "Above Average," "Average," "Below Average," "Inadequate." Rate honestly and then summarize strengths and weaknesses. The next step should be planning aimed at upgrading areas deemed in need of improvement.

A. *Appearance:* 1. Makes a good impression 2. Healthy 3. Well-Groomed

B. *Honesty:* 1. Truthful 2. Trustworthy 3. Professional Integrity

C. *Humility and Modesty:* 1. Respect for the opinion and rights of others 2. Regard for rules and regulations 3. Fraternizes with staff members 4. Avoids attitude of superiority

D. *Personality:* 1. Establishes rapport easily and quickly with adults and children 2. Friendly 3. Makes a good impression 4. Happy and cheerful 5. Tactful 6. Courteous 7. Patient 8. Enthusiastic 9. Tolerant 10. Cooperative 11. Businesslike

E. *Dependability:* 1. Prompt 2. Keeps to schedules 3. Records submitted on time 4. Keeps appointments 5. Follows through on suggestions 6. Starts tasks with a minimum waste of time 7. Senses responsibility toward: the client, the school, the profession, self

F. *Speech, language, and hearing:* 1. Voice well-modulated 2. Good articulation 3. Expresses ideas well 4. Good command of English 5. Efficient hearing

G. *Interests:* 1. Breadth of interests: Recreational, Cultural, Intellectual

H. *Professional Attitudes:* 1. Toward information: refrains from gossip toward other staff members 2. General Helpfulness and cooperation 3. Refrains from overfamiliarity 4. Self-improvement 5. Ability to recognize areas of weakness 6. Ability to work out remedies for weaknesses 7. Affiliation with professional organizations: ASHA, State SHA, Others 8. Certification in ASHA 9. Attendance at workshops 10. Attendance at conventions 11. Keeping up therapeutic competence 12. Ability to relate well to those in other disciplines: medical, dental, etc.

I. *Organization of Program:* 1. Selection of cases: Surveys, Testing, Diagnosis 2. Scheduling of classes 3. Well thought out in relation to all concerned 4. Obtaining suitable working facilities—making needs understood 5. Making the most of available facilities, effort to improve appearance of the room and make it as attractive as possible 6. Learning names of those in therapy

J. *Clinical Planning:* 1. Creativeness and originality shown in planning therapy 2. Well thought out plans and assignments 3.

Ability to motivate and stimulate participation and hold the attention and interest of those in therapy 4. Ability to shift procedures if things planned work out poorly 5. Ability to handle interruptions and to handle emergencies 6. Ability to understand and help children having behavior problems

L. *Objectivity:* 1. Willingness and ability to look at oneself and evaluate one's own assets and liabilities

COMMUNITY AGENCIES

Services provided in schools are a major source of assistance to children with communication disorders. However, they are not the only source. Many other agencies offer services to children and adults. The number of such agencies is generally dependent on the population of the community. Figure 1-2 presents possible sources of assistance to individuals. It is extremely helpful if all persons assisting the communicatively handicapped can work cooperatively. This suggests some type of formal liaison among such groups. Meetings can be arranged among heads of various community programs on a regular basis or as the need arises. Matters to be discussed can be as specific as improving methods for exchanging records of individuals, or as general as a discussion topic such as "Improving Services to the Communication Disordered in the Community." Such meetings can aid in preventing professional misunderstandings and in working toward better services for all. The SLP should continue to strive for community cooperation.

The SLP should also be aware of opportunities for children in the community. Such activities as Scouts, Little League, and Camp Fire may be indicated for all children, some in particular. In addition, awareness of such groups as Big Brother, Big Sister, Association for Retarded Children, and organizations for the physically handicapped may provide valuable resources. The SLP has a dual responsibility in such instances, not only using the various groups as resources but also making herself available for interpretation of the services she provides children.

Regardless of the competence of any professional, some children present problems beyond the individual's ability to assist. In

COMMUNICATION SERVICES ASSOCIATED WITH:	PRE SCHOOL	SCHOOL AGED	ADULT
NURSERY SCHOOL PROGRAMS	X		
EARLY INTERVENTION PROGRAMS	X		
ASSOCIATIONS FOR RETARDED CHILDREN	X	X	X
ASSOCIATIONS FOR BEHAVIORALLY HANDICAPPED	X	X	X
ASSOCIATIONS FOR PHYSICALLY HANDICAPPED	X	X	X
ASSOCIATIONS FOR LEARNING DISABLED	X	X	X
ASSOCIATIONS FOR HEARING HANDICAPPED	X	X	X
ASSOCIATIONS FOR VISUALLY HANDICAPPED	X	X	X
CHILDREN'S HOSPITALS	X	X	
VETERANS' HOSPITALS			X
OTHER HOSPITALS	X	X	X
COLLEGES AND UNIVERSITIES	X	X	X
COMMUNITY HEARING AND SPEECH AGENCIES	X	X	X
PRIVATE PRACTITIONERS	X	X	X
VOCATIONAL REHABILITATION			X
ELEMENTARY AND SECONDARY SCHOOLS		X	

Figure 1-2. Possible sources of assistance for the communicatively handicapped. From R. J. Van Hattum, Speech and Hearing Services in Schools, *Communicative Disorders*, 1977. Courtesy of Grune and Stratton.

such instances, referral to other sources is indicated. Making such referrals is an example of strength, not weakness. Every resource at the SLP's disposal must be used to assist children.

PROFESSIONAL INVOLVEMENT

Organizations

Affiliation with certain organizations is a must for the truly professional SLP. She needs to lend support to organizations which seek to promote the welfare of the exceptional individual and maintain the standards of the speech-language-hearing profession. The American Speech-Language-Hearing Association (ASHA) is a scientific and professional association whose purpose is stated in the by-laws as encouraging basic scientific study of the processes of individual human speech-language-hearing, promoting investigation of speech-language-hearing disorders, fostering improvement of therapeutic procedures with such disorders, stimulating exchange of information among persons engaged in these activities, and disseminating such information. Membership in the association is highly advisable for real professional status. Applications should be addressed to the national office, 10801 Rockville Pike, Rockville, Maryland 20852.

State organizations are closely allied to the national association. These also offer professional stimulation and deserve the active support of the persons engaged in communication disorders. Attendance at state meetings affords one the opportunity for the exchange of ideas with those in one's more immediate environment and often the chance to hear invited speakers from other localities and other disciplines as well as to learn about research in which one's colleagues are engaging.

With the growth of speech-language-hearing services, many areas have local groups or organizations where opportunity is provided the SLP to meet and discuss professional matters on a community level. Such groups allow for interchange of ideas between various employment environments, i.e. the school SLP has the opportunity to meet with clinicians working in hospital or college clinics, with resultant increased understanding and rapport with professional colleagues and help in mutual problem solving. Clinicians should avail themselves of such opportunities.

Related organizations have much to offer. Many clinicians find it stimulating to align themselves with and attend meetings of associations that include related disciplines such as the Council for Exceptional Children (CEC), its state counterpart, or others. Such affiliations help to broaden one's point of view and aid in intergroup communication and understanding.

Certification and Licensure

Those working in the various areas of speech-language-hearing should seek national and state certification and/or licensure. The American Speech-Language-Hearing-Association issues its Certificate of Clinical Competence. This certificate is granted in speech-language pathology or audiology and indicates that the holder has demonstrated ability to conduct clinical services and train others in the arts and skills of the profession and is a fully trained professional worker. A qualified individual may be certified in both areas, speech-language pathology and audiology, even though a joint certificate is not issued.

State certification is usually granted by state departments of education or public instruction. Similarly, licensure is now available in most states.

Publications

The American Speech-Language-Hearing Association publishes the following periodicals, which are invaluable to the SLP:
— *Language Speech and Hearing Services in Schools*
— *Journal of Speech and Hearing Disorders*
— *Journal of Speech and Hearing Research*
— *Asha*
— *Monographs,* which is issued irregularly
— *Directory,* which includes not only the membership list but also other pertinent information such as by-laws and code of ethics.

State organizations frequently issue periodic newsletters or journals and directories containing membership lists as well as other information that should be of interest to all in the field of communication disorders.

Conventions

National conventions are held annually at a time and place determined by the ASHA Executive Board. These are planned to stimulate exchange of information, report research, and conduct the business of the association. Short courses in various areas are offered at such times.

Many state organizations also hold annual conventions and offer similar opportunities for professional stimulation. In addition, one of the greatest dangers is that one will miss the experience of participating in meaningful decisions concerning one's own work if she does not affiliate with the professional organization and participate in the business sessions of her associations. To actually be a part of any organization one must be aware of the inner functioning, and there is no better way of achieving understanding than by attendance at business meetings and reading published reports of such meetings.

Membership

In conversation with SLPs one is often asked, "What do these associations do for me?" that is, "What have I to gain by investing my money in such organizations?" The answer might well be in the form of a question, What is an association? Dictionaries define an association as an organization of people having a common purpose and having a formal structure.

This brings to mind the adage, "A chain is only as strong as its weakest link." So one needs, so as to answer the original question, to ask still further questions: How much are you willing to give of yourself to make the association program a really vital force for the exceptional child, youth, or adult as well as for the professional worker in the field? What can be your greatest contribution? Are you going to sit on the sidelines and find fault? Are you the person who says, "Oh, let Pete do it."

Each of us recognizes that there are those who seem to have a natural talent for leadership, but it must be remembered that a leader has to have cooperation; if you are the person who feels more comfortable in other capacities, don't forget that workers, other than leaders, are also very necessary parts of the organization to which you belong. But, be sure you are not hiding your talent. Decide where you can be of assistance.

In associations, the researcher who is constantly seeking answers, the clinician who seeks clues from research for the improvement of therapy, and the professors who seek to impart this knowledge, pool efforts for a mutual cause. To reiterate, the national, state, and local associations offer opportunities for sharing and lend status to the profession. Everyone is needed to make them really function.

There is no magic wand that such organizations can wave to solve all problems that confront each individual member. One cannot expect to pay dues and immediately have a package of answers to all problems delivered to him. One cannot be an inert component of the group. He must remember that he obligates himself to activity and participation, if he is to gain membership. Too often the clinician expects the organization to solve problems that may be his own responsibility and perhaps highly individual or local and can only be solved by one's own persistent good work.

In summary, the speech-language-hearing profession is a vital, rapidly advancing one. The pioneers have carried it far. It remains for intelligent, competent, caring individuals to continue this growth to foster improved and ever expanding services to the communicatively handicapped.

STUDY ACTIVITIES

1. What specific contributions have education, psychology, and medicine made to our present methods of functioning?
2. Of what importance is the use of a single label for the professional worker?
3. Who should determine what the worker is to be called, what his function should be, and his professional conduct?
4. Is there advantage to differences of professional opinion? Explain your viewpoint.
5. Why do the authors feel an SLP has several roles?
6. Discuss some of the essential characteristics and personal qualities of a successful clinician.
7. How can the clinician give an image of the truly professional person?
8. How can a clinician coming into a school system change any

unfavorable impressions that may possibly have been created previous to his coming?
9. The American Speech-Language-Hearing Association is the official organization in the field of speech and hearing. Assume that you have been asked to influence a clinician to affiliate with this organization and its state counterpart. Present the issue.
10. It has been suggested that other disciplines may be involved in the speech-language program. Enumerate some and indicate the relationships.

REFERENCES

1. Braunstein, M. Communication Aide: A Pilot Project. *Language, Speech and Hearing Services in Schools,* 3, 32–34, 1972.
2. Cofey, C. Paraprofessionals in Speech Pathology in the Public Schools, *Journal of the Speech and Hearing Association of Virginia,* 15, 16–19, 1973.
3. Garrard, K. The Changing Role of Speech and Hearing Professionals in Public Education. *Asha,* 21, 2, 91–98, 1979.
4. Healey, W. Personal Communication, 1981.
5. Jelinek, J. A Pilot Program for Training and Utilization of Paraprofessionals in Preschools. *Language, Speech and Hearing Services in Schools,* 7, 119–123, 1976.
6. McClean, J. *The Stimulus-Shift Articulation Program,* P.O. Box 104, Northbrook, Illinois 60062: Hubbard, 1980.
7. McKee, B. *Phonemic Approximation-A Program for Correcting Lateral Sibilants and Affricates.* Hollywood: Titan Productions, 1972.
8. Mowrer, D. Baker, R. and Schutz, R. *Modification of the Frontal Lisp-Programmed Articulation Control Kit,* Tempe, Arizona: Ideas, 1970.
9. Niedermeyer, R. and Helbert, C. *Articulation Modification Program (SWRL) Speech Articulation Kit.* New York: American Book, 1971.
10. Scalero, A. and Eskeazi, C. The Use of Supportive Personnel in a Public School Speech and Language Program. *Language, Speech and Hearing Services in Schools,* 7, 150–158, 1976.
11. Van Hattum, R. Evaluating Elementary School Therapy. *Exceptional Children,* 25, 411–414, 1959.
12. Van Hattum, R. *Clinical Speech in the Schools.* Springfield: Charles C Thomas, 1969.
13. Van Hattum, R. Services of the Speech Clinician in Schools: Progress and Prospects. *Asha,* 18, 59–63, 1976.
14. Van Hattum, R. Speech and Language Services in Schools: More than Remediation. In L. Bradford (Ed), *Audio Journal in Speech Pathology.* New

York: Grune and Stratton, *4,* 1977.
15. Van Hattum, R. *Communication Disorders: An Introduction.* New York: Macmillan, 1980.
16. Van Hattum, R. Page, J. Duguay, M Baskerville, R Davis, T and Conway, L. *Taped Articulation Therapy (TAT).* Allen, Texas: DLM, in press, 1982.
17. Van Hattum, R. Page, J. Duguay, M. Baskerville, R Davis, T and Conway, L. The Speech Improvement System (SIS) Taped Program for Remediation of Articulation Problems in the Schools. *Language Speech and Hearing Services in Schools, 5,* 2, 91–97, 1974.
18. Weston, A. and Irwin, J. The Use of Paired Stimuli in the Modification of Articulation. *Journal of Perceptual Motor Skills, 32,* 947–957, 1971.

CHAPTER 2

THE SPEECH-LANGUAGE PATHOLOGIST AS A PROFESSIONAL

Rolland J. Van Hattum

Oliver M. Nikoloff

The speech-language pathologist (SLP) must be a personally competent, well-educated individual and must constantly strive for self-improvement. Additionally, to function as a true professional the specialist must display the highest level of ethical conduct and demonstrate a scientific orientation in all areas of professional function. Individuals who are receiving services must always be the major priority for the professional. In the work environment, the needs of these individuals must come before the needs of the SLP. This suggests a significant commitment; this commitment must be accepted.

When the professional accepts responsibility for altering the behavior of another human being, he or she deals not only with one aspect of behavior but with the entire individual. Although "treat the whole person" is a trite expression, and a redundant one at that (it is really impossible *not* to treat the whole person), the importance of recognizing that one is intervening in the life of another cannot be overstressed. Included among the professional functions of a speech-language pathologist are responsibilities in the area of counseling. That role *cannot* be avoided. It is important that skills in this area be developed and even more important that personal and professional limitations be recognized.

These are the three areas covered by this chapter: Ethical Conduct, Scientific Orientation, and Counseling.

ETHICAL CONDUCT

Code of Ethics

The preamble to the code of ethics of the American Speech-Language-Hearing Association states, "The preservation of the highest standards of integrity and ethical principles is vital to the successful discharge of the responsibilities of all speech-language pathologists and audiologists" (ASHA Code of Ethics, 1979). It is imperative for all clinicians to carefully study the code of ethics of the association. Copies are available by addressing the office of the American Speech-Language-Hearing Association. Some essential aspects of ethical conduct are stressed here.

Confidentiality

Respecting privileged communication is of outstanding importance. The clinician has, by the very nature of her work, information available to her concerning individuals, which consists of various records, test scores, reports of interviews with parents, clients, doctors, nurses, psychologists, research workers, and observations of teachers. All of these must be treated in a confidential way. Such material cannot be used for general information or as food for gossip. In counseling either clients or parents, the clinician may often receive direct or indirect evidence of conflict or conditions with which the individual has to contend. It is of utmost importance for the SLP to realize that most of this information was obtained by virtue of having established rapport with the person with whom she was conferring and because this individual viewed the clinician as a professional person who could be entrusted with personal information. What she learns at such times must not be divulged except as it can be used for the good of those involved. There must be fairness and a professional attitude toward all, and no person should be embarrassed or exploited. Public meeting places, including school cafeterias and faculty rooms, are no places to discuss confidential information. Neither should any child or parent be the brunt of humor or scorn. Figure 2-1 demonstrates the result of poor judgment in violating confidentiality. Professionalism and confidentiality are almost synon-

> Tuesday, November 16,
>
> ## Everybody's Column
> ## READER'S OPINIONS
>
> **Teachers' Talk Resented**
> **By L▇▇▇ Parent**
>
> Those who attended Parents Night at ▇▇▇ Senior High School Nov. 8 certainly must be interested in their children's education and improvement. Otherwise they would not have attended this event.
>
> The principals, teachers and student attendants were more than polite.
>
> This letter does not pertain to this part of the evening, but to a later incident when some of our teachers came to an establishment where we had stopped for something to eat and drink.
>
> It was a conversation even a deaf person could have heard. The teachers referred to the meeting which took place before the class sessions.
>
> One teacher laughed and said he was watching the faces of the parents and remarked that the whole thing was above their heads and he could actually see the ignorance in the faces of these people.
>
> They laughed and insulted the people they interviewed. They remarked about one parent who had a below average child in school. Instead of trying to help a child like this, they hash it over with a few beers and do nothing.
>
> Where do these people think their wages are coming from if not from school taxes paid by the ignorance parents?
>
> Next year, instead of Parents Night, they should call it Educate the Educator Night and let the parents teach them something they forgot, respect.
>
> IRATE PARENT.

Figure 2-1. Violations of professional conduct can injure public relations. Courtesy of "Everybody's Column," *The Buffalo Evening News.*

ymous. Confidential exchange can be prearranged with agencies so that one may have the benefit of information that will be of value in helping those with whom the SLP is working.

Parental Permission

The importance of having parents sign releases for medical diagnosis must be considered. In a similar way, if tape recordings or movies have been made of those in speech-language therapy, and the SLP has professional purpose for which she wishes to use these outside of therapy, it is important to obtain permission from parents and students for their use, explaining the purpose for use. The same is true if children are to participate in demonstration work or to be pictured on slides or in photographs.

Guarantees

A guarantee of a "cure" must not be made or implied. There are too many unpredictable and unknown factors in each case. "A reasonable statement of prognosis may be made, but caution must be exercised not to mislead persons served professionally to expect results that cannot be predicted from sound evidence" (ASHA Code of Ethics, 1979).

Treatment by Correspondence or Telephone

The SLP may be consulted by parents or others about problems that extend beyond the immediate school situation. She can often be very helpful in advising parents when regular clinical speech services are not available. She must, however, be sure not to give advice without first seeing the individual concerning whose problem she is advising. The code of ethics of the American Speech-Language-Hearing Association states that "An individual must not evaluate or treat individual speech-language or hearing disorders ... soley by correspondence. This does not preclude follow-up by correspondence of individuals previously seen, nor providing them with general information of an educational nature" (1979).

Ethical Relationships

Parents

Occasionally, probably because good rapport with the SLP has been established, parents ask for advice regarding matters not related to the speech-language problem or to areas in which the clinician is not qualified. The clinician may be flattered by this but must guard against offering such advice. This may be a request for recommendation of a physician or other professional person to consult. The SLP should refrain from suggesting a specific name. It is a general professional practice to suggest three alternatives.

Some parents desire to give gifts to the SLP in the spirit of appreciation. It is much safer to remain on a professional basis and not accept such gestures. This eliminates any danger of undue influence. Many school systems have established policies regarding gifts, and the SLP may indicate that she cannot accept more than "thanks" due to Board policy.

Occasionally the SLP may encounter parents or others who come with fixed ideas or complaints about various things. Sometimes such complaints may be about other school personnel. It is advisable not to discuss colleagues with them. The art of listening to complaints and handling such situations judiciously and calmly while avoiding controversy is one to cultivate. It is also a professional asset to be able to differ without becoming angry, sarcastic, or discourteous.

Children

Relationship to those in therapy must follow acceptable patterns of behavior. Clinical distance on the part of the SLP is important, especially on the part of the inexperienced clinician. A person who can achieve this is more assured of the respect of students than one who thinks and acts too much the age of the children or youths. This does not imply a rigid person, but does imply a slight difference in status. The clinician is saying, in effect, not "I am superior to you," but "in my field of specialty, I possess knowledge and skills that are superior to yours." Avoiding physical contact is one means of helping such status. Treating all on an equal basis is very essential. Firm but friendly management pays dividends.

In selection of individuals for treatment, as previously mentioned, one must give careful thought to the *why* of selection and also to the *why* of dismissal, always acting in a way that is best for the individual who needs therapy.

Co-workers

Professional attitude towards co-workers should be observed as part of the ethical code of the SLP. Most school SLPs operate on an itinerant basis and are therefore in a position where they meet many administrators, teachers, and other professional workers. For example, on the average in an urban area, the clinician may visit four schools during the week. Administrators differ in the policies they set up for their schools and staff. As the clinician travels about, she must be an adjusting individual; in addition, she must be a good listener and a very poor reporter. She should not relate what she hears and sees from one school to another. She should remain an impartial observer. If she is to maintain good working relationships, she must avoid personal controversy, seek professional discussion, and project the clinical techniques she has at her command in learning to understand the adults with whom she associates, seeking to recognize and appreciate their good qualities and skillfully finding many opportunities to foster mutual respect and cooperation.

The relationship between the SLP and other school personnel—superintendents, principals, psychologists, nurses, visiting teachers, and others—should be one of friendly give-and-take. Though these relationships will be discussed in detail in future chapters, we mention them here because it is an important function of the SLP to see that the speech-language program in the schools is well articulated with other areas.

The SLP, as all specialists, must guard against the "visiting expert posture." Classroom teachers, who are responsible for day-in, day-out educational programs, may view authoritative experts as "hit and run" specialists who deliver advice or imperatives and then leave. The SLP can do much to be viewed as a helping and supporting person by encouraging teacher suggestions for particular children as well as providing her expertise.

Other Professions

The need for mutual understanding among various medical specialists, dental specialists, audiologists, psychologists, social workers, and the SLPs is readily seen when one considers such disorders as cleft palate, voice problems, language dysfunctions, cerebral palsy, and hearing disorders. Many clinicians in the past have recognized this need and have laid foundations for interdisciplinary understanding and mutual acquaintance with services rendered. Yet, there is general agreement among these specialists that interdisciplinary communication is relatively poor, both with these individuals and ancillary services such as health departments and nursing services, and that each knows too little about what the others have to offer. This is unfortunate because many times the problems with which each is concerned are interrelated.

It is important to improve communication between these specialized areas so as to be of mutual assistance in diagnosis and treatment. In some communities, meetings have been arranged between groups representing the various specialists. Panel discussions have been conducted to create better understanding and to arrive at ideas for better communication. It is not the function of the SLP to make medical diagnosis or one that involves aspects which her training has not warranted. In turn, she may expect those in other professions not to advise in areas in which they are not qualified.

To gain and hold the respect of people in other disciplines, the SLP must be well informed. She must be aware of the need for referral, when indicated, to other specialists but not appear to make medical or dental diagnoses such as "infected tonsils" and must be prepared to listen to others when their knowledge in a particular area has something of value for her. She must know the type of information she desires from other specialists but not accept a subservient role.

Supplementing One's Income

Private Practice

Rules regarding private practice should be carefully investigated before one undertakes such a venture. Clinical certification requirements of the American Speech-Language-Hearing Association and licensure requirements in many states must be met if one is undertaking such work. It is well to refer to state and national codes of ethics before making plans to undertake such a venture. In addition to this, the SLP working in the schools needs to check to see if further rules are in effect. School systems differ in this respect, but in some communities the SLP may not act as a paid private clinician for a child or youth enrolled in speech-language therapy. The person who does elect to provide private services on a part-time basis is obligated to provide quality services and charge appropriate fees. Again, each of us represents our entire profession.

Other Outside Work

Rules regarding other outside work are among those to which all school employees are expected to conform. An example might be that all employees are required to devote their entire time during regular hours of employment for the duties to which they have been assigned. Such a rule does not apply to commitments after school hours. SLPs sometimes supplement their income with outside employment of varying kinds. In many places this is permissible. However, since this is an energy-demanding profession, one must guard against work that is too time-consuming and too strenuous or, in particular, contrary to professional image. The SLP's first obligation is to the individuals in the schools that employ her.

THE SPEECH-LANGUAGE PATHOLOGIST AS A SCIENTIFIC PRACTITIONER

Although the specialist who works in the schools will not understandably function similarly to the scientist who uses his skills in a laboratory, the program must still be scientifically oriented. This includes the use of the scientific method in all of the professional endeavors of the SLP and knowledge of terminology and procedures. In diagnostic and remedial activities, in determining the success of therapy efforts, and in adding to the individual's or the profession's store of information, scientific integrity is extremely important. Speech-language-hearing services in schools have progressed as they have because of increased commitment to this ideal. It needs to be continued and even expanded. There still remain individuals who use "hit and miss" methodology or who use one method with each person for whom they provide therapy or who do not evaluate the success or failure of their methods. There still remain individuals who do not evaluate the merits of the commercial materials they use, who do not know the reliability and validity of the tests they use, who do not adhere to the standardized methods of administration of testing materials, who are not able to interpret accurately results of testing because they have not developed sufficient familiarity with the materials they use. This is inexcusable. As mentioned previously, becoming involved in the alteration of any aspect of human behavior is a great responsibility. It should not be undertaken without the greatest possible commitment to scientific integrity. This must be a basic commitment.

The Scientific Method

The scientific method involves a systematic observation of phenomena in the most objective, unbiased manner possible. Personal opinion and prejudice must be abandoned. Fact must be separated from inference. The purpose of this is to develop a more complete and accurate understanding of a situation, relationship, or cause. Nikoloff (1969) notes that the set of rules known as the scientific method includes the following:

1. Observation of pertinent facts concerning a problem
2. Developing a hypothesis or hypotheses
3. Experimentation or testing of hypotheses
4. Generalization or conclusion

In the remedial process this could be translated into diagnosis, whereby controlled observation of behaviors (testing) leads to the development of hypotheses regarding therapeutic handling (interpretation). This is followed by testing of hypotheses through introduction of remedial measures (therapy) and finally conclusions regarding the success of therapy considered leading to further observations and the development of new hypotheses. Therapy or remediation is really an ongoing research project.

Statistical Methods

SLPs should have coursework in the area of statistics. This enables the professional to better understand research articles, to recognize the confidence they can place in reported results, to participate in research, and to better evaluate the success of programs.

Even though the clinician does have a modest background in the domain of statistics, she may need to consult with a specialist on complicated techniques. However, the basic measures of central tendency, dispersion, and correlation should be within the SLP's repertoire.

Central Tendency

The three measures used to portray the typical or "average" characteristic or person in a group are the *median,* the *mean* and the *mode.* The *median* is the midpoint in a group of measures when these are arranged from highest to lowest. Suppose the clinician has administered an articulation test to 100 children and wishes to know the typical or average number of errors for that group. By stacking the papers on a pile, placing the paper with the fewest errors on the bottom, and completing the stack with the paper or papers with the greatest number of errors on top, the task of systematic measurement has begun. To find the midpoint or halfway mark, the fiftieth and fifty-first papers need to be identified; two piles are thus separated (as are modern superhighways) by the median. The formula for finding the median is $N + 1 \div 2$ (N represents the number of persons or characteristics in the sample). In the illustration above, $100 + 1 \div 2 = 50.5$, the point halfway between the fiftieth and fifty-first papers. The median is a stable measure of central tendency; it is not affected by extremely high or low scores, and it is simple to obtain even without aid of distribution tables, desk calculators, or computers. In school settings, particularly on standardized tests of achievement, the median is the most popular descriptive measure of central tendency.

The arithmetic *mean* is obtained by summing the scores in a distribution and dividing the sum by the number of cases (N). The formula for obtaining the mean is as follows: sum of $X \div N$ (X stands for each individual score). In the illustration of 100 cases used in the preceding paragraph, each score is accumulated until the sum of the 100 articulation-error papers has been obtained. That total is then divided by 100. It is not necessary to put the scores in order using this method of calculating the mean.

The arithmetic mean is sensitive to extremely high and low scores and may portray with some distortion the "typical" or "average" case. When the mean is "pulled up" by very high scores or "pulled down" by extremely low scores, the distribution is called skewed. Despite these limitations, the arithmetic mean is preferred by statisticians because it can be used for inferential as well as descriptive purposes. By comparing the means of two groups of students, one from a suburban and one from an urban area who had been given an articulation-error test, it would be possible to infer which group averaged more errors. The median is not easily amenable to such interpretation.

The *mode* is a third measure of central tendency, but it is seldom used except as a very gross yardstick. The mode is simply the score occuring most frequently.

Measures of Dispersion

Dispersion or variability of scores in a group is sometimes of greater interest than the central tendency measures. The clinician who is giving group therapy to eight children may be more concerned about the range of different problems than the typical problem of his group.

The most popularly employed measure of variability is called the *standard deviation*. It is the companion measure to the mean, and it is measured from the mean. If a score is one standard deviation above the mean, it marks the point above which 16 percent of the scores fall (one standard deviation below the mean extends down to 16 percent). It is possible to use this measure of dispersion to calculate two or more standard deviations or parts of standard deviations. The method of obtaining the SD will not be detailed here; however, the reader who has not had a formal course in statistics should consult a statistics book for this information. Not only does the SD provide a consistent distance measure from the mean for a single distribution of scores but its properties can also be interpreted and translated for other sets of scores — there is a "standard" quality about it.

The other frequently used measure of variation is related to the median. The distribution is first divided into 100 parts, called *percentiles*. The uppermost quarter is marked by the seventy-fifth percentile, and the lowest quarter is marked by the twenty-fifth percentile. These points are called the third and first quartile. The term "interquartile range" denotes the distance between the first and third and measures the middle 50 percent of the distribution. Scores beyond the two quartiles are the more extreme or deviant scores in the distribution. It is possible, using the percentile method of description, to identify not only the quartiles but also the scores at points of the distribution.

Correlation

The other statistical question that is commonly posed by the researcher concerns the relationship between variables, the *correlation*. A typical question might concern the nature of the relationship between measured intelligence and the prevalence of language errors for a group of five year olds. To answer such a question with statistical satisfaction, measures of the variables of intelligence and language would need to be obtained on the same group of children. These two distributions of scores could then be compared, the degree of relationship determined, and an index of relationship presented. Statisticians have a number of indices that they employ to show such relationships; however, the most commonly employed is called the Pearson product moment correlation coefficient (r). This index is calculated basically by using paired scores for individuals. Again, the detailed explanation of the computation can be found in any elementary statistics text.

The Pearson r as an index ranges from $+1.0$ to -1.0. An $r = +1.0$ indicates perfect positive relationship, or "going-togetherness" or correlation. In this illustration of perfect positive correlation, the child who scored highest on the intelligence test also scored highest on the language test, and every other child maintained the same rank and distance on both scales. If the child who was highest on the intelligence test scored lowest on the language test and every child reversed the position he held on the intelligence test, the r would equal -1.0. In real life, perfect positive or perfect negative relationships exist only under the most unusual circumstances. An $r = .0$ indicates no relationship between variables. For instance, toe length and scholastic aptitude have consistently shown no relationship. Between an r of 0 and 1 all gradations of relationship can exist. The researcher, naturally, prefers to discover a high relationship between variables because predictions can be made with greater accuracy and confidence and cause and effect relationships more readily inferred. One needs to be particularly cautious, however, in concluding that *cause-and-effect* relationships necessarily exist merely because a high correlation is found. An illustration of jumping to conclusions may be shown in the widely publicized correlation between car ownership and low grades in some high schools studied. Many newspapers (and educators who should know better) immediately assumed that car ownership by high school students caused low grades. Before this conclusion can be reached, many other questions need to be answered. How does the scholastic aptitude of the car owners compare to that of non–car owners? If, as a group, the car owners have lower IQs than the non–car owners, then the cause of the low grades needs to be recalculated.

A high statistical correlation between domineering mothers and stuttering children may be shown to exist, but to demonstrate that the mothers cause the stuttering would require much additional information.

Although the previous section provides a brief review of several measures of central tendency, dispersion, and correlation, the serious researcher needs much more knowledge in this area to function in a competent fashion.

Validity, Reliability, and Standardization

Knowledge of statistical measures helps the SLP understand how much confidence can be placed in the testing instruments she uses. Three important aspects of test construction and administration are *validity, reliability,* and *standardization*.

Tests compare individuals with other individuals on selected aspects of behavior. Generally we want to know how an individual compares with others in the population; specifically, whether the person is within normal limits or not. To test the entire population would be unrealistic. Thus, attempts are made to select a representative *part* of the population to serve as representative of the total population. The larger the sample drawn from the population the more likely the sample will accurately represent the total population. The clinician should read the information on *standardization* very carefully. Standardization describes how the instrument was constructed and normed. Similarly, information on *validity* and *reliability* should be thoroughly reviewed. Validity indicates the extent to which the test measures what it purports to measure. Reliability is the extent to which the test results would be duplicated if repeated.

In the area of diagnosis, "good" scores are not high scores, they are accurate scores. This involves using reliable, valid instruments and following correct procedures in administration. Similarly, "bad" scores are not low scores. Rather, they are those lacking in accuracy.

Sampling

A feature of both standardization and research that is intimately related to the measurement process is known as the *sampling* problem. Almost never does the researcher have opportunity (because of time, cost, or availability) to observe or measure the complete population that is to be studied. The SLP who wishes to determine the prevalence in percent of children in his school system who have voice problems may not be able to interview every one of 3,000 pupils. Instead, he may have to be satisfied to interview 100 children who represent adequately the entire school population.

The process of sample selection is based on the premise that if a fair and unbiased selection method is employed, a small group can be representative of the entire population.

Two systems of sampling are commonly employed. The least complicated is called *random sampling;* this method is typically used when little is known about the population. If 3,000 children form the population of a school system from which 100 are to be randomly selected, all children's names from the attendance roster could be placed on slips of paper, placed in a wastebasket and shaken, and 100 drawn from the container. A random selection for ascertaining the prevalence of voice problems could thus be obtained.

The essential quality involved in the selection process is that everyone of the 3,000 children had an equal chance to be selected. A more efficient method for obtaining the names of the 100 children is by use of a table of random numbers — a set of numbers that serves the same purpose as drawing names from a wastebasket.

The second sampling technique, *restricted sampling*, includes stratified, quota, and selective methods. A stratified sample from 3,000 children might prescribe random selection of ten children at each grade level. Because of known characteristics of a graded school organization, the researcher might want his sample to include an equal number from each grade.

It is quite likely that there are more children in the elementary grades than in the twelfth grade (sixteen year olds who drop out reduce the upper grade population), and a quota sampling method might be employed that called for twelve sixth graders and eight twelfth graders to be chosen.

Selective sampling would be employed if a particular characteristic were thought to be associated with voice problems in the school population. From the school medical records, all children with frequent colds might form a group from which the 100 would be randomly chosen.

The determination of the size of the sample is dependent on a number of factors. The representativeness of each respondent, the difficulty of obtaining accurate responses, and the size of the entire population are among the most important considerations. The SLP would be wise to seek the advice of a statistically sophisticated person before research is begun that employs sampling techniques. A basic flaw in much otherwise adequate research design is the use of biased or inadequate sampling techniques.

One Person Research

In 1964, Jerger labelled the informal theoretical method as one of the most exciting developments in contemporary behavioral research. In addition to "one person research" this also has been called "one subject research." Jerger describes this method as consisting of precisely controlled observation on a single individual, experimental manipulation of behavior, and the search for meaningful functional relationships among actual data. This method is in contrast to formal theory construction, classical hypothesis-testing, and statistical inferences regarding averages.

Research

Nikoloff (1969) describes the purpose of research as improving understanding and the intensive investigation of a problem. Although most SLPs will not engage in large research projects, they should participate in efforts at understanding their own methods and procedures and in investigating intensively various aspects of their programs. The activities of the SLP might include experimenting with various methods of case finding case selection, or scheduling. The purpose of this research is not for publication or to share with others unless unusual results are determined. Rather, it is to provide information for program improvement.

Other types of information that should be carefully collected and tabulated relate to statistical data regarding services provided and the success of these services.

Enough stress cannot be placed on scientific function. In its absence, the individual is not a true professional.

THE SPEECH-LANGUAGE PATHOLOGIST AS A COUNSELOR

There are some who question whether there are areas of counseling specific to work with the speech-language handicapped child that could not be better handled by a child psychologist or psychiatrist. There are those who seriously question the advisability of counseling as a legitimate function of the SLP, and there are those who express concern that the clinician may not recognize when psychological or psychiatric treatment is indicated. There are SLPs who feel they are not equipped to handle such an activity. Such concerns have been expressed many times and have been debated at length. Yet, counseling has many dimensions. At its basic level it includes a talk before the Parent-Teacher Association on the nature of speech-language defects, or a discussion with a parent group on the development of speech and language. It is also counseling when the clinician suggests to a parent that some pressure be removed from the child. In actuality, counseling exists along a continuum. At one end of the continuum is group information giving. A step away is the giving of specific advice to a parent. The next step is discussion regarding a child. Further along is counseling a parent regarding a child's communication disorder. The other end of the continuum is the actual providing of counseling services to a child or a parent. The question is not whether the clinician *should* provide counseling. She *does*, to some degree. It is the SLP's responsibility to continually improve skills in counseling techniques and to recognize limitations along the continuum.

Mange (1969) points out that most of the real controversy regarding the clinician's ability to provide counseling relates to the area of emotional adjustment counseling. Many of the adjustment problems of children with speech-language disabilities are strongly associated with reactions resulting from the disability. The SLP is uniquely qualified by training and experience to assess the influence of emotional, organic, perceptual, and habit patterns and to detect the elements of commonality in the behavioral responses that are present. Reluctance to speak, use of very short verbal responses requiring few words, verbal hostility and aggressiveness, circumlocutions, and a host of other patterns of substitution, avoidance, and procrastination are often present. Such self-defeating patterns of behavior are useful as focal points for the counseling approach.

Those who feel that counseling should only be attempted by persons specifically trained in these techniques argue that potential harm to the person is an ever present threat. There is merit to this argument, and the clinician must never extend beyond her competency. Further, she herself should seek competent professional advice should the slightest doubt arise in her mind. In addition, speech-language-hearing function provides the basic responsibility for the SLP. SLPs should not rival psychologists in their actions. Counseling activities should be conducted as a part of the speech-language remedial program.

Human beings, especially children, are gregarious and social beings who seek out those contacts which provide satisfying relationships. Indeed, the development of a stable personality and an adequate self-concept requires the repeated contact and experience of extensive verbal relationships with others. Those which are most satisfying are with warm and responsive friends who provide stimulation and personal acceptance. More counseling is done by the layman than by all professionals combined. It is done because people do seek close personal relationships with others. It is the normal and necessary result of these relationships. To be a friend; to converse, suggest, discuss, and explore ideas, problems, and solutions; to do these things with a group or with one other is the essence of counseling. When the effect is a change of feeling and attitude, a change of behavior or an adjustment for a more effective life, the goals of counseling are achieved. The SLP who spends many hours with the child, in individual and small group settings, cannot deny the counseling relationship. Instead, limitations should be recognized and skills developed as an efficient tool in the improvement of the child's speech-language and emotional adjustment.

The Public School Setting

The training regimen of most SLPs in a university clinical setting deviates in at least one important way from the setting of the school clinician. In the training program, one or both parents frequently accompany the child and are included in discussions of the progress of therapy as well as analysis of the interactions of parent and child. These opportunities are generally quite extensive and are required for every child accepted in the therapy program. The university setting also includes opportunities for gathering rather complete case histories, observation of parent-child interaction, medical evaluation, and psychological diagnosis including both intellectual and emotional aspects. These necessitate close contact with professionals in other fields. Fortunately, these relationships are particularly productive because of the mutual understandings developed by continuing association as a team, working towards solutions to mutual questions and problems.

The public school setting is seldom as permissive as to time, case load, and resources. Consequently the approach taught in its totality in the training program is seldom possible of complete achievement, in the public school setting, for every child included in the program. Selection of those to be included in the counseling program and subjective judgments of the relative worth of certain information must be made. The responsibility for these decisions rests upon the clinician almost entirely. There are, however, occasions when the observations of other teachers and of school special service personnel and community agencies can provide many helpful insights. In some instances, pupil personnel files may contain other significant and useful information pertinent to an understanding of the child, his speech, and his behavior. Each of these sources should be explored. All too often, however, the clinician must rely on her own analysis and judgment because few school systems possess sufficient psychological and diagnostic resources necessary for objective decisions.

The school counseling setting also carries with it the attitudes built up by children and parents that relate to all parts of the school function. When counseling opportunities are provided to parents, the SLP may develop a closer relationship with the home than any of the other school personnel. Frequently questions such as these are asked: Will Johnny be promoted? Why doesn't his teacher like him? How can I get him to bring home his arithmetic work? and a host of others of similar nature. Most of these are not within the province or responsibility of the clinician. They are, however, vehicles for better understanding and counseling relating to behavior, school achievement, and speech-language therapy. Certain other aspects of the school setting with an important bearing on the counseling program will be discussed in the following sections.

The Speech-Language Pathologist in Counseling

Three important and distinguishable areas are included within the counseling function of the SLP: emotional adjustment counseling of the child, parent counseling, and educational counseling. Although the clinician must work with a variety of different persons and in somewhat different settings for the areas mentioned, the techniques and approaches of counseling should be directed toward stimulation of independent constructive behavior, toward alteration of noxious environmental factors, and toward improved social relationships and increased efficiency of total school performance.

Counseling of the Child with a Speech-Language Problem

The SLP frequently meets and recognizes adjustment problems that are secondary to the speech-language disorder, i.e. they result from listener and self-reactions to the deviant speech-language pattern. Certain listener reactions and attempts to correct the defective pattern are easily sensed by the child and quickly internalized. Although corrective attempts by adults, including the SLP, may be tolerated with little overt reaction, they hold great potential for inadequate development of the self-concept.

Avoidance

Many children resort to avoidance learning in which any speech-language attempts likely to elicit negative reactions are inhibited. The SLP most frequently deals with avoidance behavior that tends towards denial or superficial acknowledgment of the problem, towards withdrawal from situations likely to require speech-language, and towards expressions of hostility and aggressiveness.

An alert third grade teacher reported the development of avoidance behavior in Jim, a boy whose articulation errors were very noticeable to his classmates.

> Several times Jim told me he had a cold and no voice when he was supposed to give a report. At first I excused him, but then I arranged for Jim to see the nurse. She found nothing unusual and told him so. I was quite sure his reports were done so I talked with him about his feelings when talking to the group. He seemed somewhat relieved that I knew his desire to keep silent, but soon after he began to be absent whenever he was due to report. Each time he sent his written report to me with an older brother. We finally began to make progress only when we arranged it so he could use pictures and exhibits or write on the blackboard at the same time he was talking. He seems to get along better when attention is directed towards the materials he uses rather than towards himself. His reports are always very brief, he almost never looks at the children, and he seems to do everything possible to direct attention away from himself — but at least he is now talking a little more.

Secondary Symptoms

There are also many children with both general and specific types of avoidance resulting from other deviations associated with cleft lip, protruding teeth, or cerebral palsy, for example. Varying forms of this behavior in the speech-language handicapped child are so frequent that the term "secondary," as used to explain the symptom patterns of stuttering, can be extended to include associated behavior patterns in articulation, voice, other speech disorders, and language deviations. *Secondary symptoms* are learned behaviors that, although not a part of the symptomatology of the basic problem, result from it and add to the severity. For example, a child with a cleft palate may cover her mouth when speaking or a child with poor speech associated with cerebral palsy may refuse to speak before any one other than family.

It is the clinician's task to stimulate development of constructive behavior that permits the intrinsic rewards of speech and language to be experienced more frequently, while the self-destructive avoidance behavior is reduced.

Techniques and Approaches to Counseling

Withdrawal and Hostility

There is a tendency for the layman to suggest that the symptoms of withdrawal and hostility be explained verbally and that the child be told that others really do accept him despite the speech-language deviation. Advice, admonition, and exhortation to participate and to feel more positively toward others is then advised. The SLP, however, recognizes that the child's behavior is a result and an expression of attitudes and feelings and that the cause and effect relationship seen by others is almost never applied to one's own behavior through such a direct approach. "Bootstrap psychology," with its "get hold of yourself and act differently" orientation, has not proven to be effective counseling. The child may understand all the logical reasons for behaving in a different fashion, yet he experiences negative emotional reactions and responds with behavior symptomatic of them. He understands that it is wrong to steal, that it is immature to cry, and that fighting with others is inappropriate—yet he does these things, not because of his understanding, but because of his feelings.

Children and adults typically react to stimuli on the basis of their emotional impact first rather than to the actual content of the stimulus. To point out that one has made an error, that one is lazy, that one is acting "like a baby," or that one may have forgotten something he should have remembered is likely to elicit an emotional reaction that may be defensive or hostile. Positive learning is not enhanced under these conditions.

> Kevin, a third grade boy with a persistent lateral lisp, was a case in point. Although his mental abilities were considerably above his group, Kevin experienced continuing correction by his parents in every aspect of his behavior. When things went well and he performed as desired, little was said and few verbal rewards were offered, but when he experienced some difficulty his parents were overly quick to correct. Kevin generalized these corrective attempts to his elementary teacher and particularly to the speech therapy situation. His usual reaction included crying. If the situation continued, he would often become very resistive and hostile to the point of striking the clinician. After this he would frequently explain that he had made a mistake and he didn't want to cry but that he just couldn't help it. Behavior only improved after he experienced role-playing situations in which errors and mistakes were deliberately included as part of the roles to be acted. From this point, tolerance of his own errors increased, and he moved ahead to assume responsibility for his own actions.

Nondirective Counseling

Some of the most helpful information relating to adjustment counseling is contained in the writings of Rogers (1942). Rogers feels that the ability to improve his or her adjustment is present in each individual. His exposition points up the movement of the client from expressions of feeling concerning the problem, expression of faint positive impulses, the development of insight and self-acceptance, consideration impulses, the development of action, and ultimately, initiation of positive, constructive behavior. This progression is basically similar in all forms of adjustment counseling situations, whether the client is speech-language handicapped or has other problems. These steps can be used as a rough guide to progress in the counseling relationship. They are extremely interesting to observe and analyze, but it should be recognized that progress is the normal outgrowth of the relationship between the clinician and the student. The relationship permits emotional catharsis and expression of feelings without threat of reprisal or negative reaction by the counselor. In addition, it must provide an atmosphere of true acceptance by the counselor. Improvement occurs because the individual is able to examine and "feel" his behavior without the emotional concomitants, and he is able to experience reactions more fitting the situations encountered. It assumes a desire to be accepted and valued by others. Improved, effective behavior results from self-direction rather than from direct manipulation and instruction by the counselor. The emphasis for counseling the speech-language handicapped lies in the areas of reactions to the speech or language disability and to the social experiences encountered. It is a communication and an exploration of these feelings and attitudes without the actual presence of the external threat encountered in real-life situations. In this situation the clinician is always the objective listener, never the evaluator, never the judge. By work or facial expression he should not convey messages of surprise, amazement, embarrassment, or displeasure.

The SLP should verbally reward and reinforce improved behavior as soon as the child can accept it, by noting the improved reactions of others to the new behavior. This procedure can often reduce the tendency toward ignoring the cause and effect relationship so important in social contacts. If the child fails to realize that others react to him because of the way he behaves, it is very likely that he will increase his negative social attitudes, which, in turn, will be quickly reinforced. The mechanism of role-playing, to be described, is one of the most effective means of pointing up the cause and effect importance in human contacts at the affective or feeling level.

Catharsis

Experiences with children suggest that the discussion approach to counseling can be helpful to some speech-language handicapped children of school age, particularly at the later elementary and secondary levels. It has been surprising to see the open expression of feelings towards family, teachers, and classmates and the acquisition of simple insights that develop. John, with a precocious younger sister who possessed classic female verbal skills, was one of these children.

For many therapy sessions, John seemed to resent the female clinician's frequent talking. He also showed much resentment towards his sister. These points appeared often in the counseling sessions until one day he exploded with a verbal torrent of abuse that included both sister and clinician. He then said, "You should go to speech class, too—and my sister, too." While the clinician searched her own speech pattern for some little defect, he added, "You talk too much."

Another boy, Fred, who told the clinician about his feelings during severe stuttering, commented in the following way:

> When I just told you about it, it didn't seem quite so bad. It felt bad when it happened, but now I don't think it would be so bad if it happened all over again.

Unfortunately, however, for many children the progress of counseling often bogs down at the point of catharsis and expression of feelings when only verbal discussion is used. Catharsis alone is generally insufficient to achieve adequate emotional adjustment. It must be followed by an active trial and use of new modes of behavior and by experiencing new reactions to otherwise disturbing situations.

Discussion

One of the direct approaches to the solution of some specific and isolated problems causing conflict is through mutual discussions and analysis of that problem with the SLP. The technique has been used by many school mental health workers and guidance counselors, especially for those problems which are school centered. Problems centering around behavior at recess, hostile behavior towards a classmate, and difficult relationships with a specific teacher are examples. The clinician and child attempt an objective analysis of the problem, the long-term effect of such continued behavior, and alternate types of behavior that might be employed. This approach operates at the verbal level and usually must be supplemented with experiences at the feeling level.

Role-playing

Another approach that is generally more effective than verbal discussion and direct approaches makes use of the techniques of role-playing. These techniques are also used in sociodrama and psychodrama. They hold extremely high interest for all age levels and provide a vehicle for breaking the habit patterns of stereotyped emotional and behavioral responses. In role-playing, the SLP structures situations that may deal with problems common to the group or that are specific to one of the children. They may revolve around uncomfortable social situations such as being late for an important meeting, difficult parent-child situations, or other emotion-producing situations.

Children are allowed to select or are assigned the roles of parent, teacher, child, and other important persons in the scene to be enacted. No dialogue is supplied; instead, the general situation is outlined and the lines are elicited spontaneously according to the child's perception of the situation. When the brief scene is completed there is discussion of the ways in which each person reacted to the others. Was the person liked by the group or was he disliked? What words or tone of voice was used that made him liked or disliked? Did he seem angry and hostile, or was he friendly and complimentary? When he played the role of being angry, how did the person to whom he was talking behave? Is this the way most people behave when they are angry or when someone attacks them through words? What phrases and words does he often use by habit that have positive effects on the listener? Are there some that are habitually used which produce negative effects? This type of analysis can and should be extended to actions of a nonverbal nature as well. By analyzing the roles in this way, both the SLP and the children gain considerable insight into the way people react to specific types of behavior. Roles are frequently reversed, either by choice of the child or by judicious assignment of the clinician. At certain points in the counseling program it may be advisable for the inhibited child to play the role of the dominant teacher and parent.

Role-playing also makes possible the trial use of new forms of behavior. Many of these are suggested by the group or occasionally by the SLP. As more varying roles are attempted by each child, there is greater freedom of behavior and greater emotional insight into those forms of behavior which are most satisfying. It is usually preferable to present a choice of roles to the child so that he will have the experience of making his own decisions. Many children do not seem to understand that life presents numerous alternatives. Instead, they seem to feel that they are compelled to act in a specific and often harmful way. The simple method of presenting choices provides stimulation for the child to seek out the alternatives that are always present, to assist in the alleviation of stereotyped responses, and to avoid that "locked-in," trapped feeling common to many poorly adjusted children.

Referral

The SLP will also encounter children whose emotional problems go far beyond those relating to their speech-language disability. It is essential to recognize when the total psychological and environmental picture is so harmful that attempts at adjustment counseling are insufficient. Responsibility must be assumed by the clinician for consultation with the school psychologist and, likely, referral of such children to other agencies and services specifically designed to deal with them. When in doubt about the severity of the problem, it is imperative to seek all possible means for professional evaluation. It is indefensible to delay or block treatment of serious emotional problems through the provision of superficial and/or infrequent counseling sessions.

It is extremely fortunate that public schools within the past decade have made marked progress in the provision of services for evaluation and treatment of exceptional children, including those with emotional adjustment difficulties. Increasing numbers of special education programs use well-trained itinerant mental health workers, classroom or "crisis" teachers of the emotionally disturbed and personality matching of children and teachers. In many communities there are also child guidance clinic programs, family service agencies, and other professional workers who can be of great assistance. Use of these resources when indicated is an essential element of all quality programs.

Counseling Parents of Children with Speech-Language Problems

Although many authors have discussed and advocated direct counseling of the parents of children with speech-language handicaps, the most convincing evidence of value was presented a number of years ago in a study by Wood (1946). In his study, the speech of the children with functional articulation defects whose parents received adjustment counseling made significantly greater improvement than that of a control group whose parents did not receive counseling. Even if there is no immediate effect on the communication of the child, there are often many benefits that accrue to a counseling program, particularly in relationship to the improved emotional climate in the home and between the home and school.

The SLP can be an extremely effective liaison between school and home through a carefully conducted parent counseling program. As SLPs and school administrators experience more of the beneficial effects of parent counseling there is greater expectation that the clinician should have training and skill in this important area. Counseling is no longer an optional accessory; it is becoming a required activity of the effective clinician in many school systems. Numerous school administrators have expressed their conviction that programs with close and continuing parent contact are one of their most valuable public relations tools. Parents who are aware of the school's interest in their child become enthusiastic and supportive, despite some academic and social problems that the child may experience.

It is also true that school programs involving parents are presented with the opportunity to impair public relations very significantly if carried on with any degree of disinterest, disorganization, or incompetence. Consequently, there is often some administrative reluctance to permit extensive parent contacts until the clinician has proven to be competent in this type of activity.

Those SLPs with large case loads cannot expect to provide continuing counseling opportunities to parents of more than a very few children. Therefore, it is necessary to select those to be included on some practical basis. The condition of limited openings has made some systems formulate exceedingly restrictive criteria for inclusion, such as the necessity for both parents to be in attendance at all sessions. Such restrictions are neither required nor practical. It is important, however, to center these counseling opportunities on the mothers because of their major influence on the development of the child's attitudes and emotions. Those to be selected should be those whose relationship with their child tends to produce speech-language anxiety and inhibitory speech-language behavior. In making this judgment, it is essential to be concerned with the relationship between the parent and child rather than between the parent and the SLP. Scheduling of at least one afternoon or evening group session per week is necessary, with other periods of time available for individual parents to schedule conferences with the SLP as either may desire. It is extremely important to set up a regular schedule of group meetings early in the school year without leaving the matter to chance and conflict with other meeting dates.

A few simple facts regarding parents, SLPs, and the counseling relationship are of value.

1. No parent can be completely objective and rational about her child or herself.
2. Objective observations of the SLP about either the child or the parent have a reason for being discussed only if some benefit will accrue. The counseling relationship has no place for utterance of subjective observations, facts, and other erudite analyses to satisfy the SLP's needs.
3. Parents as well as children will respond best to the SLP who has both sincerity and competency.
4. The counseling relationship always has the potential for expression of the feeling of parental guilt and the use of defense techniques.
5. Most parents are very unfamiliar with the terminology of speech-language-hearing and require an explanation of complex ideas with simple vocabulary.

The Initial Contact with Parents

Contact with parents on an "in person" or at least an "in voice" basis, rather than through the use of parent letters, which are routinely duplicated with space for the insertion of parent and names, is strongly urged. Personal contact offers some advantages that can avoid barriers to a good counseling relationship. The initial contact should provide information about specific arrangements that the SLP desires to make with the parent, and it must also provide for a response to potential fears or concerns of the parent. Some parents, after reaching the point of reasonable security in the counseling sessions, have related an intense feeling of anxiety after the initial contact relating to the "real reasons" for the counseling sessions. One felt that counseling was a prelude to assignment of her child to a class for the retarded, while another thought the sessions were a type of compulsory night school and that she would in some way be graded on her performance.

Parents and teachers, when approached by a specialist, often automatically assume a "problem set" born from past experiences in which the specialist expressed or conveyed some element of blame or incompetence. Defensive reactions are normal under these conditions. Unfortunately, these reactions direct one's attentions to rationalizations and explanations and make it very difficult to develop understanding of a speech-language problem and effective approaches. Consequently, it is important not only to minimize these implications but also to actually build the self-image of the parent or teacher. The SLP should also recognize that seeming lack of parental interest may really reflect genuine inability to cope with the problem or fears associated with the need to interact with educated individuals (also, we always outnumber them).

If problem sets are displayed in the opening moments of clinician and parent or teacher contact, the visit should be limited to information gathering with questions directed to the parent or teacher designed to elicit her perception of the problem and the course of action that she may feel is important. The SLP can assist the respondent in formulating constructive thought by suggesting two or more major alternatives from which the person may choose. For example, the teacher or parent may be asked if, in her judgment, speech errors persist because of a basic inability to hear differences between phonemes or because the child's habitual manner of producing speech developed strongly before fine discriminations were possible. Questions phrased in this manner show respect for the opinions and judgments of the parent and teacher, which will make their involvement in the therapy program much easier.

Information Sharing

Counseling sessions can effectively include information giving by the SLP in addition to less formally structured opportunities for catharsis and discussion. Specific information relating to a child's particular speech-language problem is almost routinely requested by parents and should be provided in a simple, yet complete manner. Some carefully selected reference material can be used for study and later recall by parents in their own homes. Materials of greatest benefit are the small booklets designed for use by the speech-language handicapped. Some SLPs produce their own. Many clinicians and schools find it very helpful to have a supply of these booklets available for passout or sale to parents when appropriate. As the counseling sessions progress, there is less need for information giving. As the parents feel more secure, they will concern themselves more and more with problems that are real to them centering around their own feelings and techniques for aiding their children.

In addition to the information that should be available for parents about their child's specific speech-language and behavior condition, it is helpful to communicate three major ideas early in the counseling sequence. First, few parents have an awareness of the complexity of speech-language function or of human behavior. Consequently, there is the tendency to feel that the child should be able to alter his speech-language or behavior pattern simply by being instructed to do so. Parents have also been frustrated in their own direct attempts to alter the situation with this approach and may feel that the child is resistive or negative. A small amount of judicious explanation of the complex functions of encoding, decoding, association, memory, motor, and feedback components of speech can sometimes be helpful in relieving parents of their feelings of frustration and failure.

The second major concept relates to the effect of habit patterns on the maintenance and persistence of behavior once it is learned. Proper understanding of this aspect of learning not only helps the parent understand the discouraging persistence of the disorder but, more significantly, is also an effective inducement for the parents to plan realistic and frequent rewards for altered speech-language patterns. One mother pointed up the problems of many parents when she said, "I couldn't understand why he'd keep on doing it the wrong way. I tried to correct him over and over again, but it didn't seem to help. I accepted the good things that he did as a matter of course, but always criticized the things I didn't like." This mother began to use a planned program of occasional verbal rewards when her son made attempts to alter his speech-language. The results were almost immediately apparent as shown by heightened interest in therapy and rapid improvement in the child's speech-language patterns.

Third, it is essential to provide an overview of the course of the therapy program as it relates to the parent's own child. This must include basic oral explanation of the major aspects of the type of speech-language problem presented: stuttering, articulation, voice, language, or problems accompanying various organic conditions. It should include an explanation of the reasons for any special diagnostic assessments requested and a discussion of the structure and function of the speech musculature appropriate to the specific disorder. Booklets and selected references, previously mentioned, are an excellent supplement and extension of the oral explanation.

Dealing with Parents' Questions

As the counseling meetings continue, there will be many topics of significance that will be discussed. Parent concerns often relate to a fear of criticism and ridicule by the child's playmates and by the family's relatives and social contacts; expression of varying forms and degrees of guilt, inadequacy, and failure; problems of selecting and evaluating competent medical advice and treatment; the fear of retardation or significant emotional disturbance; lack of understanding by the teacher; vocational prospects for their child; educational achievement questions; social relationship skills; and myriad other concerns. It is neither possible nor desirable to supply answers to many of these questions. Rather, it is essential to accept the concerns as real and to permit the parent to express the problem, and then progress towards a self-answer. Role-playing experiences, as previously described, are often very effective at this point. Many parents seem to first become aware that they can actually guide and manipulate the experiences of their child in a constructive manner several meetings after the first expression of their concerns.

There are, of course, some parents who are more likely to play the "take charge" role and who operate on the basis of "any action is better than nothing." The group process may be especially helpful in developing insight for these parents, since such an impulsive mode of operation is frequently subject to serious error. These are usually obvious to the other parents and provide much opportunity for group discussion.

Perhaps the most beneficial effect of the parent-counseling effort is the resultant sense of being freed from the imprisoning walls of culture and society and its many judgments upon others. This sense of personal freedom and worth can be communicated to the speech-language handicapped child only when the important people in the environment possess it themselves.

The Parents' Roles in Therapy

There are some differing opinions as to the efficacy of using the parent as a direct helper in the speech-language program. It seems very likely that the disagreement arises because it is so difficult to generalize about parents when involved in such a role. Many SLPs who have attempted to use the parent as an aide have quickly found that the procedure may be quite harmful unless very carefully structured. As an example, one clinician, after the lapse of nearly two weeks when the child was ill, found that the parent had used the time at home by teaching and habituating a seriously distorted phoneme. Similarly, another mother provided ear training work with her child when she possessed a "tin ear" with very little ability to make accurate discriminations of even gross auditory stimuli. The result, as could be forecast, was heightened auditory confusion and habituation of error, which caused the child to reject all such training.

Despite these and certain other problems, much success can be found in using the parent as an aide when the SLP understands those areas in which the parent can be most effective. It is often helpful to explain that there are two major divisions of the therapy program. First, the SLP works toward the *elicitation* of new and correct communication behavior. The parent can and should do very little in this first phase. The understandings and approaches here are too delicate to permit anyone other than the SLP to attempt. Second, the program works towards *habituation* of new and correct communication behavior.

Actual listing of activities in these two major divisions makes it explicit to the parent that techniques directed towards eliciting new speech-language patterns are highly skilled functions of the SLP. It also points up the critical and important role that the parent can play in stimulating use and habituation of the newly acquired patterns. It then becomes apparent that the SLP cannot go much beyond the first division of activities within the brief period each week that is available in the school therapy schedule.

Parents often inquire about the availability of additional therapy opportunities including camps and special schools. Usually this reflects an increased interest in providing all that is possible for their child. Similar inquiries are also made relating to medical and surgical evaluation and treatment. Competent advice in these areas depends upon a knowledge of resources, which can only be gained by extensive contact with other professional personnel.

In summary, the true professional receives many satisfactions. However, she or he, in turn, must function as competently, ethically, and scientifically as possible. The students must be viewed not only as speech, language, or hearing handicapped but also as a total individual. In this regard the need for various levels of counseling children or parents must be recognized and competencies developed to meet appropriate needs.

STUDY ACTIVITIES

1. Do you feel ethical codes are to protect the profession or the recipient of services. Why?
2. If speech-language services are part of the educational program, why should parental permission be obtained?
3. What are the disadvantages of the SLP accepting employment that is not consistent with a professional image?
4. Why should the SLP be interested in research?
5. How can she use research to improve her clinical program?
6. Why would the clinician do research if the clinician does not

plan to publish the results?
7. What areas of research are most lacking in the clinical speech field?
8. Why is it that speech-language handicapped children with emotional problems find it so difficult to concentrate on altering their communication patterns?
9. What signs are frequently present in behavior of children and parents which suggest that the discussion is approaching an emotionally sensitive area?
10. If it is true that children have a strong desire to be accepted by others, why do some with emotional maladjustments persist in behavior unacceptable to others?

REFERENCES

1. American Speech-Language-Hearing Association, *Code of Ethics.* 10801 Rockville Pike, Rockville, Maryland 20852, 1979.
2. Mange, C. The Speech Clinician as a Counselor. In R. Van Hattum (Ed.), *Clinical Speech in the Schools.* Springfield: Thomas, 1969.
3. Nikoloff, O. The Speech Clinician as a Researcher. In R. Van Hattum (Ed.), *Clinical Speech in the Schools.* Springfield: Thomas, 1969.
4. Rogers, C. *Counselling and Psychotherapy.* Boston: Houghton, 1942.
5. Wood, K. Parental Maladjustment and Functional Articulation Defects in Children, *Journal of Speech and Hearing Disorders, 11,* 255–275, 1946.

Chapter 3

THE SPEECH-LANGUAGE PATHOLOGIST AS A MEMBER OF THE EDUCATIONAL TEAM

Frederick E. Garbee

The role of the speech-language pathologist in the schools is paramount in providing for the needs of the individual pupil with a communication disorder or delayed speech-language development. During this current time of revolutionary changes, prompted primarily by implementation of the Education for All Handicapped Children Act of 1975 (Public Law 94-142), the role of the speech-language pathologist in the schools has expanded and broadened to assist the school more than ever in accomplishing its commitment to education in the community. Since the largest population of individuals in the schools with handicapping conditions is comprised of individuals with communication disorders in language, speech, and hearing, it is evident that the role of the speech-language pathologist is a leadership role. With this leadership role, however, there is an increased necessity for clarification of responsibilities, cooperative planning with other educators and parents, coordinated programming with instructional staff, administrators, and support personnel, and of course, accountability. In other words, the educational team is an important vehicle in this cooperative and coordinated effort.

Focus of the educational team is on the pupil. The pupil with an inability to speak or understand others effectively may have substantial difficulty in learning, social growth, personal adjustment, and self-image. As an essential member of the school's educational team, the speech-language pathologist is a most vital individual in identifying, assessing, educational planning, program implementing, and evaluating the individual with a communication disorder. In each of these areas of educational involvement for the individual student, the speech-language pathologist demonstrates commitment to education.

COMMITMENT TO EDUCATION IN OUR SCHOOLS AND COMMUNITIES

The school's commitment to education embraces an ideal of the best education possible for every citizen, including individuals with communication disorders. This commitment includes an interest in the extent and quality of education at all levels. It encompasses achieving competence in skills, e.g. reading and mathematics, as well as general competence such as ability to work cooperatively towards group goals, development of problem-solving skills, flexibility in behavior and thought, and creativity.

In order to fulfill this commitment to education, schools are assigned the systematic development of intellectual, social, and vocational competence of the individual child. Also, the effective school is always concerned with the promotion of physical and mental health as well as satisfying human relationships in a setting of moral and ethical values. Teaching must be based upon the best that is known about human development and the understanding and application of learning concepts.

An important study by the Educational Policies Commission of the National Education Association stated these basic areas as essential to a good educational program:

1. The objectives of self-realization
2. The objectives of human relationship
3. The objectives of economic efficiency
4. The objectives of civic responsibility[1]

An even more specific statement of the role of the public school is found in the conference statement of the 1956 White House Conference on Education, which encompasses the following points:

> 1. The fundamental skills of communication—reading, writing, spelling—as well as other elements of effective oral and written expression; the arithmetical skills, including problem solving. While schools

---

[1]Educational Policies Commission, *The Purposes of Education in American Democracy* (Washington, D.C., N.E.A., 1938).

are doing the best job in their history in teaching these skills, continuous improvement is desirable and necessary.
2. Appreciation for our democratic heritage.
3. Civic rights and responsibilities and knowledge of American institutions.
4. Respect for and appreciation of human values and for the beliefs of others.
5. Ability to think and evaluate constructively and creatively.
6. Effective work habits and self-discipline.
7. Social competency as a contributing member of his family and community.
8. Ethical behavior based on a sense of moral and spiritual values.
9. Intellectual curiosity and eagerness for lifelong learning.
10. Esthetic appreciation and self-expression in the arts.
11. Physical and mental health.
12. Wise use of time, including constructive leisure pursuits.
13. Understanding of the physical world and man's relation to it as represented through basic knowledge of the science.
14. An awareness of our relationships with the world community.[2]

The object of the educative process in our schools is to assist the child by increasing his power to communicate, to understand, and to live effectively and meaningfully with his fellows, to emphasize what is possessed in common and what makes a community possible.

While the common characteristics of people make a community possible, it is their uncommon qualities that make it better. Leadership, variety, innovation, and progress, to a great extent, come from individuality. As a part of our commitment to the educative process of children, our educational purpose must be understood in the broad framework of our convictions concerning the worth of the individual and the importance of individual fulfillment.

PUBLIC SCHOOLS AND THEIR ROLES IN EDUCATION

Just what is the nature of a school system? What is this employment environment in which the competent speech-language pathologist is to work?

Actually, the citizens in each state in the United States hold the

---

[2]The Committee for *The White House Conference on Education* (Washington, D.C., U.S. Government Printing Office, 1956, pp. 91–92).

key to the realities and potentialities of education. They elect the legislators who, representing the citizens, determine the enactment of laws pertaining to education. In most local communities the citizens select the members of the board of education. In many communities citizens' committees have been organized to assist the local school board and the staff with studies, problems, and issues.

The board of education in the local community represents the people of the school district and county on matters pertaining to the schools, yet it does not administer school affairs. The chief functions of the board are to select a well-qualified administrator and assign him or her the responsibility of operating the educational program and to determine policies in developing and carrying out the program.

A good board of education distinguishes between its responsibilities as a policy-making body and the superintendent's (administrator's) responsibility as its executive officer. The board should guarantee freedom for expression of local ideas and freedom for tailoring school programs to fit local needs. The board also does not limit itself to business and financial affairs alone but also considers educational issues and policies brought to it by the superintendent. The board establishes personnel policies wherein the superintendent represents the board in negotiating with the staff of the schools. The superintendent makes all personnel recommendations for the board's consideration, including employment, promotion, and dismissal.

The administrator or superintendent of schools is usually the secretary and executive officer of the board. He executes the policies formulated and adopted by the board. Ideally, he is the educational leader in the community. He should provide leadership in facing issues and solving problems in building an effective school system. The administrator must be efficient in making decisions, organizing, planning, communicating, influencing, coordinating, and evaluating the many aspects of the educational process.

The staff of a school system likely includes professional members such as teachers, principals, supervisors, psychologists, speech-language pathologists, social workers, audiologist, and counselors as well as custodians, bus drivers, and clerical and secretarial staff.

In effective school systems the staff cooperates with the superintendent and the board and through a cooperative endeavor promotes developing policies and planning in carrying out a good program. In planning and providing for good schools this teamwork and coordination are extremely important.

The organization and the administration of education in this country vary greatly from state to state and often among communities within the same state. The similarities appear to outweigh the differences, however.

THE FEDERAL GOVERNMENT'S COMMITMENT TO EDUCATION

The organization and administration of education in the United States continue to be local prerogatives. However, two legislative milestones and state and national litigation affirming handicapped children's rights to a free appropriate public education have enhanced Congressional and U.S. Department of Education (formerly Health, Education and Welfare) involvement, particularly during the 1970s and continuing into the 1980s. An excellent and succinct discussion of legislation and court action pertaining to the handicapped is published in *National Incentives in Special Education, A History of Legislative and Court Action.*[3]

Even though Congress provided for a facility for the deaf in Kentucky in 1827 and Gallaudet College for the deaf and blind in 1864, it was not until 1954 that Congress again recognized the need for aid to education for handicapped children on a national basis. At that time a program of grants was enacted (Public Law 83-531) for institutions of higher learning and state agencies for cooperative support of educational research, surveys, and demonstration for dissemination of information from educational research. Also, the N.D.E.A. Act of 1958 was a "landmark" legislation because it set a precedent and trend for categorical aid for the handicapped. Legislative support accelerated from that point. In 1964, Public Law 88-164 added federal support for training teachers of the

---

[3]David P. Riley, Herbert D. Nash, and J. T. Hunt, National Association of State Directors of Special Education (1201 Sixteenth Street, Northwest, Washington, D.C., 20036, November, 1978).

hard-of-hearing, speech impaired, and visually impaired, at the same time creating a Division of Handicapped Children and Youth in the Department of Health, Education and Welfare. In 1965, Public Law 89-313 amended Title I of the Elementary and Secondary Education Act (E.S.E.A.) and established grants to state agencies to assist handicapped children in state-operated or supported schools. In 1966 the National Advisory Committee on Handicapped Children was created. In 1967, Public Law 90-247 enacted further E.S.E.A. amendments benefiting programs for the communication handicapped including (1) the development of regional resource centers; (2) a program of recruitment and information; (3) expansion of the media program to include all handicapped children; (4) centers and services for deaf/blind children; (5) program provisions for the handicapped under Title III of E.S.E.A.; (6) increased institution funds; (7) research and demonstration funds; and (8) changes in and increased funding of Title VI grants. In 1968, the Handicapped Children's Early Education Assistance Act became law, establishing experimental preschool and early education programs for the handicapped.

During the early 1970s, Congress paid increased attention to the handicapped. Public Law 93-112, the Vocational Rehabilitation Act of 1973, containing Section 504, gave priority to "individuals with most severe handicaps." In 1974 Congress enlarged authorized funding for the education of the handicapped from $100 million to $600 million (Public Law 93-380). On November 28, 1975, President Gerald Ford signed into law the Education for All Handicapped Children Act (Public Law 94-142). The intent of this act is to provide a free appropriate public education for all handicapped children between the ages of three and twenty-one by 1980. This landmark act (Public Law 94-142) is inevitably having a far-reaching impact on special education and related services throughout the nation.

Shirley Hufstedler, the nation's first cabinet-level Education Secretary, states the position of federal concern very well in her July, 1980, presentation at the National Education Association's Annual Conference (1980) in Los Angeles when she pleaded . . . not to turn back the calendar . . . to simpler times . . . , which she labeled "a form of edited amnesia" point of view that ignores the generations of minority children who were denied equal education and the handicapped children who were excluded from public schools.[4]

The federal committment to education may also be strengthened by the creation in 1980 of the Department of Education and by increasing federal financial assistance to education by 73 percent since 1977.

The topic of "federal commitment" would not be complete without calling attention to special interest groups and coalitions that have had great influence in creating new concepts in current federal legislation. Decidedly the legislative, judicial, and executive branches of federal government have moved and are continuing to move towards providing resources and benefits for the handicapped in an equitable distribution. Through effectual administration and enforcement, these benefits and resources will become reality for school-age individuals with communication disorders.

In the federal Department of Education an Assistant Secretary for Special Education and Rehabilitative Services is stipulated; therefore giving substantial impetus and attention to programs for the handicapped including the communication handicapped (*see* Fig. 3-1).

THE STATE'S COMMITMENT TO EDUCATION

The major responsibility for implementing education is found in the states rather than in the federal government. However, the federal Education for All Handicapped Children Act of 1975 (Public Law 94-142) and the Vocational Rehabilitation Act of 1973, Section 504 (Public Law 93-112), have had broad significance in assuring that all states adequately provide for all handicapped individuals according to federal statutes and regulations. The people of each state make the basic policies and framework for education through their constitutional provisions and laws enacted by their legislatures. State boards of education have been established by most states to determine statewide policies and rules and regulations relating to the operation of the schools. A chief state school officer (state superintendent of schools or director of instruction) has been provided by all states. He or she usually serves as executive officer of the state board. A state department of education,

---

[4]*Los Angeles Times*, "Shun the Past, Look to the Future, Teachers Told, 6 July 1980, pp. 3, 22.

Speech-Language Pathologist as Member Educational Team   79

DEPARTMENT OF EDUCATION

```
                    ┌──────────────────────┐
                    │      SECRETARY       │
                    ├──────────────────────┤
                    │   UNDER SECRETARY    │
                    └──────────────────────┘
```

- INTERGOVERNMENTAL ADVISORY COUNCIL ON EDUCATION
- FEDERAL INTERAGENCY COMMITTEE ON EDUCATION

- OFFICE OF BILINGUAL EDUCATION AND MINORITY LANGUAGES AFFAIRS
- GENERAL COUNSEL
- INSPECTOR GENERAL
- OFFICE OF NON-PUBLIC EDUCATION

- MANAGEMENT AND BUDGET
- PLANNING, EVALUATION AND POLICY DEVELOPMENT
- CONGRESSIONAL RELATIONS
- PUBLIC INFORMATION

- ASSISTANT SECRETARY FOR CIVIL RIGHTS
- ASSISTANT SECRETARY FOR ELEMENTARY AND SECONDARY EDUCATION
- ASSISTANT SECRETARY FOR POSTSECONDARY EDUCATION
- ASSISTANT SECRETARY FOR EDUCATIONAL RESEARCH AND IMPROVEMENT

- ASSISTANT SECRETARY FOR VOCATIONAL AND ADULT EDUCATION
- ADMINISTRATOR OF EDUCATION FOR OVERSEAS DEPENDENTS
- ASSISTANT SECRETARY FOR SPECIAL EDUCATION AND REHABILITATIVE SERVICES

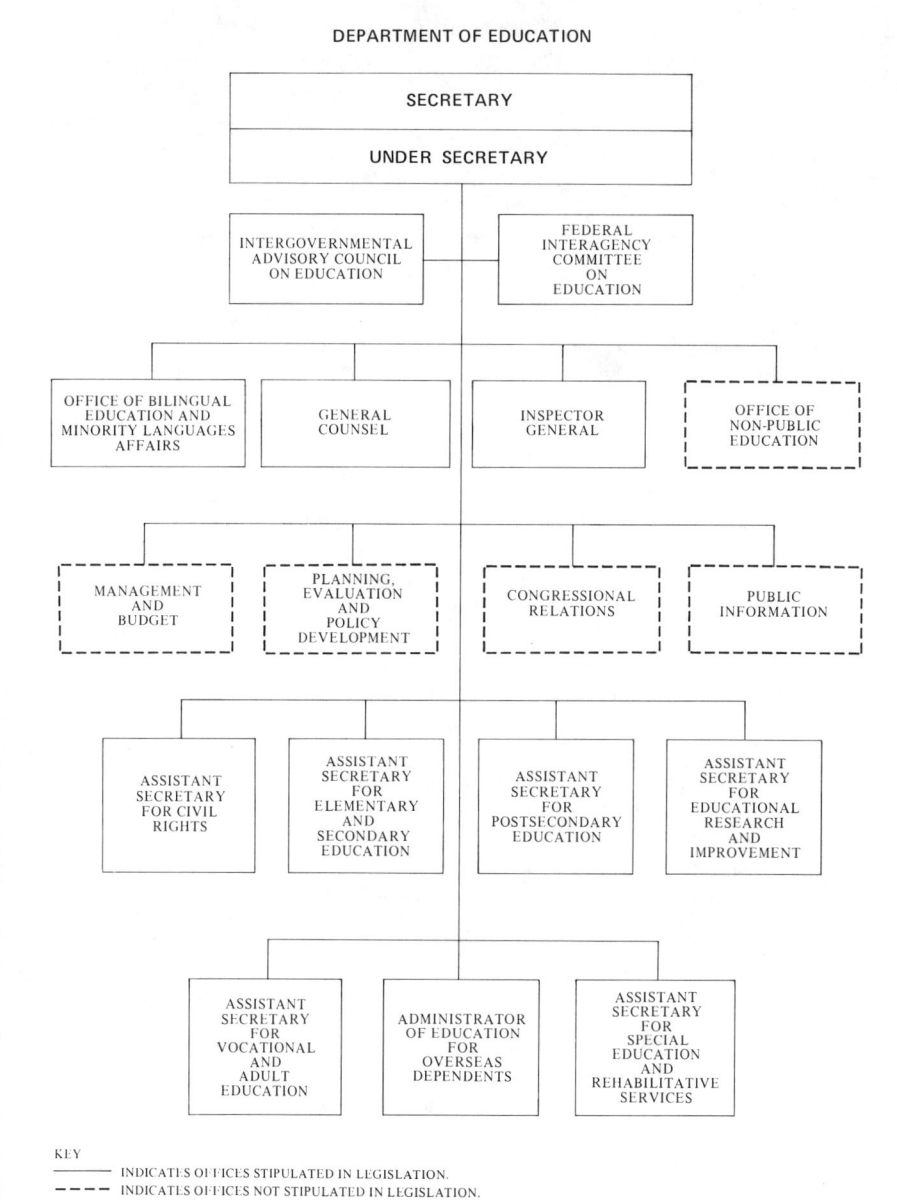

KEY
——— INDICATES OFFICES STIPULATED IN LEGISLATION.
- - - INDICATES OFFICES NOT STIPULATED IN LEGISLATION.

Figure 3-1. Organization of the United States Department of Education (1980).

i.e. state educational agency, (SEA) is responsible to the chief state school officer, and through him or her to the state board in providing leadership, developing policies and regulations, and carrying out research and studies relating to the educational program.

Within the provisions of Public Law 94-142 (1975), the state educational agency also has responsibility for an annual plan to be approved by the U.S. Education Department, Assistant Secretary for Special Education and Rehabilitation Services, Office of Special Education, to include the following:

1. Certification of the annual program plan for the state by the state educational agency and attorney general.
2. Procedures which insure that public hearings, public notice of the public hearings, reasonable opportunity for interested parties throughout the state to participate in public hearings, review of public comments before adopting the annual plan, and publication and availability of the approved annual state plan.
3. Information which shows that the State has in effect a policy which insures that all handicapped children have the right to a free appropriate public education within the age ranges and timelines within the scope of the statute and regulations of Public Law 94-142.
4. Policies and procedures to insure that the State will undertake or has undertaken a goal of providing full educational opportunity to all handicapped children aged birth through twenty-one, including timetables and, adequate facilities, personnel and services.
5. Established priorities for serving individuals, i.e., eligible for a free appropriate public education, not receiving any education, individuals with most severe handicaps who are receiving an inadequate education.
6. Identification, location and assessment of handicapped children.
7. Confidentiality of personally identifiable information.
8. Individualized education programs (I.E.P.'s) as implemented by each public agency, e.g., school districts, and, information showing each public agency establishes, reviews, and revises the I.E.P. according to federal regulations.
9. Procedural safeguards including due process procedures for parents and children, e.g. opportunity to examine records, independent educational evaluation, prior notice and parent consent, impartial due process hearing, hearing rights, appeal procedures, civil action, timelines, and convenience of hearings and reviews, child's status during proceedings, surrogate parents, protection in assessment procedures and placement procedures, the least restrictive environment for the pupil, and, confidentiality of information.
10. Procedures which insure the least restrictive environment for each handicapped child in the state.

11. Protection in assessment procedures.
12. Policies and procedures of private schools in the state.
13. Control of funds and property.
14. Prohibiting of comingling of federal and state funds.
15. Assurance that the programs for the handicapped throughout the state show nondiscrimination and also employment of handicapped individuals.
16. Assurance that procedures are established for consultation with individuals involved in or concerned with the education of handicapped children, including handicapped individuals and parents of handicapped children.
17. Insure that funds received under any other federal program are used by the state only in a manner consistent with the goal of providing free appropriate public education for all handicapped children.

The speech-language pathologist in the schools should be familiar with the state plan to know state priorities and implications for the speech-language program, and to remain abreast of the scope and extent of the many aspects of the special education program in the state.

In addition to the requirements of an annual plan, state educational agencies are (1) responsible for all educational programs for handicapped children administered within the state; (2) responsible to undertake monitoring and evaluating activities to assure compliance of all public agencies within the state with federal statutes and regulations for educating handicapped children; (3) responsible for adopting complaint procedures; (4) responsible for proper usage of federal funds for state administration and local educational agency programming; (5) responsible for establishing a state advisory panel on the education of handicapped children; (6) responsible for an annual report including information on children served and criteria for counting children; (7) responsible for a comprehensive system of personnel development; and, (8) responsible for keeping records to assure the correctness and verification of reports and proper disbursement of funds provided in Public Law 94-142.

The Role Of A State Consultant

Even though a consultant of a state educational agency or state department of education is not ordinarily a member of the educational team providing direct services to children, he or she has an important role in contributing professionally to sound programming for communication impaired children. Most state departments of education employ consultants in speech, language, and hearing. Consultants in speech-language-hearing (speech pathology and audiology or hearing education) in state departments of education or state educational agencies have among their duties the following:

1. Providing statewide consultative services and technical assistance to all counties and school districts needing assistance.
2. Cooperating and participating in district, county, regional, and state conferences and in projects pertaining to meeting the needs of children with speech-language-hearing handicaps.
3. Promoting an understanding of sound professional criteria and the procedures used in establishing and maintaining public school programs for speech-language handicapped pupils.
4. Identifying needs and areas for development and improvement in the state's programs for the speech-language-hearing handicapped as an outgrowth of objective study, research, and observation.
5. Promoting and assisting in establishing and organizing programs in locales where programs are nonexistent or in need of expansion.
6. Explaining state and federal level policies, standards, and regulations.
7. Evaluating objectively speech-language-hearing services throughout the state.
8. Working closely with college and university personnel responsible for the preparation of competent speech-language pathologists and placing primary importance on keeping the colleges and universities informed of public school needs, objectives, and unique characteristics.
9. Encouraging and delineating sound professional standards, competencies, and practices for all speech-language pathologists.
10. Working with professional organizations to promote the enhancement of research and services for children with speech, language, and hearing handicaps.
11. Serving as an advocate within the department of education on behalf of the speech-language-hearing handicapped children in the schools.
12. Preparing information for dissemination that will assist those responsible for helping children with speech-language-hearing disorders.

13. Participating in school program reviews to monitor and review program compliance and quality delivery of services.
14. Approving program plans from local educational agencies.

LOCAL AND INTERMEDIATE EDUCATIONAL AGENCIES

The Local School District or Local Educational Agency (LEA)

Local school districts or educational agencies have been provided by all states. Some states have fewer than 100; others have over 5,000 districts. The small school districts established in the early days of the country are definitely on the decline; however, local autonomy continues to be a cherished element in public education in the smaller (as well as larger) districts. The smaller districts are being replaced in many parts of the country by more comprehensive, larger, unified districts.

The local system is responsible for the organization and implementation of school programs within its area. Within the boundaries of state and federal legal provisions, the people in each local school system determine directly or indirectly the essence of the educational program. The people of the area usually elect a lay board of education to determine policies. The board selects a superintendent of schools who is the administrator. On his recommendations, the needed staff is appointed to operate the schools.

The individual school in the local school system is organized to carry out an instructional program for students and mandated and permissive special education programs and related services. A principal is usually the local administrator. Sometimes in small districts the superintendent serves as the principal of the school. The principal is the main spokesperson for the school in the local community. It is very important for the speech-language pathologist and the school principal to understand one another's roles and functions. They can be of great assistance to one another in helping the child with a communication disorder.

The better school programs always make energetic efforts to know thoroughly the wide variation in interests, needs, and abilities existing among their pupils. They constantly redefine and reappraise their goals and objectives in terms of the changing needs of the community. The effective school also evaluates the outcomes of its program in terms of the educational development of individual pupils and the successes of its graduates. It strives to improve its methods for encouraging the development and success of individual pupils in many dimensions. In providing a staff, materials of instruction, and services and physical facilities, it insures, along with good service, the maximum progress of each pupil towards his specific educational goals.

No two schools are exactly alike. This is also true of all school systems. The speech-language pathologist should be realistic in her conceptualization of the public schools and be aware of the many idiosyncracies in organization from one program or system to another.

In many parts of the nation the trend seems to be to have the speech-language pathologist work directly under the supervision of a director of special services or special education. In other school systems she may be supervised by the director of pupil personnel services. The speech-language pathologist should be alert to policies in a school system that give her the prerogatives and flexibilities necessary to carry out a good clinical program of thorough assessment as well as speech-language-hearing therapy for the pupil with a communication disorder.

The Intermediate Agency in the Schools

In many states the intermediate unit for schools, often known as the county schools office, performs a valuable coordinating function. It usually provides leadership and services to certain or all districts in the area. It also compiles and transmits important information on the schools' programs. These intermediate units may cross county lines. Many of the large counties employ county speech-language and hearing consultants or coordinators. Their responsibilities may include the following:

1. Planning professional meetings to better coordinate efforts and upgrade services to children with speech-hearing-language disorders. Each year specific meetings may be coordinated for all concerned with the speech-language-hearing programs, i.e. a countywide orientation meet-

ing for all new personnel and administrators, an all-day study conference, monthly area institutes for district speech-language pathologists, meetings with personnel from the state department of education, other county offices, and those who work in community centers. Additional professional and working committee meetings or task forces are held as needed and requested.
2. Working closely with the state department of education and clarifying state policies, standards, and regulations for school districts.
3. Working with school district personnel, upon request, in a joint evaluation of their speech-language-hearing program for the purpose of improvement of service and better integration with the total school program.
4. Giving consultative service to those concerned with speech-language-hearing programs in areas such as legal aspects, scheduling and organization of programs, assessment of children, parent conferences, criteria for placement, therapy, and coordinative responsibilities.
5. Assisting school districts in planning and establishing new speech-language-hearing programs and in expanding programs already in existence.
6. Coordinating the publication of a county speech-language-hearing communication exchange, guidebooks, films and filmstrips, and other speech-language-hearing projects and materials requested by the professional.
7. Coordinating joint research projects involving school districts and colleges and universities within their boundaries, the state department of education, other county school offices, and professional organizations.
8. Assisting small school districts in identifying and evaluating children with speech-language-hearing disorders; holding conferences with administrators, parents, and teachers, and when indicated, making referrals to community facilities.
9. Planning with local colleges and universities for the education and orientation of students who plan to work in school speech-language-hearing programs.
10. Working closely with professional organizations.
11. Serving on state program review teams.

Roles of School Personnel

The Role of the School Administrator

Leadership and cooperation from school administrators and supervisors are extremely crucial to the success and effectiveness of the speech-language-hearing program. Ideally, school administrators will do the following to ensure that pupils with speech-language-hearing handicaps are given the help they need:

1. Encourage communication among their staff members, including the speech-language pathologist. Through bulletins, memoranda, and other media of communication within the school system, e.g. discussion at staff meetings, elucidation of the speech-language pathologist's services including the nature, scope, and availability of her services may encourage a better flow of information among staff members concerning individual students with whom the speech-language pathologist is extending services. Support and endorsement of the school administrator are important.

2. Keep informed regarding the roles of the SLP. The well-informed administrator keeps himself up to date on the philosophy and nature of speech-language pathology as it relates to the service of the speech clinician in his school system. By conferring with the clinician, maintaining mutual professional respect, and sharing ideas, he keeps informed of this complementary service to individuals with communication impairments in his school or school system.

3. Support development and expansion of the speech-language-hearing program. The effective administrator acknowledges the importance of special programs as well as programs for the majority of pupils in his school. His support manifests itself in his pursuing all avenues possible in obtaining financial support for programs, upholding the best recommended professional standards, and encouraging improvement and enhancement of programs when needs exist.

4. Urge and assist SLPs to attend local, state, and national professional conferences to increase their professional growth and effectiveness. In-service training and professional development contribute to upgrading and perfecting needed services to the communication-impaired pupils with whom the clinician works. The administrator may be of valuable assistance to the program by being sympathetic to in-service activities, representing the SLP in getting board approval for participation in conferences, and recommending financial support for such endeavors.

5. Encourage classroom teachers to participate in the speech-language-hearing program. Ask the classroom teachers to cooperate with the SLP when children need to be scheduled for therapy or need special assessment by the clinician or other specialists. Let the teacher know she is a valuable member of the professional team in understanding and alleviating the child's communication disorder. Encourage the teacher to take the initiative in contacting the clinician when a need exists for a better understanding of any individual child. Suggest to teachers that they air freely their needs in meeting the special needs of the communication-impaired child.

6. Seek support for adequate local financing of the program. The effective administrator studies the financial adequacies and inadequacies of speech-language-hearing program. He recommends augmentation of the support

of the program, if needed, and furnishes specific evidence for that which is needed. He never permits financial inadequacies to defeat his program until all avenues of local, state, and federal support have been exhausted.

7. Help secure and maintain community understanding and acceptance of the program. Furnishing the board of education with information about the nature and scope of the speech-language-hearing program and sending press releases to local papers are helpful in keeping the community informed. Encouraging the SLP to meet with parent and teacher groups is desirable. Upholding the highest standards in speech-language therapy services to students needing the help is probably the most effective way to maintain acceptance of the program.

8. Support study and research on a school district and county level. Research delving into the merits of various practices and procedures in surveying, assessment, and therapy may call attention to areas needing improvement in the program. Studies showing specific results of therapy or the extent of needs in the school system may contribute information needed in supporting and perpetuating the speech-language habilitation and rehabilitation program. An ongoing alertness to study, research, and evaluation of the program is vital in a progressive program.

The initial success of the speech-language-hearing program depends, to a great extent, on the superintendent's support. It is important that he show interest in this program as in any other phase of educational programs offered by the school system. He needs to interpret the program accurately to the board of education and seek its support. Understanding and support are equally important in informing the community, classroom teachers, supervisors, other administrators, and specialists throughout the school system.

The continued success of the speech-language-hearing program depends considerably on the cooperation of the school principal. She can support the program in these ways:

1. Participate as a required member of the "I.E.P. team." This participation should be active involvement in "I.E.P. team" meetings.
2. Assure quiet and adequate facilities in the school where assessment and therapy can be provided with few interruptions.
3. Visit therapeutic sessions and confer with the speech-language pathologist as frequently as with teachers and other school personnel.
4. Cooperate with the speech-language pathologist in scheduling children for therapy and in seeing that the schedule is maintained.
5. Provide the opportunities for the speech-language pathologist to meet with parent and teacher groups to explain the purposes and goals of the speech-language program.

6. Make it apparent to everyone concerned that the speech-language pathologist is an essential member of the school staff.
7. Keep well informed about the speech-language program so that he or she can accurately and realistically discuss it with members of the community.

The principal is sometimes the immediate supervisor of the speech-language pathologist. She is very often the most direct liaison with the classroom teacher. Most often she is the real spokesperson in the community of closest proximity for all of her school's programs and activities. It is therefore very essential for the speech-language pathologist and principal to understand, appreciate, and support one another's roles and functions.

Other administrative personnel in the public schools, including directors of special education, supervisors of speech-language-hearing program specialists, resource specialists, and elementary and secondary supervisors in charge of all special programs, play vital roles in ensuring that speech-language services in their schools are effective. The people in these positions should work closely with the speech-language pathologist. Whenever a speech-language pathologist is employed in a specific school system she should familiarize herself with the availability of these professional staff members. District policies vary in assignments of these individuals, but in almost every instance a close working relationship with the speech-language pathologist is necessary and advantageous. In working with the speech-language pathologist, duties of these other professional personnel include the following:

1. Carrying out policies concerning speech-language-hearing services as they relate to the total school program; these policies should clearly reflect the professional objectives and standards of the field of speech-language pathology and audiology.
2. Serve as liaison between the speech-language pathologist and other school administrators when appropriate.
3. Coordinate and use the services of all personnel available in the school system with the services of the speech-language pathologist as much as is feasible.
4. Assist the speech-language pathologist in obtaining adequate materials, equipment, and working facilities.
5. Help provide secretarial assistance for the speech-language pathologist.

The supervisor of speech-language-hearing services contributes to the efficiency of the school's program in the following ways:

1. Provides specialized staff assistance to speech-language pathologists and to other personnel concerned in the development, coordination, and maintenance of the speech-language-hearing program.
2. Acts as administrator for speech-language pathologists.
3. Serves as a consultant to line and staff personnel in the regular school program.
4. Furnishes specialized technical assistance in the assessment, selection, and effective use of specific instructional and clinical materials, equipment, and supplies.
5. Assists in conducting research to improve the program.
6. Participates in the preparation of resource materials.
7. Participates in the promotion of in-service professional growth, teacher training, and personnel activities such as employment and evaluation of speech-language pathologists.
8. Carries out policies established by the local school system and the state board of education (through the state educational agency).
9. Functions as liaison representative of his administrative office in committees, conferences, and meetings related to speech-language-hearing (for lay and professional groups).

When personnel and services of different school systems are shared, all administrators concerned should understand their roles and make maximum use of the services and personnel. Conferences to clarify procedures should be held during the beginning stages of the program, whenever policy changes occur, and whenever new personnel are added to the program.

The Role of the Classroom Teacher

The classroom teacher, of course, greatly influences the development of a child who has a speech or language disorder. Motivating the child to improve his speech and language and incorporating well-planned objectives for speech and language development in classroom curricula and activities are vital goals the classroom teacher should seek.

To qualify as an effective classroom teacher for the speech, language or hearing handicapped child, the teacher should do the following:

1. Accept the child and help his classmates accept him.
2. Make sure that the classroom invites communication.
3. Foster good relationships among the children and be cooperative with the school's staff members.
4. Be an active, involved member of the child's "I.E.P. team."

5. Take the necessary steps to make her own speech and voice worthy of imitation.
6. Hear accurately the speech and language errors her children make.
7. Have accurate knowledge of how the sounds of our speech are produced and how our language is organized.
8. Create a good communication environment for speech and language improvement.
9. Be cognizant of the values of speech, language, and hearing services.
10. Be able to identify students in her class who need the speech-language pathologist's services.
11. Understand normal speech and language development and concepts including phonology, morphology, syntax, semantics, and pragmatics.
12. Be well informed on how to incorporate the objectives of the speech-language-hearing program with the objectives of the regular classroom curricula.

Appropriate times for scheduling children in the therapy sessions should be arranged as a cooperative endeavor between the classroom teacher and the speech-language pathologist. If possible, children should be scheduled for speech-language therapy sessions so that they can continue to participate in the mainstream of school activities. Denying children opportunities to participate in these activities may make them feel resentful, isolated, different, or penalized because of their speech-language impairment. However, if the child has a severe handicap, speech-language therapy may be more valuable than any other school subject or activity scheduled at a conflicting time. Care should be taken to always give top priority to placing the student in the least restrictive environment at school.

The role of the regular and special classroom teachers of handicapped children is expanded within the provisions of Public Law 94-142. "The child's teacher" is to be a participant in meetings to develop, review, and revise a handicapped child's individualized education program (I.E.P.). For a handicapped child who is receiving special education, the "teacher" could be the child's special education teacher. If the child's only handicap is a speech disorder, the "teacher" could be the speech-language pathologist. For a speech-language handicapped child who is being considered for placement in special education, the "teacher" could be the pupil's regular teacher, or a teacher qualified to provide education in the type of program in which the child may be placed, or both. If the pupil is not in school or has more than one teacher (as in secondary schools), the local educational agency may designate which teacher will participate in the I.E.P. meetings. For the child to reap the full benefits of Public Law 94-142 provisions, the receiving teacher should be included in drafting and planning the I.E.P. for the child. The receiving teacher plays a key role in assuring successful mainstreaming.

The Role of the Parent(s)

The role of the parent on the educational team is indeed important. The parent's role should never be overlooked in an effective speech-language program in the school. Not only does the parent provide the professional team with information but he or she also contributes insight into the interpersonal (parent, peer, sibling) relationships and an infinite number of variables in understanding the many facets of the child's development.

Hoffman and Hoffman (1966), in their *Review of Child Development Research,* synthesize findings that clearly point out not only the influences of parents on children and their development but also the dynamics of parental participation in the child's maturational processes. In other words, evidence is available to show that the speech-language pathologist must always include the parent on the team in habilitating, rehabilitating, and educating the communicatively handicapped child.

Parents are a part of the team in the following ways:

1. Contributing information to the speech-language pathologist and other school personnel about the child during the assessment process and during the meetings devoted to I.E.P. development.
2. Helping solve family psychological problems, which may contribute to the child's disorder.
3. Assisting the speech-language pathologist in carrying out therapeutic and other clinical goals for the child when appropriate.
4. Helping the child "carry over" the accomplishments of his or her therapy.
5. Contributing to the child's self-concept, identity, and maturation.
6. Cooperating with school personnel in the educative-rehabilitative process.

Parents may function on the educational team by writing communications, telephoning, and attending I.E.P. meetings and other conferences. Conferences may include those with the speech-language pathologist and (1) parent(s), (2) parent and child, (3) parent, child, and teacher, (4) parent and teacher, (5) counselor, parent and child, (6) parent and administrator, (7) teacher, or any other combination deemed helpful in the education (regular and special) of the individual student with a communication disorder.

Parent participation has been made more important than ever through Public Law 94-142 mandates. For example, the following federal regulations point out the attention currently given to parent participation in I.E.P. meetings:

300.345 **Parent participation.**

(a) Each public agency shall take steps to insure that one or both of the parents of the handicapped child are present at each meeting or are afforded the opportunity to participate, including:

(1) Notifying parents of the meeting early enough to insure that they will have an opportunity to attend; and

(2) Scheduling the meeting at a mutually agreed on time and place.

(b) The notice under paragraph (a)(1) of this section must indicate the purpose, time, and location of the meeting, and who will be in attendance.

(c) If neither parent can attend, the public agency shall use other methods to insure parent participation, including individual or conference telephone calls.

(d) A meeting may be conducted without a parent in attendance if the public agency is unable to convince the parents that they should attend. In this case the public agency must have a record of its attempts to arrange a mutually agreed on time and place such as:

(1) Detailed records of telephone calls made or attempted and the results of those calls.

(2) Copies of correspondence sent to the parents and any responses received, and

(3) Detailed records of visits made to the parent's home or place of employment and the results of those visits.

(e) The public agency shall take whatever action is necessary to insure that the parent understands the proceedings at a meeting, including arranging for an interpreter for parents who are deaf or whose native language is other than English.

(f) The public agency shall give the parent, on request, a copy of the individualized education program.

(20 U.S.C. 1401(19); 1412 (2) (B), (4), (6); 1414(a)(5).)

Comment. The notice in paragraph (a) could also inform parents that they may bring other people to the meeting. As indicated in paragraph (c), the procedure used to notify parents (whether oral or written or both) is left to the discretion of the agency, but the agency must keep a record of its efforts to contact parents.[5]

The parent(s) is an equal partner in working with members of the "I.E.P. Team" in developing the child's individualized education program (I.E.P.). The parent is also a valuable resource and supporter in achieving goals and objectives in the I.E.P. for the child with a communication disorder.

The Role of the Speech-Language Pathologist in Providing a Speech-Language Program in the School

The child's ability to preserve and use his individuality is enhanced by his effectiveness in communicating, especially in the use of speech and language.

Through communication a child both conveys and interprets feelings and thoughts as he interacts with other individuals. In the process of communication, language becomes the all-encompassing construct of symbols used to represent experiences, thoughts, and feelings, and a child needs language if he is to comprehend the language of others and express his ideas through the medium of speech and language. Teaching accurate speech and language to the child, therefore, is a vital aspect of a good language development program and important to meeting the child's total communication needs (a role shared by teacher and speech-language pathologist).

To understand and help the child with a communication disorder, his maturation, cognition, physical condition, hearing, motivation, psychosexual development, environment, social behavior, and emotional development must be understood. All perceptual and cognitive aspects of the individual need to be carefully considered. Achieving this goal in the educational setting of the school demands coordination and unity of an educational team. The speech-language pathologist must receive cooperation from and extend cooperation to parents, teachers, psychologists, nurses, school administrators, and other school personnel if her services are to be effective.

The primary purpose of speech-language programs in the schools is to provide a thorough identification-assessment-educational/therapeutic-planning-implementation-and-evaluation-program for

---

[5]*Federal Register,* Vol. 42, No 163, Tuesday, August 23, 1977, 45CFR, Section 121a.345, page 42490. (Effective November 21, 1980, all federal regulations designated as 45CFR, Part 121a, are redesignated as 34CFR, Part 300)

94 Speech-Language Programming in the Schools

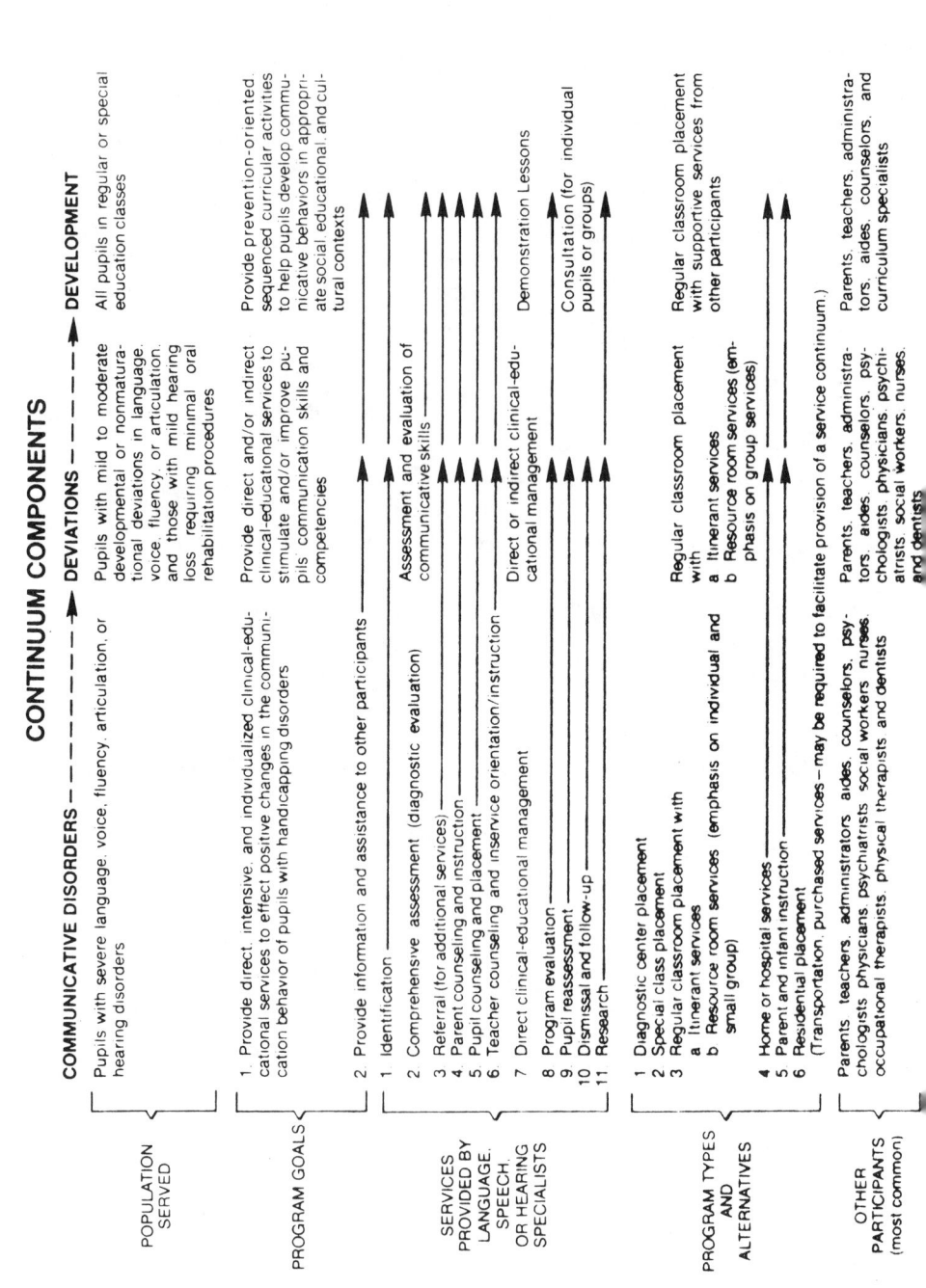

Figure 3-2. The continuum of language, speech, and hearing services for children and youth. From N. Coates et al., *Standards and Guidelines for Comprehensive Language, Speech and Hearing Programs in the Schools*, 1974. Courtesy of American Speech and Hearing Association.

each individual with a speech or language disorder. In meeting the individual's needs, coordination of services, cooperation and understanding of school personnel, parents, and the pupil are all extremely important.

The role of speech-language pathologist is pivotal in the school's speech-language program. The scope of the services that may be provided by the speech-language pathologist may be thought of as a continuum of services as shown in Figure 3-2 by Coates and others.

Garrard (1979) delves into the changing roles of the speech-language pathologist in the schools and relates these roles to the influences of Public Law 94-142 and program alternatives. She discusses a fusion of educational services and its feasibility (Figure 3–3). The Education for All Handicapped Children Act (Public Law 94-142, 1975) includes speech pathology as a related service and defines speech pathology as follows:

Speech pathology includes:

(i) Identification of children with speech or language disorders;
(ii) Diagnosis and appraisal of specific speech or language disorders;
(iii) Referral for medical or other professional attention necessary for

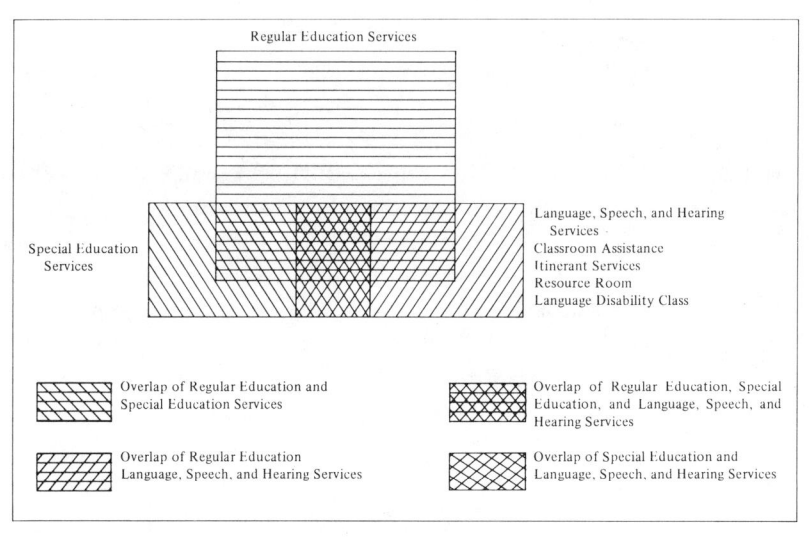

Figure 3-3. A broad view of communication development, an alternative placement model, and an education team approach demand a fusion of educational services. From K. Garrard, The Changing Role of Speech and Hearing Professionals in Public Education, *Asha, 21(2):*93, 1979. Courtesy of American Speech–Language–Hearing Association.

the habilitation of speech or language disorders;
- (iv) Provisions of speech and language services for the habilitation or prevention of communicative disorders;
- (v) Counseling and guidance of parents, children, and teachers regarding speech and language disorders.[6]

A comment in these federal regulations states that appropriate administrative and supervisory activities that are necessary for program planning, management, and evaluation may be included in this and other related services. The federal regulations also clarify services by stating that "special education . . . includes speech pathology . . . if the service consists of specially designed instruction, at no cost to the parents, to meet the unique needs of a handicapped child, and is considered 'special education' rather than a 'related service' under state standards."[7]

Of course, relevant to the role of the speech-language pathologist in the schools is the Public Law 94–142 regulation definition of "speech impaired": "Speech impaired' means a communication disorder, such as stuttering, impaired articulation, a language impairment, or a voice impairment, which adversely affects a child' educational performance.'"[8]

The U.S. Department of Education's Office of Special Education has developed additional clarification of this definition of "speech impaired" as related to the concept of the impairment adversely affecting educational performance. (Refer to Appendix A: U.S. Office of Education, DAS Information Bulletin #66, 3 July 1980.)

The individual who has the luxury of establishing her program in the schools as a speech-language pathologist should examine the excellent details in the "Comprehensive Assessment and Service Evaluation Information System for Language, Speech and Hearing Programs" developed by the American Speech-Language-Hearing Association (Supported in part by funds provided by DHEW, Office of Education, Grant No. G007701877, 1980 Revision). The CASE project is an information system that collects, stores, and allows for

---

[6]*Federal Register,* Vol. 42, No. 163, August 23, 1977, Section 121a. 13(b)(12), and 121a.14(a)(2), page 42480.

[7]*Federal Register,* Vol. 42, No. 163, August 23, 1977, Section 121a.13(b)(12), and 121a.14(a)(2), page 42480.

[8]*Federal Register,* Vol. 42, No.163, August 23, 1977, Section 121a.5(b)(10), pages 42478–42479.

retrieval of language, speech, and hearing student and program information. The CASE Information System Manual could serve as a comprehensive guide of essential elements or components in a school speech, language, and hearing program. (Refer to Appendix B: CASE, 1980 Revision.)

The success of a school's speech-language program may very much depend on the competencies possessed by the speech-language pathologists serving that school.

As stated by the Council for Exceptional Children, the following competencies must be assured in the speech-language pathologist:

> 1. Knowledge of goals, general organization and procedures for achieving these goals, and the basic issues in public education.
> 2. Knowledge of the school's responsibilities and of the way the responsibilities of the speech and hearing specialist relate to this broader framework.
> 3. Awareness of the precise contributions that the speech and hearing program makes to the total educational program.
> 4. Preparation for participation in activities usually associated with speech and hearing programs in the schools; for example, conferring with parents and teachers, conducting speech and hearing surveys, preparing reports.[9]

These competencies should complement the competencies specified in meeting the certification requirements established by the American Speech-Language-Hearing Association and state certification boards or commissions. Standards for effective oral communication also contribute to enhancing the competencies of SLPs. (Refer to Appendix C: Standards For Effective Oral Communication Programs.)

The role of the speech-language pathologist in the public schools is a vital one. All speech-language pathologists are obligated to uphold the best professional standards, a responsibility that involves their assisting the school system in which they are working to establish policies and procedures that will provide for speech and language programs that effectively meet the needs of the children being served.

Among responsibilities of the speech-language pathologist is knowing how to make the special speech and language program

---

[9]Professional Standards Project Report, *Professional Standards for Personnel in the Education of Exceptional Children* (The Council for Exceptional Children, Washington, D.C., 1966).

objectives further those of the regular school program. This means cooperating with teachers and administrators in scheduling speech-language services, always notifying appropriate school personnel of changes in schedules, and attending faculty meetings to keep well informed regarding school policies and procedures.

Another important responsibility of the speech-language pathologist is making proper referrals to other professional personnel within the school program or in the community. Many children with speech-language and/or hearing handicaps also have physical, educational, psychological, and social problems that require the services of a physician, psychologist or psychiatrist, social worker, counselor, nurse, or audiologist, to name a few. If medical assistance is needed, this should be received before any therapeutic goals are established.

Focus On The Individualized Education Program (I.E.P.)

The role of the speech-language pathologist on the educational team is not an easy one. She must continually make her unique objectives and capabilities known. She is a specialist with skills geared to appraising and assessing the child with a communication handicap. One of her major goals is to use assessment findings to guide in eradicating the child's communication disorder in a therapeutic setting. In accomplishing this goal the speech-language pathologist, along with professional colleagues and parents, must complement the other educational processes in the child's total development.

The student's individualized education program (I.E.P.), then, is the focal point of all concerned, including its development and its implementation. In 1977 the National Advisory Committee on the Handicapped devoted its entire *Annual Report* to "The Individualized Education Program: Key to an Appropriate Education for the Handicapped Child." The Committee supports the following propositions, which may very well guide the speech-language pathologist in developing and completing a pupil's I.E.P.:

> 1. That the individualized education program is an invaluable education tool which should be fully and unreservedly used by every school in the Nation, with every handicapped child;

2. That the IEP should be seen as concerning the whole child, in all aspects of his or her life—outside of school as well as in it, and bearing on physical and emotional as well as intellectual needs;

3. That the preparation of each IEP should be an interdisciplinary effort, with appropriate participation by every member of the staff who can make a substantial contribution;

4. That every effort should be made to involve parents both in the development of IEPs and in their implementation; and

5. That school officials should demonstrate their understanding of the importance of IEPs by establishing priorities, special in-service training programs, teacher schedules, and resource allocation procedures that recognize the needs involved and assure optimum results.[10]

The speech-language pathologist is a unique member of the I.E.P. team in that she may provide services to the pupil who has only a communication disorder or the pupil who may be handicapped in other ways, e.g. mentally retarded, cerebral palsied, severely emotionally disturbed, or autistic. This overlapping role of the pathologist fits well in the model suggested by Garrard in Figure 3-3. It also imposes on the speech-language pathologist the responsibility to be skilled and knowledgeable about the communication disorders superimposed on other exceptionalities.

The individualized education program (I.E.P.) has a number of purposes and functions, which include the following:

1. The IEP meeting serves as a communication vehicle between parents and school personnel, and enables them, as equal participants, to jointly decide upon what the child's needs are, what will be provided, and what the anticipated outcomes may be.

2. The IEP itself serves as the focal point for resolving any differences between the parents and the school; first through the meeting and second, if necessary, through the procedural protections that are available to the parents.

3. The IEP sets forth in writing a commitment of resources necessary to enable a handicapped child to receive needed special education and related services.

4. The IEP is a management tool that is used to insure that each handicapped child is provided special education and related services appropriate to his/her special learning needs.

5. The IEP is a compliance/monitoring document which may be used by monitoring personnel from each governmental level to determine whether a handicapped child is actually receiving the free appropriate public

---

[10]National Advisory Committee on the Handicapped, *Annual Report*, 9, 1977.

education agreed to by the parents and the school.

6. The IEP serves as an evaluation device for use in determining the extent of the child's progress toward meeting the projected outcomes. (NOTE: The law does not require that teachers or other school personnel be held accountable if a handicapped child does not achieve the goals and objectives set forth in his/her IEP. See §121a.349.)[11]

Because federal statutes and regulations are very specific concerning requirements of the "Individualized Education Program" (I.E.P.), the speech-language pathologist should be very familiar with them.

The statute and federal regulations pertaining to the individualized education program (I.E.P.) include the following excerpt from Public Law 94–142:

> (19) The term "Individualized education program" means a written statement for each handicapped child developed in any meeting by a representative of the local educational agency or an intermediate educational unit who shall be qualified to provide, or supervise the provision of, specially designed instruction to meet the unique needs of handicapped children, the teacher, the parents or guardian of such child, and, whenever appropriate, such child, which statement shall include (A) a statement of the present levels of educational performance of such child, (B) a statement of annual goals, including short-term instructional objectives, (C) a statement of the specific educational services to be provided to such child, and the extent to which such child will be able to participate in regular educational programs, (D) the projected date for initiation and anticipated duration of such services, and (E) appropriate objective criteria and evaluation procedures and schedules for determing, on at least an annual basis, whether instructional objectives are being achieved.

The following is an excerpt from federal regulations, P.L. 94–142 (August 23, 1977):

> INDIVIDUALIZED EDUCATION PROGRAMS
> § 300.340 **Definition.**
>
> As used in this part, the term "individualized education program" means a written statement for a handicapped child that is developed and implemented in accordance with §§300.341–300.349.
> (20 U.S.C. 1401(19).)
>
> § 300.341 **State educational agency responsibility.**

---

[11]U.S. Education Department, Office of Special Education, DAS Information Bulletin #64, Policy paper on IEPs, page 3, May 23, 1980.

(a) *Public agencies.* The State educational agency shall insure that each public agency develops and implements an individualized education program for each of its handicapped children.
(b) *Private schools and facilities.* The State educational agency shall insure that an individualized education program is developed and implemented for each handicapped child who:
(1) Is placed in or referred to a private school or facility by a public agency; or
(2) Is enrolled in a parochial or other private school and receives special education or related services from a public agency.
(20 U.S.C. 1412 (4), (6); 1413(a)(4).)
Comment: This section applies to all public agencies, including other State agencies (e.g., departments of mental health and welfare), which provide special education to a handicapped child either directly, by contract or through other arrangements. Thus, if a State welfare agency contracts with a private school or facility to provide special education to a handicapped child, that agency would be responsible for insuring that an individualized education program is developed for the child.

§ 300.342 When individualized education programs must be in effect.

(a) On October 1, 1977, and at the beginning of each school year thereafter, each public agency shall have in effect an individualized education program for every handicapped child who is receiving special education from that agency.
(b) An individualized education program must:
(1) Be in effect before special education and related services are provided to a child; and
(2) Be implemented as soon as possible following the meetings under § 300.343.
(20 U.S.C. 1412 (2) (B), (4), (6); 1414 (a) (5); Pub. L. 94–142, Sec. 8(c) (1975).)
Comment. Under paragraph (b) (2), it is expected that a handicapped child's individualized education program (IEP) will be implemented immediately following the meetings under § 300.343. An exception to this would be (1) when the meetings occur during the summer or a vacation period, or (2) where there are circumstances which require a short delay (e.g., working out transportation arrangements). However, there can be no undue delay in providing special education and related services to the child.

§ 300.343 Meetings.

(a) *General.* Each public agency is responsible for initiating and conducting meetings for the purpose of developing, reviewing, and revising a handicapped child's individualized education program.
(b) *Handicapped children currently served.* If the public agency has determined that a handicapped child will receive special education during

school year 1977–1978, a meeting must be held early enough to insure that an individualized education program is developed by October 1, 1977.

(c) *Other handicapped children.* For a handicapped child who is not included under paragraph (b) of this action, a meeting must be held within thirty calendar days of a determination that the child needs special education and related services.

(d) *Review.* Each public agency shall initiate and conduct meetings to periodically review each child's individualized education program and if appropriate revise its provisions. A meeting must be held for this purpose at least once a year.

(20 U.S.C. 1412 (2) (B), (4), (6); 1414 (a) (5).)

Comment. The dates on which agencies must have individualized education programs (IEPs) in effect are specified in §300.342 (October 1, 1977), and the beginning of each school year thereafter). However, except for new handicapped children (i.e., those evaluated and determined to need special education after October 1, 1977), the timing of meetings to develop, review, and revise IEPs is left to the discretion of each agency.

In order to have IEPs in effect by the dates in §300.342, agencies could hold meetings at the end of the school year or during the summer preceding those dates. In meeting the October 1, 1977 timeline, meetings could be conducted up through the October 1 date. Thereafter, meetings may be held any time throughout the year, as long as IEPs are in effect at the beginning of each school year.

The statute requires agencies to hold a meeting at least once each year in order to review, and if appropriate revise, each child's IEP. The timing of those meetings could be on the anniversary date of the last IEP meeting on the child, but this is left to the discretion of the agency.

§ 300.344 Participants in meetings.

(a) *General.* The public agency shall insure that each meeting includes the following participants:

(1) A representative of the public agency, other than the child's teacher, who is qualified to provide, or supervise the provision of, special education.
(2) The child's teacher.
(3) One or both of the child's parents, subject to §300.345.
(4) The child, where appropriate.
(5) Other individuals at the discretion of the parent or agency.

(b) *Evaluation personnel.* For a handicapped child who has been evaluated for the first time, the public agency shall insure:

(1) That a member of the evaluation team participates in the meeting; or
(2) That the representative of the public agency, the child's teacher, or some other person is present at the meeting, who is knowledgeable about the evaluation procedures used with the child and is familiar with the results of the evaluation.

(20 U.S.C. 1401(19); 1412 (2) (B), (4), (6); 1414(a) (5).)

Comment. 1. In deciding which teacher will participate in meetings on a child's individualized education program, the agency may wish to consider the following possibilities:
(a) For a handicapped child who is receiving special education, the "teacher" could be the child's special education teacher. If the child's handicap is a speech impairment, the "teacher" could be the speech-language pathologist.
(b) For a handicapped child who is being considered for placement in special education, the "teacher" could be the child's regular teacher, or a teacher qualified to provide education in the type of program in which the child may be placed, or both.
(c) If the child is not in school or has more than one teacher, the agency may designate which teacher will participate in the meeting.
2. Either the teacher or the agency representative should be qualified in the area of the child's suspected disability.
3. For a child whose primary handicap is a speech impairment, the evaluation personnel participating under paragraph (b) (1) of this section would normally be the speech-language pathologist.

§ 300.345 Parent participation.

(a) Each public agency shall take steps to insure that one or both of the parents of the handicapped child are present at each meeting or are afforded the opportunity to participate, including:
(1) Notifying parents of the meeting early enough to insure that they will have an opportunity to attend; and
(2) Scheduling the meeting at a mutually agreed on time and place.
(b) The notice under paragraph (a) (1) of this section must indicate the purpose, time, and location of the meeting, and who will be in attendance.
(c) If neither parent can attend, the public agency shall use other methods to insure parent participation, including individual or conference telephone calls.
(d) A meeting may be conducted without a parent in attendance if the public agency is unable to convince the parents that they should attend. In this case the public agency must have a record of its attempts to arrange a mutually agreed on time and place such as:
(1) Detailed records of telephone calls made or attempted and the results of those calls.
(2) Copies of correspondence sent to the parents and any responses received, and
(3) Detailed records of visits made to the parent's home or place of employment and the results of those visits.
(e) The public agency shall take whatever action is necessary to insure that the parent understands the proceedings at a meeting, including arranging for an interpreter for parents who are deaf or whose native language is other than English.

(f) The public agency shall give the parent, on request, a copy of the individualized education program.
(20 U.S.C. 1401(19); 1412 (2) (B), (4), (6); 1414 (a) (5).)

Comment. The notice in paragraph (a) could also inform parents that they may bring other people to the meeting. As indicated in paragraph (c), the procedure used to notify parents (whether oral or written or both) is left to the discretion of the agency, but the agency must keep a record of its efforts to contact parents.

§ 300.346 Content of individualized education program.

The individualized education program for each child must include:
(a) A statement of the child's present levels of educational performance;
(b) A statement of annual goals, including short term instructional objectives;
(c) A statement of the specific special education and related services to be provided to the child, and the extent to which the child will be able to participate in regular educational programs;
(d) The projected dates for initiation of services and the anticipated duration of the services; and
(e) Appropriate objective criteria and evaluation procedures and schedules for determining, on at least an annual basis, whether the short term instructional objectives are being achieved.
(20 U.S.C. 1401(19); 1412 (2) (B), (4), (6), 1414(a) (5); Senate Report No. 94–168, p. 11 (1975).)

§ 300.347 Private school placements.

(a) *Developing individualized education programs.* (1) Before a public agency places a handicapped child in, or refers a child to, a private school or facility, the agency shall initiate and conduct a meeting to develop an individualized education program for the child in accordance with § 121a.343.
(2) The agency shall insure that a representative of the private school facility attends the meeting. If the representative cannot attend, the agency shall use other methods to insure participation by the private school or facility, including individual or conference telephone calls.
(3) The public agency shall also develop an individualized educational program for each handicapped child who was placed in a private school or facility by the agency before the effective date of these regulations.
(b) *Reviewing and revising individualized education programs.* (1) After a handicapped child enters a private school or facility, any meetings to review and revise the child's individualized education program may be initiated and conducted by the private school or facility at the discretion of the public agency.
(2) If the private school or facility initiates and conducts these meetings, the public agency shall insure that the parents and an agency representative:

(i) Are involved in any decision about the child's individualized education program; and

(ii) Agree to any proposed changes in the program before those changes are implemented.

(c) *Responsibility.* Even if a private school or facility implements a child's individualized education program, responsibility for compliance with this part remains with the public agency and the State educational agency. (20 U.S.C. 1413(a) (4) (B).)

§ 300.348 Handicapped children in parochial or other private schools.

If a handicapped child is enrolled in a parochial or other private school and receives special education or related services from a public agency, the public agency shall:

(a) Initiate and conduct meetings to develop, review, and revise an individualized education program for the child, in accordance with § 300.343; and

(b) Insure that a representative of the parochial or other private school attends each meeting. If the representative cannot attend, the agency shall use other methods to insure participation by the private school, including individual or conference telephone calls.

(20 U.S.C. 1413(a) (4) (A).)

§ 300.349 Individualized education program—accountability.

Each public agency must provide special education and related services to a handicapped child in accordance with an individualized education program. However, Part B of the Act does not require that any agency, teacher, or other person be held accountable if a child does not achieve the growth projected in the annual goals and objectives.

(20 U.S.C. 1412(2) (B); 1414(a) (5), (6); Cong. Rec. at H 7152 (daily ed., July 21, 1975).)

Comment. This section is intended to relieve concerns that the individualized education program constitutes a guarantee by the public agency and the teacher that a child will progress at a specified rate. However, this section does not relieve agencies and teachers from making good faith efforts to assist the child in achieving the objectives and goals listed in the individualized education program. Further, the section does not limit a parent's right to complain and ask for revisions of the child's program, or to invoke due process procedures, if the parent feels that these efforts are not being made.

Several questions occur rather often concerning the involvement of the speech-language pathologist in the I.E.P. process:

1. If a child's primary handicap is a speech impairment, must the child's regular teacher attend the I.E.P. meeting? No. A speech-language

pathologist would usually serve as the child's "teacher." The regular teacher could attend at the option of the school. However, some member of the "I.E.P. team" must be a qualified speech-language pathologist. (U.S. Education Department, Office of Special Education, DAS Information Bulletin #64, May 23, 1980, p. 14, 17, 24 and 25)

2. If a child is enrolled in a special education class because of a primary handicap and also receives speech-language pathology services, should both specialists attend the I.E.P. meeting?

In general the answer is yes.The special education teacher must attend the meeting. The speech-language pathologist could either (1) participate in the meeting itself, or (2) provide a written recommendation concerning the nature, frequency, and amount of services to be provided to the child. (DAS information Bulletin #64, p. 14)

3. For a child with a suspected speech impairment, who represents the evaluation team (assessment team) at the I.E.P. meeting?

In general, a speech-language pathologist would be the most appropriate person. For many children whose primary handicap is a speech impairment, there may be no other evaluation personnel involved. The comment following Section 121a.532 (Evaluation procedures) states:

Children who have a speech impairment as their primary handicap may not need a complete battery of assessments (e.g., psychological, physical, or adaptive behavior). However, a qualified speech-language pathologist would (1) evaluate each speech impaired child using procedures that are appropriate for the diagnosis and appraisal of speech and language disorders, and (2) where necessary, make referrals for additional assessments needed to make an appropriate placement decision.

(DAS Information Bulletin #64, p. 17)

4. Does the IEP list all special education and related services needed or only those available in the public agency?

Each public agency must provide a free appropriate public education to all handicapped children under its jurisdiction.

Therefore, the IEP for an individual handicapped child must include all of the specific special education and related services needed by the child—as determined by the child's current evaluation. This means that the services must be listed in the IEP even if they are not available in the local agency, and must be provided by the agency through contract or other arrangements. (DAS Information Bulletin #64, p.24–25)

Other questions have been succinctly stated and answered by Dublinske and Healey (*Asha*, March 1978, p. 188–205). These questions and answers should be required reading for all speech-language pathologists to foster their understanding of Public Law 94–142 and implications for implementation. Besides including pertinent questions on the I.E.P., additional coverage is made (pages 197–199) concerning procedural safeguards (due process) and confidentiality. All of these topics identify extensive responsibilities of the school's speech-language pathologist. Appendix D enumerates one school system's procedural safeguards and parents' rights. The speech-language pathologist must adhere to and promote these procedures.

Guidance is often sought concerning a format for the pupil's I.E.P. Two examples are given in Appendix E. The first model I.E.P. format is from the American Speech-Language-Hearing Association's CASE project (1980 Revision). The second is an example used by a large school system serving both large and small communities.

SUMMARY

The speech-language pathologist plays a vital role in assisting the school in meeting its responsibilities of providing the best possible education for each individual. The speech-language pathologist must understand the nature of the school system in which he or she functions. The board of education represents the people of the school district, yet it does not administer school affairs. This responsibility is delegated to the administrative staff headed by the superintendent.

Although the organization and administration of school programs may vary from one school district to another, certain similarities exist. For example, it is the state's major responsibility to provide education for its citizens rather than the federal government's. Since the enactment of Public Law 94-142 the federal government, working through state implementation, has expanded its role with programmatic and funding provisions.

The local school district has the most direct responsibility for the school program. The local board of education employs a superintendent and school principals. The principal is usually the local school administrator and is most directly responsible for the speech-language program. The speech-language pathologist should work closely with the school principal and be well informed in the area of local policies.

The importance of the classroom teacher and parent cannot be overstated. The classroom teacher, parent, and speech-language pathologist have separate but joint roles in the development of good speech and language for all children.

Finally, in addition to school administrators and teachers, other specialists function as important members of the educational team. In addition to psychologists, nurses, and social workers, parents play vital roles. Cooperation and coordination of all of the members of the team make it possible to develop a meaningful and useful I.E.P. to meet the child' educational needs.

The wise speech-language pathologist not only understand his or her role as a member of the educational team but also understands, respects, uses and complements to the fullest advantage other members of the team so as to assist each child in achieving his or her potential.

STUDY ACTIVITIES

1. What are the relative responsibilities of the state and federal governments in special education?
2. In what ways has this changed in recent years?
3. What is the relationship of the state department of education with local school districts?
4. Define "I.E.P." and explain the contents of an "I.E.P."
5. Why should the speech-language pathologist be familiar with local board policies?
6. How can the relationship between the speech-language pathologist and school principal affect the clinical speech-language program?
7. What contributes to a good working relationship between the speech-language pathologist and the parent?
8. What factors should be considered by the "IEP team" in determining if a speech impairment "adversely affects educational performance"?
9. According to federal regulations, how inclusive is the definition of "speech pathology."
10. Who serves on the "IEP team" and what is the role of each member?

REFERENCES

1. Ainsworth, s. The Speech Clinician in Public Schools: Participant or Separatist? *Asha, 7,* 495–503, December, 1965.
2. Ainsworth, S. *Speech Correction Methods, A Manual of Speech Therapy and Public School Procedures.* Englewood Cliffs: Prentice-Hall, 1948.
3. American Speech and Hearing Association, Steer, M. (Project Director) and Darley, F. (Ed.). Public School Speech and Hearing Services. *Journal of Speech and Hearing Disorders, Monograph Supplement 8,* June, 1961.
4. Black, M.E. *Speech Correction in the Schools.* Englewood Cliffs: Prentice-Hall, 1964.
5. Brickman, W.W. *Educational Systems in the United States.* New York: Center for Applied Research in Education, 1964.
6. Bruner, J.S. *The Process of Education.* Cambridge, Harvard University Press, 1960.
7. Burr, J.B. Coffield, W., Jenson, T.J., and Neagley, R.L. *Elementary School Administration.* Boston: Allyn & Bacon, 1963.
8. Campbell, B. *Sixty-three Tested Practices in School Community Relations.* New York: Bureau of Publications, Columbia University, 1954.
9. Coates, N.H. Standards and Guidelines for Comprehensive Language, Speech and Hearing in the Schools. Washington, D.C.,: American Speech and Hearing Association, 1973-1974.
10. Dean, S.E. *Elementary School Organizations and Administration.* Washington, D.C.: U.S. Govt. Print. Office, Dept. HEW Bulletin 11, 1960.
11. Educational Policies Commission. *Education for All American Children.* Washington D.C., N.E.A., 1948.
12. Eisenson, J. and Ogilvie, M. *Speech Correction in the Schools, 2nd ed.* New York: Macmillan, 1963.
13. Elementary School Organization, Purposes, Patterns, Perspectives. *The National Elementary School Principal, 61,* December, 1961.
14. Garrard, K.R. The Changing Role of Speech and Hearing Professionals in Public Education. *Asha, 21, Z,* 98, 1979.
15. Garbee, F.E. Audiological Services in the Schools. Santa Anna, California: Orange County Department of Education, 1979.
16. Garbee, F.E. The California Program for Speech and Hearing Handicapped School Children. Sacramento: Bulletin 33, California State Department of Education, December, 1964 (rev. 1967).
17. Hansen, K.H. *Philosophy for American Education.* Englewood Cliffs: Prentice-Hall, 1960.
18. Hoffman, M.L. and Hoffman, L.W. *Review of Child Development Research.* New York: Russell Sage, 1964, (Vol. 1), 1966 (Vol. 2).
19. James, T.H. et al. *Excellence in Administration: The Dynamics of Leadership.* Stanford: Stanford University Press, 1963.
20. Johnston, H. *A Philosophy of Education.* New York: McGraw-Hill, 1963.
21. Milisen, R. The Incidence of Speech Disorders. In L. Travis (Ed.), *Handbook of Speech Pathology.* New York, Appleton, 1957.

22. Milisen, R. The Public Schools as a Site for Speech and Hearing. *The Speech Teacher, 12,* January, 1963.
23. Morphet, E.L., Johns, R.L., and Reller, T.L. *Educational Administration — Concepts, Practices, and Issues.* Englewood Cliffs, Prentice-Hall, 1959.
24. Powers, M.H., What Makes an Effective Public School Speech Therapist? *Journal of Speech and Hearing Disorders, 21,* 463-467, December, 1956.
25. Services and Functions of Speech and Hearing Specialists in Public Schools. *Asha, 4,* 90-100, April, 1962.
26. Smith, E.W., Krouse, W.S., Jr., and Atkinson, M.M. *The Educator's Encyclopedia.* Englewood Cliffs, Prentice-Hall, 1961.
27. The Speech Clinician's Role in the Public School. *Asha, 6,* 189-191, June, 1964.
28. Van Hattum, R.J. Elementary School Therapy *Exceptional Children, 25,* 411-415, May, 1959.
29. Willey N.R. An Examination of Public School Speech and Hearing Therapy Facilities. *Exceptional Children, 28,* 723-727, November, 1961.
30. Williams, S.W. *Educational Administration in Secondary Schools.* New York: Holt, 1964.

Public Law 94-142 Resources

1. 1. Abeson, A. and Zettel, J. The End of the Quiet Revolution: The Education for All Handicapped Children Act of 1975. *Exceptional Children,* 114-128, October, 1977.
2. *A Guide to Understanding the Education for All Handicapped Children Act (PL 94-142): Questions and Answers on the Federal Law and Regulations.* American Federation of Teachers AFL-CIO, Dupont Circle N.W., Washington, D.C. 20036. Item 435 ($5.00 for 100 copies).
3. *A Teacher's Reference Guide to P.L. 94-142.* National Education Association, 1978. 1201 16th Street, N.W., Washington, D.C. 20036.
4. *An Analysis of Public Law 94-142.* Washington, D.C., National Assoc. of State Directors of Special Education, 1976 ($2.00).
5. *Clarification of P.L. 94-142 for the Classroom Teacher,* 1978. Publications Office Research for Better Schools, Inc., 1700 Market Street, Philadelphia, PA 19103.
6. *Education of the Handicapped Litigation Brough Under P.L. 94-142 and Section 504.* NASDSE, November, 1978, Washington, D.C.
7. Education of Handicapped Children, P.L. 94-142 Regulations, *Federal Register,* Vol. 42, No. 163, August 23, 1977.
8. *Education of the Handicapped:* A biweekly newsletter on Federal Legislation, programs and funding for special education. Capitol Publications, Inc., Suite G-12, 2430 Pennsylvania Ave., N.W., Washington, D.C. 20037. The annual subscription rate is $105.
9. *Handicapped American Reports:* A biweekly newsletter. Handicapped American Reports, 2626 Pennsylvania Ave., N.W., Washington, D.C. 20037.

10. *The Handicapped, the Teacher and the Law,* 1978. A filmstrip package from National Education Association, 1201 16th St., N.W. Washington, D.C. 20036 (202— 833-4336.
11. *IEP Packet.* Foundation for Exceptional Children, 1920 Association Dr., Reston, VA 22091 ($65).
12. *Implementating Procedural Safeguards.* Filmstrip. Council for Exceptional Children, 1920 Association Dr., Reston, VA 22091, #167 ($90).
13. Non-Discrimination on the Basis of Handicap (Section 504). *Federal Register, 42,* May 4, 1977.
14. *Preparing for the IEP Meeting.* Council for Exceptional Children. 1920 Association Dr., Reston, VA 22091, #188 ($35).
15. *Primer on Due Process.* Council for Exceptional Children. 1920 Association Dr., Reston VA 22091, #104 ($4.95).
16. Zettel, J.T. and Abeson, A. The Right to a Free Appropriate Public Education. In *The Courts and Education,* NSSE Yearbook, Part I, 1978. Chicago.
17. P.L. 94–142 Developing the Individualized Education Program. *Asha,* 380, May, 1978.
18. Privacy Rights of Parents and Students Final Rule on Education Records. *Federal Register, 41,* June 17, 1976.
19. *Questions and Answers on P.L. 94–142.* Washington, D.C.: National Association of State Directors of Special Education, 1976.
20. *Section 504 of the Rehabilitation Act of 1973 Fact Sheet,* March, 1978. Brochure: Department of Health Education and Welfare. Office of the Secretary, Office of Civil Rights, Washington, D.C. 20201.

OTHER IEP RESOURCES*

Conducting the Annual Program Review: Midwest Regional Resource Center

This handbook is divided into three parts; an annual review meeting guide and worksheet, a chairperson's manual, and a resource/reference section. 1978, 66 pages. Available through:
ERIC Document Reproduction Service
Computer Microfilm International, Corp.
2020 14th Street, North P.O. Box 190
Arlington, VA 22201

Developing Effective Individualized Education Programs for Severely Handicapped Children and Youth: Norris G. Haring

---

*The following selected resources were compiled and produced by the Midwest Regional Resource Center, Drake University, Des Moines, Iowa, October, 1979:

This document, a product of the topical conference, was designed to be a source of relevant and current information. The overview includes information of the development of the IEP and multi-agency interactional, cooperative model for SEAs, LEAs, and centers for severely handicapped children and youth. Additional information covers the following areas: motor skills, perceptual skills, daily living skills, communication skills, social skills, cognitive skills, occupational education, and interdisciplinary teaming. 1977, 342 pages, $10.95.
Special Press
Department R
724 S. Roosevelt Ave.
Columbus, Ohio 43209

Educators Self-Teaching Guide to Individualized Instructional Programs: R. Dunn and K. Dunn

1975, 335 pages, $10.95
Parker Publishing Company
% Prentice-Hall, Inc.
Englewood Cliffs, N.J. 07632

Guide to Trainers: A Resource for Workshops on Developing Individual Education Programs: Michael Norman

This 152 page trainer's manual provides state and local education agency personnel with a simulation training process and materials for use with planning committees to improve their abilities in developing IEPs. 1977, $3.00 per copy or $2.50 each in quantity of 10 or more, prepaid.
National Association of State Directors of Special Education
1201 16th St., NW
Washington, D. C. 20036
202/833-4193

Individualized Education Plans (IEPs), A Trainer's Guide

This workshop not only focuses on developing IEPs to comply with P.L. 94-142, but more closely with IEP *Implementation Strategies.* The goals of this workshop are to provide general information on the overall process of instructional programming; to provide an opportunity for participants to apply IEP

skills in the development of an IEP for an identified student; and to supply information and materials for a team to use in training others to develop IEPs. Material used for training is included in this workshop as well as training options or ways to use the content of the training package. 1977.
California Regional Resource Center
600 South Commonwealth Ave, Suite 1304
Los Angeles, California 90005

The Individualized Education Program: A Team Approach: Midwest Regional Resource Center and Mary Green

Designed as a two day staff development workshop on the IEP process, the goal of this inservice training package is to develop the skills necessary to participate as an effective member of an IEP team. 1978, 163 pages. Available through:
ERIC Document Reproduction Service
Computer Microfilm International, Corp.
2020 14th St., North P. O. Box 190
Arlington, VA 22201
Order No. 168 292 Microfilm $.83 Papercopy $6.32 plus postage

Individualized Educational Programming Emphasizing IEPs for Very Young and for Severely Handicapped Learners (An IEP on IEP!): Anne Langstaff Pasanella, Cara B. Volkmor, Mary Male, Marilyn Stem

A programmed manual is designed to instruct special educators in the development of IEPs. Sections include: IEP overview, present levels of performance, long-range goals, annual objective, placement alternatives, special education services, evaluation and annual review, short-term objectives and learning steps, instructional strategies and techniques, materials and resources, progress checks, and appendices. 1977, 286 pages.
California Regional Resource Center
600 Commonwealth Ave., Suite 1304
University of Southern California
Los Angeles, CA 90005

Individualized Eudcational Programming (IEP): A Child Study Team Process: Judy A. Schrag

This workshop kit contains a filmstrip, cassette, leader's guide

and participant manual. Objectives focus on training participants to design, implement, and evaluate IEPs and to understand the roles and reponsibilities of child study team members. This workshop kit may be completed in one to three hours. 1977, $49.95.
Learning Concepts
2501 N. Lamar
Austin, Texas 78705
800/531-5004

The Intent of the IEP

This set of 57 color slides, cassette and script provides an overview of the IEP for parent groups and others explaining P. L. 94-142 and its impact on handicapped children. Congressman Albert Quie discusses the congressional intent behind the IEP. 1977. $75.00.
National Association of State Directors of Special Education
1201 Sixteenth Street, NW
Washington, DC 20036
202/833-4193

IEP Man

This set of 60 animated slides and a cassette depicts a step-by-step analysis of placement committee procedures for developing an IEP. 1977, $75.00
National Association of State Directors of Special Education
1201 Sixteenth Street, NW
Washington, DC 20036
202/833-4193

Implementation of the Individualized Education Program: A Teacher's Perspective

1979, 106 pages, cost not available.
Mid-East Regional Resource Center
George Washington University
1901 Pennsylvania Ave. N.W.
Suite 505
Washington, D. C. 20006
202/676-7200

Individual Education Program for Handicapped Children

This set of three color filmstrips, cassettes, instruction sheets, and a copy of "A Primer on Individualized Education Programs for Handicapped Children" provides a step-by-step procedure for developing IEPs, for inservice training purposes. 1978. $65.00.
Council for Exceptional Children
1920 Association Drive
Reston, VA 22091
800/336-3728

A Primer of Individualized Education Programs for Handicapped Children: Scott Torres

This 60 page document is organized around the development of an IEP. Each section is arranged in sequential order to provide the reader with the necessary information to develop, implement, and monitor an individualized education program for every handicapped child who requires special education and related services. 1977, 60 pages, $4.95.
Council for Exceptional Children
1920 Association Drive
Reston, Va 22091
800/336-3728

Reading in Individualized Education Programs: Robert Piazza and Irving Newman

Present a compilation of already published article on the general subject of mainstreaming. Provides the reader with a good overview and basic understanding of this concept. 1978, 209 pages, $8.75.
Special Learning Corporation
42 Boston Road
Guilford, CT 06437

APPENDIX 3A
DEPARTMENT OF HEALTH, EDUCATION, AND WELFARE
OFFICE OF EDUCATION
Washington, D.C. 20202

July 8, 1980

Our Reference: DAS Information Bulletin #66

INFORMAL LETTER TO CHIEF STATE SCHOOL OFFICERS, STATE DIRECTORS OF SPECIAL EDUCATION, STATE COORDINATORS OF PART B OF EHA, AND STATE COORDINATORS OF ESEA I HANDICAPPED PROGRAM (P.L. 89-313)

Subject: Clairfication of the Term "Adversely Affects Educational Performance" as It Is Used in the Part B Definition of "Speech Impaired" Handicapped Children

We have been asked for a policy clarification of the term "adversely affects educational performance" as it is used in the Part B definition of "speech impaired" handicapped children (Section 121a.5(b)(10)).

Attached is a copy of a recent letter sent by the Division of Assistance to States in response to an inquiry from the American Speech-Language-Hearing Association. We hope you will find this letter helpful in determining eligibility of children with communication disorders for special education and related services.

Sincerely,

Garry L. McDaniels
Director
Division of Assistance to States
Office of Special Education

Attachment

DEPARTMENT OF HEALTH, EDUCATION, AND WELFARE
OFFICE OF EDUCATION
Washington, D.C. 20202

May 30, 1980

Mr. Stan Dublinske, Director
School Services Program
American Speech-Language
 & Hearing Association
10801 Rockville Pike
Rockville, Maryland 20852

Dear Mr. Dublinske:

Recently, you requested a policy interpretation of the term "adversely affects educational performance" as it relates to speech impaired children. You indicated that the American Speech-Language-Hearing Association (ASHA) has received reports that some State and local educational agencies are requiring educational assessments of all speech impaired children as part of the evaluation process in order to determine their eligibility for special education and related services.

The broad issue raised in your inquiry is whether the definition of "speech impaired" in the regulations implementing the Education of the Handicapped Act, Part B (as amended by P.L. 94-142) is interpreted to mean that children with communicative disorders who have no other handicapping condition are ineligible for services as "handicapped children" unless educational assessments indicate concomitant problems in academic achievement. An interpretation is needed because "educational performance" is not specifically defined in the Part B regulations. However, the standard for determining whether a child fits into any of the categories of handicaps listed in the Act and regulations is that the impairment "adversely affects a child's educational preformance." Under Section 602 (1) of the Act, a child with one of the listed impairments must need special education to be a "handicapped child." For children who need a "related service" but no other special education services, the Part B regulations in section 121a.14 (a) (2) allow a State to consider that service as "special education," bringing those children within the scope of the Act.

I agree that an interpretation which denies needed services to speech impaired children who have no problem in academic performance is unreasonably restrictive in effect and inconsistent with the intent of the Act and regulations.

There is strong support in the Act and regulations for a broad construction of the term "educational performance." By its terms, the Act affords some services (and encourages States to provide more) to infants and preschoolers with the kinds of handicapping conditions listed in the statute. "Speech impaired" is one of those categories of handicapping conditions. Obviously, assessments of academic performance (through standardized achievement tests in subject matter areas) would be inappropriate or inconclusive if administered to many such children. The meaning of "educational performance" cannot be limited to showing of discrepancies in age/grade performance in academic subject-matter areas.

The extent of a child's mastery of the basic skill of effective oral communication is clearly includable within the standard of "educational performance" set by the regulations. Therefore, a speech/language impairment necessarily adversely affects educational performance when the communication disorder is judged sufficiently severe to require the provision of speech pathology services to the child.

The process for determining a child's disabilities and need for educational services is described in Sections 121a.530-533 of the Part B regulations. These evaluation and placement procedures contemplate that the diagnosis and appraisal of communicative disorders as handicapping conditions would be the responsibility of a qualified speech-language pathologist (*see also* the definition of "speech pathology" in Section 121a.13 (b) (12)).

Section 121a.432 sets minimum requirements for the evaluation procedures that public educational agencies administer.

Section 121a.532 (f) indicates the possible range of areas for assessment (i.e., health, vision, hearing, social-emotional status, general intelligence, academic performance, communicative status, and motor abilities). However, the "comment" following this section states:

> Children who have a speech impairment as their primary handicap may not need a complete battery of assessments (e.g., psychological, physical or adaptive behavior). However, a qualified speech-language pathologist would (1) evaluate each speech impaired child using procedures that are appropriate for diagnosis and appraisal of speech and language disorders, and (2) where necessary, make referrals for additional assessments needed to make an appropriate decision.

The "multisource" requirement of Section 121a.533 (a) (1) makes public agencies responsible for using information from a variety of sources in interpreting evaluation data and making placement decisions. Listed sources include ". . .aptitude and achievement tests, teacher recommendations, physical condition, social or cultural background and adaptive behavior." Following this section is a "comment" which clarifies the multisource requirement in relation to speech-language children:

> Paragraph (a) (1) includes a list of sources that may be used by a public agency in making placement decisions. The agency would not have to use all the sources in every instance. . .For example, while all the named sources would have to be used for a child whose suspected disability is mental retardation, *they would not be necessary for certain other handicapped children, such as a child who has a severe articulation disorder as his primary handicap*. For such a child, the speech-language pathologist, in complying with the multi-source requirement, might use (1) *a standardized test of articulation and* (2) *observation of the child's articulation in conversational speech.* (Emphasis added)

Any public agency requirements which impose procedures more extensive or stringent than those in the Federal regulations must be scrutinized in light of these clarifying comments. It is clear that, in establishing the existence of a speech/language impairment that is "handicapping" in Part B terms, a professional judgement is required. The basis for that judgment is the child's performance on formal and/or informal measures of linguistic competence and performance, rather than heavy reliance on the results of academic achievement testing. The impact of the child's communicative status on academic performance is not deemed the sole or even the primary determinant of the child's need for special educational services. It is the communicative status — and professional judgments made in regard to assessments of communicative abilities — which has overriding significance.

In the event that the speech-language pathologist establishes through appropriate appraisal procedures the existence of a speech/language impairment, the determination of the child's status as a "handicapped child" cannot be conditioned on a requirement that there must be a concurrent deficiency in academic performance.

It was not the intent of the Act to reduce services to handicapped children. The practice which you have brought to our attention could have that kind of negative effect. I appreciate your inquiry on behalf of children with speech/language impairment and trust that this response has made clear the Office's position on this issue.

Sincerely,

Edwin W. Martin
Acting Assistant Secretary
for Special Education & Rehabilitative Services

cc: Garry McDaniels
    Jack Jones
    Tom Irvin
    Bill Tyrrell
    Jerry Vlasak

APPENDIX 3B

CASE INFORMATION SYSTEM
FLOW CHART

STUDENT MANAGEMENT
LEVEL

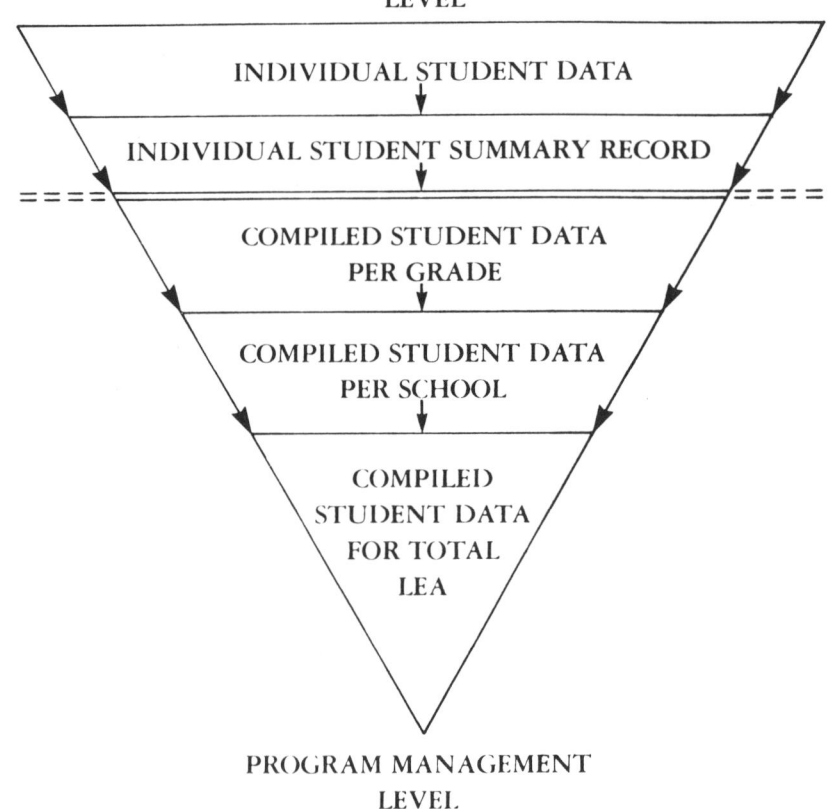

INDIVIDUAL STUDENT DATA

INDIVIDUAL STUDENT SUMMARY RECORD

COMPILED STUDENT DATA
PER GRADE

COMPILED STUDENT DATA
PER SCHOOL

COMPILED
STUDENT DATA
FOR TOTAL
LEA

PROGRAM MANAGEMENT
LEVEL

DESCRIPTION OF THE
CASE PROGRAM MANAGEMENT SYSTEM

PROCESS	FORM NAME	PURPOSE	WHEN COMPLETED	COMPLETED BY	COPIES TO	DATA FLOWS TO
STUDENT INFORMATION	GRADE LIST FOR REPORTING SCREENING RESULTS (SI-1)	To furnish a listing by grade of the students screened for communication disorders and the overall results of each screening	Each time a student is referred/screened	Speech-language pathologist. Audiologist or Designee	Classroom teacher Principal LSH supervisor	Screening Results (SI-2)
	SCREENING RESULTS (SI-2)	To provide, by grade and school, unduplicated counts of students screened for LSH disorders and the results of these screenings	Each time counts are to be computed for students screened, but at least annually	Speech-language pathologist. Audiologist or Designee	LSH supervisor Principal	Summary of Language, Speech and Hearing Services (SI-8)
	ASSESSMENT RESULTS (SI-3)	To provide, by grade and school, unduplicated counts of students with communication disorders, communication differences, and no apparent communication problems based on assessment results	Whenever counts are computed of student assessment results, but at least annually	Speech-language pathologist. Audiologist. LSH supervisor or Designee	LSH supervisor Principal	School Summary of Communication Disorders/Differences Population (SI-5)
	PLACEMENT REPORT (SI-4)	To provide, by grade and school, unduplicated counts of students: • receiving intervention for single and multiple communication disorders/differences • requiring, but not receiving, intervention for communication disorders/differences	Whenever counts are computed of student placement results, but at least annually	Speech-language pathologist. Audiologist. LSH supervisor or Designee	LSH supervisor Principal	School Summary of Communication Disorders/Differences Population (SI-5)

DESCRIPTION OF THE
CASE PROGRAM MANAGEMENT SYSTEM (continued)

SCHOOL SUMMARY OF COMMUNICATION DISORDERS/ DIFFERENCES POPULATION (SI-5)	To provide, by grade and school, unduplicated counts of students: • identified with communication disorders/differences • placed for communication disorders/differences	Whenever counts are computed of student assessment and placement results, but at least annually	Speech-language pathologist, Audiologist, LSH supervisor or Designee	LSH supervisor Principal	LEA Summary of Communication Disorders/Differences Population (SI-6)
LEA SUMMARY COMMUNICATION DISORDERS/DIFFERENCES POPULATION (SI-6)	To provide a school district summary of unduplicated counts of students: • identified with communication disorders/differences • placed for communication differences	Whenever counts are computed of student assessment and placement results, but at least annually	LSH supervisor	LSH supervisor	Summary of Language, Speech and Hearing Services (SI-8)
END OF PERIOD SERVICE STATUS REPORT (SI-7)	To provide, by grade and school, unduplicated counts of students' status at the end of the service period	At end of service period or at least annually	Speech-language pathologist, Audiologist, LSH supervisor or Designee	LSH supervisor	Summary of Language, Speech and Hearing Services (SI-8)
SUMMARY OF LANGUAGE, SPEECH AND HEARING SERVICES (SI-8)	To summarize LSH program student information and to develop unduplicated counts of students served in various service capacities	Whenever complete summaries of student information are compiled, but at least annually	LSH supervisor	Director of Special Education	Not applicable
PROGRAM FUNDING SOURCES (CA-1)	To provide a breakdown of funding sources and amount of funding for the LSH program	At the beginning of each fiscal year or budget period	LSH supervisor or Designee	LSH supervisor, Director of Special Education and/or Other administrative personnel	Program Budget and Expenditure Report (CA-2) Staff Information Analysis and Time Distribution Report (CA-4)
COST ANALYSIS (not included)					

APPENDIX 3C
DESCRIPTION OF THE
CASE PROGRAM MANAGEMENT SYSTEM

PROCESS	FORM NAME	PURPOSE	WHEN COMPLETED	COMPLETED BY	COPIES TO	DATA FLOWS TO
	PROGRAM BUDGET AND EXPENDITURE REPORT (CA-2)	To provide a breakdown of budgeted and expended costs for the LSH program	At the beginning and end of each fiscal year or budget period	LSH supervisor or Designee	LSH supervisor, Director of Special Education and/or Other administrative personnel	Not applicable
	MONTHLY STAFF TIME DISTRIBUTION REPORT (CA-3)	To provide a distribution of LSH service activities by hours that each staff member worked	Daily for each month of service	Speech language pathologist Audiologist and LSH supervisor	LSH supervisor	Staff Information Analysis and Time Distribution Report (CA-4)
	STAFF INFORMATION ANALYSIS AND TIME DISTRIBUTION REPORT (CA-4)	To provide a breakdown of costs of LSH service activities per staff member	At the end of each fiscal year or budget period	*Section I* Speech-language pathologist, Audiologist, LSH supervisor and/or Other Personnel *Section II-V* LSH supervisor or Designee	LSH supervisor	Cost Allocation of Aggregate Staff Hours (CA-5)
	COST ALLOCATION AND AGGREGATE STAFF HOURS REPORT (CA-5)	To provide a breakdown of individual and aggregate staff costs for direct and indirect service activities	At the end of each fiscal year or budget period	LSH supervisor or Designee	LSH supervisor, Director of Special Education and/or Other administrative personnel	Program Budget and Expenditure Report (CA-2) Expenditure Allocation Summary Report (CA-6)

DESCRIPTION OF THE
CASE PROGRAM MANAGEMENT SYSTEM (continued)

	EXPENDITURE ALLOCATION SUMMARY REPORT (CA-6)	To provide a breakdown of type of LSH program and direct service activity costs	At the end of each fiscal year or budget period	LSH supervisor or Designee	LSH supervisor, Director of Special Education and/or Other administrative personnel	Program Budget and Expenditure Report (CA-2)
SPECIAL REPORTS (not included)	EQUIPMENT AND MATERIALS SUPPLIES REQUISITION (SR-1)	To describe, justify, and maintain records of requisitions for equipment and materials/supplies for the LSH program(s) To provide a mechanism for distributing costs and planning budgets for equipment and materials/supplies for the LSH program(s)	Each time equipment and materials/supplies are requested	Speech language pathologist Audiologist	LSH supervisor	Program Budget and Expenditure Report (CA-2) Cost Summary of Equipment and Materials/Supplies Requisition (SR-2)
	COST SUMMARY OF EQUIPMENT/ SUPPLIES REQUISITION (SR-2)	To provide a breakdown of requested funds and actual expenditures for equipment and materials/supplies by LSH program area and service activity	At the end of each fiscal year or budget period	LSH supervisor or Designee (in conjunction with accountant)	LSH supervisor, Director of Special Education and/or Other administrative personnel	Program Budget and Expenditure Report (CA-2) Expenditure Allocation Summary Report (CA-6)
	FACILITIES INFORMATION SURVEY FORM (SR-3)	To provide information of the adequacy of the physical facilities used for the LSH program(s)	Annually	Facility survey team speech-language pathologists, audiologists, LSH supervisor and other members)	LSH supervisor, Director of Special Education and/or Other administrative personnel	Program Budget and Expenditure Report (CA-2)

DESCRIPTION OF THE
CASE PROGRAM MANAGEMENT SYSTEM (continued)

PROCESS	FORM NAME	PURPOSE	WHEN COMPLETED	COMPLETED BY	COPIES TO	DATA FLOWS TO
STUDENT IDENTIFICATION	STUDENT INDENTIFICATION RECORD (1)	To record all relevant student identification information on a single page	At Referral, Screening or Assessment	Speech-language pathologist, Audiologist, Parent/guardian or Designee	Student LSH file LSH supervisor	Student Management Forms (1-15)
PARENT CONTACT	PARENTAL CONTACT RECORD (2)	To maintain a chronological record of parental contacts throughout all phases of service provided in the language, speech and hearing program	Following each parental contact (telephone, written, personal)	Speech-language pathologist and/or Audiologist	Student LSH file	Student Register (14)
REFERRAL	REFERRAL FORM (3)	To document that a referral is being made and to maintain a record of referrals for screening and/or assessment	Whenever a student is referred for LSH screening and/or assessment	Teacher, Parent/guardian or Other school/ health personnel	Student LSH file	Student Register (14) Grade List for Reporting Screening Results (SI-1)
SCREENING	SCREENING FORM (4)	To record information obtained during language, speech and hearing screening	During or after a student is screened for language, speech and/or hearing problems	Speech-language pathologist and/or Audiologist	Student LSH file School file Referral source Parent/guardian	Student Register (14) Grade List for Reporting Screening Results (SI-1)

DESCRIPTION OF THE
CASE PROGRAM MANAGEMENT SYSTEM (continued)

ASSESSMENT	LANGUAGE, SPEECH AND HEARING CASE HISTORY FORM (5)	To obtain a brief case history of the student prior to the delivery of further language, speech and hearing services	Before or after assessment	Parent/guardian	Student LSH file	Not applicable
	COMPREHENSIVE CASE HISTORY (6) (NOT INCLUDED)	To obtain a comprehensive history of the student's development as part of the complete assessment process	Before or after assessment	Speech-language pathologist	Student LSH file	Not applicable
	AUDIOLOGIC ASSESSMENT FORM (7)	To record the presence or absence of audiologic problems, the results of a complete differential diagnostic assessment, and recommendations for further service	During or after completion of an audiologic assessment	Audiologist	Student LSH file	Student Summary Record (13) Student Register (14)
	LANGUAGE AND SPEECH SUMMARY ASSESSMENT FORM (8)	To record the results of all diagnostic assessment information relevant to the language and speech behaviors of a student, including names of test instruments used, test results and conclusions and recommendations for further services)	During or after completion of a language and/or speech assessment	Speech-language pathologist	Student LSH file Assessment/ placement team	Student Summary Record (13) Student Register (14)

DESCRIPTION OF THE
CASE STUDENT MANAGEMENT SYSTEM (continued)

PROCESS	FORM NAME	PURPOSE	WHEN COMPLETED	COMPLETED BY	COPIES TO	DATA FLOWS TO
PLACEMENT	INDIVIDUALIZED EDUCATION PROGRAM (9)	To provide a record of the Individualized Education Program plan for each student in the language, speech and hearing program	Before each placement decision is made Whenever a student's program goals/objectives are changed At the time student progress is recorded	Assessment/placement team	Student LSH file Each specialist serving student Parent/guardian LSH supervisor Director of Special Education	Student Summary Record (13) Student Register (14)
INTERVENTION	INTERVENTION SESSION SUMMARY (10) INTERVENTION RECORD FORM (11A) INTERVENTION SCORE SHEET (11B)	To provide two alternative procedures to systematically record and evaluate performance of students in the language, speech and hearing program	During each session in which student performance data is recorded	Speech-language pathologist or Designee	Student LSH file	End of Period Progress Report (12)
	END OF PERIOD PROGRESS REPORT (12)	To provide a record of services delivered, progress achieved, status, and recommendations for each student in the language, speech and hearing program to teachers, parents, etc.	At the end of each reporting period or when student is dismissed or transfers out of the school district	Speech-language pathologist and/or Audiologist	Student LSH file Parent/guardian Teacher(s) Other specialists serving student	Student Summary Record (13) Student Register (14)

DESCRIPTION OF THE
CASE PROGRAM MANAGEMENT SYSTEM (continued)

CASE COORDINATION	STUDENT SUMMARY RECORD (13)	To maintain a cumulative record of service for each student in the language, speech and hearing program. To inform language, speech and hearing administrative supervisory personnel of changes in student information or status. To provide administrative/supervisory and LSH staff with a means for compiling student data that can be used to help make program management decisions	At Assessment, Placement, End of Period or whenever these processes are repeated	Speech-language pathologist, Audiologist or Designee	Student LSH file Speech-language pathologist Audiologist LSH supervisor	Assessment Results (SI-3) Placement Results (SI-4) End of Period Service Status Report (SI-7)
	STUDENT REGISTER (14)	To record summary information on Referral, Screening, Assessment, Placement and End of Period for all students with communication disorders. To assist the speech-language pathologist and/or audiologist to monitor the status of students in the LSH program	Each time information on Referral, Screening, Assessment, Placement and End of Period. Progress is recorded for each student in the LSH program	Speech-language pathologist, Audiologist or Designee	Speech-language pathologist and/or Audiologist	Not applicable
	STUDENT MASTER RECORD OF SPECIAL EDUCATION SERVICES (15)	To maintain a cumulative record of special education services provided to a student within and/or outside the school district	Each time assessment and/or intervention is initiated and at conclusion of services	Case coordinator or Designee	Student's school file Director of Special Education	Not applicable

APPENDIX 3D*

STANDARDS FOR EFFECTIVE ORAL COMMUNICATION PROGRAMS

Prepared by American Speech-Language-Hearing Association and Speech Communication Association

Adequate oral communication frequently determines an individual's educational, social and vocational success. Yet, American education has typically neglected formal instruction in the basic skills of speaking and listening. It is important that state and local education agencies implement the most effective oral communication programs possible.

The following standards for oral communication were developed by representatives of the Speech Communication Association and the American Speech-Language-Hearing Association.

If effective oral communication programs are going to be developed, all components of the recommended standards must be considered. Implementation of these standards will facilitate development of adequate and appropriate oral communication necessary for educational, social and vocational success.

DEFINITION

Oral Communication: the process of interacting through heard and spoken messages in a variety of situations.

Effective oral communication is a learned behavior, involving the following processes:
1. Speaking in a variety of educational and social situations: Speaking involves, but is not limited to, arranging and producing messages through the use of voice, articulation, vocabulary, syntax and non-verbal cues (e.g., gesture, facial expression, vocal cues) appropriate to the speaker and listeners.
2. Listening in a variety of educational and social situations: Listening involves, but is not limited to, hearing, perceiving, discriminating, interpreting, synthesizing, evaluating, organizing and remembering information from verbal and non-verbal messages.

BASIC ASSUMPTIONS

1. Oral communication behaviors of students can be improved through direct instruction.
2. Oral communication instruction emphasizes the interactive nature of speaking and listening.
3. Oral communication instruction addresses the everyday communication needs of students and includes emphasis on the classroom as a practical communication environment.
4. There is a wide range of communication competence among speakers of the same language.
5. Communication competence is not dependent upon use of a particular form of language.
6. A primary goal of oral communication instruction is to increase the students' repertoire and use of effective speaking and listening behavior.
7. Oral communication programs provide instruction based on a coordinated developmental continuum of skills, pre-school through adult.
8. Oral communication skills can be enhanced by using parents, supportive personnel, and appropriate instructional technology.

---

*From *Asha*, December, 1979. Courtesy of the American Speech—Language—Hearing Association.

AN EFFECTIVE COMMUNICATION PROGRAM HAS THE FOLLOWING CHARACTERISTICS: TEACHING/LEARNING

1. The oral communication program is based on current theory and research in speech and language development, psycholinguistics, rhetorical and communication theory, communication disorders, speech science, and related fields of study.
2. Oral communication instruction is a clearly identifiable part of the curriculum.
3. Oral communication instruction is systematically related to reading and writing instruction and to instruction in the various content areas.
4. The relevant academic, personal and social experiences of students provide core subject matter for the oral communication program.
5. Oral communication instruction provides a wide range of speaking and listening experience, in order to develop effective communication skills appropriate to:
   a. a range of situations: e.g., informal to formal, interpersonal to mass communication
   b. a range of purposes: e.g., informing, learning, persuading, evaluating messages, facilitating social interaction, sharing feelings, imaginative and creative expression
   c. a range of audiences: e.g., classmates, teachers, peers, employers, family, community
   d. a range of communication forms: e.g., conversation, group discussion, interview, drama, debate, public speaking, oral interpretation
   e. a range of speaking styles: impromptu, extemporaneous, and reading from manuscript
6. The oral communication program provides class time for systematic instruction in oral communication skills e.g., critical listening, selecting, arranging and presenting messages, giving and receiving constructive feedback, non-verbal communication, etc.
7. The oral communication program includes development of adequate and appropriate language, articulation, voice, fluency and listening skills necessary for success in educational, career and social situations through regular classroom instruction, co-curricular activities, and speech-language pathology and audiology services.
8. Oral communication program instruction encourages and provides appropriate opportunities for the reticent student (e.g., one who is excessively fearful in speaking situations), to participate more effectively in oral communication.

SUPPORT

1. Oral communication instruction is provided by individuals adequately trained in oral communication and/or communication disorders as evidence by appropriate certification.
2. Individuals responsible for oral communication instruction receive continuing education on theories, research and instruction relevant to communication.
3. Individuals responsible for oral communication instruction participate actively in conventions, meetings, publications, and other activities of communication professionals.
4. The oral communication program includes a system for training classroom teachers to identify and refer students who do not have adequate listening and speaking skills, or are reticent, to those qualified individuals who can best meet the needs of the student through further assessment and/or instruction.
5. Teachers in all curriculum areas receive information on appropriate methods for a) using oral communication to facilitate instruction, and b) using the subject matter to improve students oral communication skills.

6. Parent and community groups are informed about and provided with appropriate materials for effective involvement in the oral communication program.
7. The oral communication program is facilitated by availability and use of appropriate instructional materials, equipment and facilities.

ASSESSMENT AND EVALUATION

1. The oral communication program is based on a school-wide assessment of the speaking and listening needs of students.
2. Speaking and listening needs of students will be determined by qualified personnel utilizing appropriate evaluation tools for the skills to be assessed, and educational levels of students being assessed.
3. Evaluation of student progress in oral communication is based upon a variety of data including observations, self-evaluations, listeners responses to messages, and formal tests.
4. Evaluation of students' oral communication encourages, rather than discourages, students' desires to communicate by emphasizing those behaviors which students can improve, thus enhancing their ability to do so.
5. Evaluation of the total oral communication program is based on achievement of acceptable levels of oral communication skill determined by continuous monitoring of student progress in speaking and listening, use of standardized and criterion-referenced tests, audience-based rating scales, and other appropriate instruments.

APPENDIX 3E
OFFICE OF THE LOS ANGELES COUNTY SUPERINTENDENT OF SCHOOLS
DIVISION OF SPECIAL EDUCATION
ANNUAL NOTIFICATION
PARENT RIGHTS AND PROCEDURAL SAFEGUARDS

I. *PARENTS HAVE A RIGHT TO:*
   A. Attend and assist in all planning conferences and to be notified in advance of all such meetings.
   B. Question decisions regarding identification, assessment and placement (see separate Appeal Procedures).
   C. Review with appropriate interpretation and request copies of pupil records which are maintained in a secure and confidential manner. Any fee is only copying cost. Pupil records are maintained in the school office and in the central office.
   D. Challenge content of pupil record if thought to be inaccurate, misleading or a violation of privacy. Records may be changed if parent and school agree to do so. An appeals process may be used if necessary. Complete procedures are available upon request. Upon request, receive a list of types of records maintained on the pupil.

II. *SEPARATE PARENT INFORMED CONSENTS ARE REQUIRED FOR:*
    (CONSENTS MAY BE REVOKED AT ANY TIME)
   A. Pupil assessment such as psychological, audiological and language/speech upon which educational placement decisions are made. Separate consents are required for placement/service.
   B. Administration of medication/physical examination/treatment/immunizations at school.
   C. Absence for religious exercise and/or instruction in a place away from school property and after the pupil has attended school for a minimum day.
   D. Corporal punishment; approval shall be in force for the school year in which it is submitted and may be withdrawn by the parent at any time. The County Superintendent of Schools also enforces a policy prohibiting the use of corporal punishment without specific approval of the administrator of the Division.

III. *UNLESS PARENTS INDICATE OBJECTIONS IN WRITING, WE MAY:*
   A. Release directory information from pupil record. This is limited to: name, address, telephone, birthdate and place of birth, major field of study, participation in approved sports and activities, weight and height of members of athletic teams, dates of attendance, degrees and awards received and the most recent previous public or private school attended by the pupil.
   B. Release appropriate information regarding handicapped pupils to the California State Department of Education as required.

C. Include the pupil in instruction in health, family life and sex education. If a course in sex education or family life education in which reproductive organs and their functions are described, illustrated or discussed, is planned at some future time, you will be notified of your rights to inspect and review materials prior to the holding of the course. Written consent is not required but written objection based upon religious or moral grounds shall be honored for the pupil. This section does not apply to words or pictures in any science, hygiene or health text book.
D. Screen for vision and hearing as required in Education Code 49452 and in the area of speech, language. Such screenings are used to identify a need for assessment. Conduct routine measurement of classroom progress.

IV. *PARENTS SHOULD KNOW THAT:*
A. When a pupil moves to a new school district, records will be forwarded upon that district's request:
B. Three years after the pupil leaves a county operated program, the following information is kept as a permanent pupil record: identification information, subjects taken, grades, credits, levels of completion or graduation, immunization record, accident reports, involving litigation, permission for professional use of pupils' stills or motion pictures and, in the case of permanently disabled pupils, the most recent verification of disability. Other data is destroyed.
C. When a pupil reaches adult status, (s)he assumes rights of consent and access to records. Sixteen year old pupils have the right to review their records.
D. If the pupil is suspended, parents will be informed within 24 hours of the suspension and their rights. Regulations about pupil discipline may be reviewed in the school office.
E. There are justifiable reasons for excused pupil absence. (Information available from school principal)
F. They are required to inform the school of any medication the pupil is taking regularly. Forms will be provided for this purpose.
G. If the pupil is eligible for a full day special education class and there is no appropriate public school program, parents have the right to apply for private school tuition payment. This application is made through the school district of residence.
H. If they believe this office is not in compliance with federal or state law or regulation, they may file a complaint with the State Superintendent of Schools. Complaint procedures include the right to informal review by the Superintendent or his designee and a hearing before the Board if requested. A copy of complete compliance/appeal procedures will be provided upon receipt of a complaint.
I. Copies of policies, regulations and procedures are available for inspection in the principal's office, the area office or the central office of the Special Education Division of the Office of the Los Angeles County Superintendent

of Schools.

THE LAW REQUIRES THAT WE HAVE A SIGNED COPY OF THIS NOTIFICATION IN EACH PUPIL'S FILE. IF YOU WOULD LIKE TO DISCUSS ANY OF THE ABOVE ITEMS BEFORE SIGNING, PLEASE CONTACT THE SCHOOL PRINCIPAL

I have read and/or had the above information explained to me and I understand its meaning as it relates to my rights and those of the pupil.

_____   _____
Signature of Parent or person acting as   Signature of Adult pupil
parent (please specify)

_____
Date

PLEASE RETURN THE SIGNED SECOND COPY TO SCHOOL AND KEEP THE WHITE COPY FOR YOUR RECORDS. THANK YOU.

INDIVIDUALIZED EDUCATION PROGRAM (IEP) (9)

Date IEP Developed

Month	Day	Year

1. Student Name (Last, First, Middle Initial) 2. Student Number 3. Grade/Educational Setting

4. Teacher's Name (Last, First) 5. School Name

I. IEP DEVELOPMENT INFORMATION

1. Case Coordinator's Name (Last, First) 2. IEP Approved by

3. IEP Entry Date 4. IEP Exit Date 5. Follow up/Review Date(s)

Month	Day	Year	Month	Day	Year	Month	Day	Year	Month	Day	Year

6. Persons Developing IEP 7. Persons Implementing IEP

Name	Position	Name	Position
6.1		7.1	
6.2		7.2	
6.3		7.3	
6.4		7.4	
6.5		7.5	

II. ASSESSMENT INFORMATION

Test Instrument(s)	Date	Results	Examiner

Student Name _____

III. SPECIAL EDUCATION AND RELATED SERVICES NEEDED

1. Service Area	2. Placement Model	3. Type of Session		4. Number of Sessions Per Week	5. Length of Each Session		6. Subtotal/Per Week	
Code	Code	Individual (Check)	Group (No. in Group)		Hours	Minutes	Hours	Minutes

7. Total Sessions/Week

8. Total Time Per Week

9. % Time in Spec. Ed.

10. % Time in Reg. Ed.

Service Area Code:
A = Articulation Disorder
L = Language Disorder
V = Voice Disorder
F = Fluency Disorder
H = Hearing Impairment
Cdf = Communication Difference
VH = Visually Handicapped
MR = Mentally Retarded

ED = Emotionally Disturbed
OH = Orthopedically Handicapped
OHI = Other Health Impaired
DB = Deaf-blind
MH = Multi-handicapped
LD = Learning Disabilities
Other (specify) _____

Placement Model Code:
1 = Regular classroom (consultation)
2 = Follow-up/maintenance
3 = Support services (itinerant or school based)
4 = Resource room
5 = Special self-contained classroom
6 = Special school (day or residential)
7 = Hospital or homebound
8 = Other (specify) _____

IV. PLACEMENT JUSTIFICATION

Student Name _____

V. PRESENT LEVELS OF PERFORMANCE

VI. NEED STATEMENTS

VII. ANNUAL GOALS
_____ Signature (Parent or guardian)

Student Name _____

VIII. INSTRUCTIONAL OBJECTIVES

1. Service Area Code	2. Goal Number	3. Instructional Objectives	4. Recommendations	5. Status Report Code	6. Comments or Revision

Service Area Code:
- CD/LS = Communication Disorder (language and/or speech)
- MR = Mentally Retarded
- HH = Hard of Hearing
- D = Deaf
- VH = Visually Handicapped
- ED = Emotionally Disturbed
- OH = Orthopedically Handicapped
- OHI = Other Health Impaired
- DB = Deaf-blind
- MH = Multi-handicapped
- LD = Learning Disabilities
- Other (specify) _____

Status Report Code:
- A = According to Schedule
- B = Not Begun
- C = Completed
- D = Delayed
- E = Eliminated
- R = Revised
- PC = Partially Completed

OFFICE OF THE LOS ANGELES COUNTY SUPERINTENDENT OF SCHOOLS
DIVISION OF SPECIAL EDUCATION
ELIGIBILITY AND PLANNING CONFERENCE REPORT/ INDIVIDUAL EDUCATIONAL PLAN

☐ Initial IEP/Program Change
☐ Review of IEP (date) _____
☐ Supplementary Service(s)
☐ Triannual IEP
☐ LES ☐ NES (as applicable)

NAME	DISTRICT	DATE
BIRTHDATE	PRINCIPAL ADMINISTRATIVE UNIT	SCHOOL GRADE OR LEVEL PLACEMENT

After discussing educational alternatives, the Eligibility and Planning Committee makes the following recommendations:
I. EDUCATIONAL ALTERNATIVE

☐ Return to district for placement
☐ Special day class: Specify County *program* and *school*: _____

☐ Transfer from parallel program: From _____
☐ Placement changed from one county-operated program to another, indicate:
from _____ to _____
☐ Extent of participation in regular class activities or with other regular class pupils: _____

☐ Individual instruction : (Describe) _____

☐ Other: (Specify) _____

DATE OF ENROLLMENT	PROJECTED DURATION OF PLACEMENT	DATE OF REVIEW OF EDUCATIONAL PLAN
LAST DATE OF ENROLLMENT	REASON FOR TERMINATION (INCLUDE PLACEMENT RECOMMENDATIONS AS APPROPRIATE)	

II. OTHER SPECIAL EDUCATION SERVICES to be provided by County Eligibility has been determined:

☐ Adapted Physical Education . . . . From _____ To _____
☐ Remedial Language/Speech/Hearing . . . . From _____ To _____
   Estimate frequency of service _____
☐ _____ From _____ To _____
☐ _____ From _____ To _____
☐ _____ From _____ To _____
☐ _____ From _____ To _____

III. JUSTIFICATION FOR EDUCATIONAL ALTERNATIVE(S) AND SERVICE(S) SELECTED. Include a summary of handicapping condition(s), list alternatives discussed and rejected.

IV. GENERAL COMMENTS. Include specific alternative means for a secondary pupil to meet graduation proficiency standards. Include provisions for return to regular education and career education as appropriate.

OFFICE OF THE LOS ANGELES COUNTY SUPERINTENDENT OF SCHOOLS
DIVISION OF SPECIAL EDUCATION

INDIVIDUAL EDUCATIONAL PLAN

NAME OF PUPIL		BIRTHDATE	DATE
NOTE LEVELS OF EDUCATIONAL PERFORMANCE IN AREAS RELATING TO SPECIAL NEEDS. SUCH DATA SHOULD INCLUDE STRENGTHS AND WEAKNESSES (i.e. ACADEMIC, SOCIAL-ADAPTIVE, PSYCHO-MOTOR, PRE-VOCATIONAL, SELF-HELP, LANGUAGE, INTELLECTUAL, MEDICAL, LES, NES)	GOAL NUMBER	LIST ANNUAL GOALS AND SHORT TERM OBJECTIVES INCLUDE MEASUREMENT CRITERIA AND RELATE TO PERFORMANCE LEVELS	SERVICE PROVIDED BY (USE SOURCE CODE)
		GOAL .... OBJECTIVE(S)	
		GOAL .... OBJECTIVE(S)	
		GOAL .... OBJECTIVE(S)	

NOTE: A pupil's individual program includes all areas of the curriculum appropriate to his/her level(s) of functioning. The above goals and objectives are written in priority areas of instruction to ameliorate the effects of the handicapping condition(s).

DIRECTIONS: Under Column 1 headings indicate (1) Examiner/Source*; (2) Assessment Date (where applicable); (3) Data supporting functional descriptions/strengths and weaknesses. Where appropriate, include information from the classroom observation and parent input.

*SOURCE ABBREVIATION CODE:
Pa = Parent
A = Administrator
Au = Audiologist
LSS = Language/Speech Specialist
PS = Program Specialist
Outside = Agency/Medical Report
Psyc. = Psychologist
APE = Adapted Physical Education
T = Teacher
Nu = School Nurse
SDi. = District

OFFICE OF THE LOS ANGELES COUNTY SUPERINTENDENT OF SCHOOLS
DIVISION OF SPECIAL EDUCATION

ELIGIBILITY AND PLANNING CONFERENCE REPORT — INDIVIDUAL EDUCATIONAL PLAN

NAME	BIRTHDATE	DATE

V. It is the professional judgment of this committee that recommendations are based on adequate assessment data and are appropriate to the implementation of the Individual Educational Plan. For enrolled pupils, the undersigned assume responsibility for implementation and monitoring of the individual pupil's plan as specified.

ADMINISTRATOR**	DATE	SCHOOL NURSE	DATE
SPECIAL EDUCATION TEACHER	DATE	PROGRAM SPECIALIST	DATE
SCHOOL PSYCHOLOGIST	DATE	AUDIOLOGIST/PHYSICIAN/OTHER	DATE
LANGUAGE AND SPEECH SPECIALIST	DATE	DISTRICT REPRESENTATIVE	DATE
INTERPRETER/OTHER	DATE	OTHER (SPECIFY)	DATE
TEACHER SPECIALIST (SPECIFY)	DATE	OTHER (SPECIFY)	DATE

VI. PARENT/PUPIL PARTICIPATION
   RIGHTS/NOTIFICATIONS

   CHECK BELOW TO VERIFY THAT PARENT HAS BEEN GIVEN OR WILL BE SENT THE FOLLOWING:
   ☐ INDIVIDUAL EDUCATIONAL PLAN/APPEAL PROCEDURES (SEE REVERSE SIDE OF THIS FORM)
   ☐ PARENT RIGHTS AND PROCEDURAL SAFEGUARDS   SIGNED COPY TO BE IN PUPIL FILE (ANNUAL NOTICE)
   ☐ MEETING HELD AT PARENT'S REQUEST WITHOUT ADVANCE WRITTEN NOTICE

Signature of parent, legal guardian or person acting as parent indicates participation, not necessarily agreement.

SIGNATURE OF PARENT, LEGAL GUARDIAN OR PERSON ACTING AS PARENT	DATE	SIGNATURE OF PUPIL	DATE
THE FOLLOWING DOCUMENTS EFFORTS TO CONTACT PARENTS. (SPECIFY DATES, PERSON(S) MAKING CONTACT, COMMENTS.)			

DISSENTING MEMBER: PRINT NAME, ASTERISK AND ATTACH RATIONALE INCLUDING SPECIFIC RECOMMENDATIONS.
**MUST BE IN COMPLIANCE WITH CAC TITLE 5 AND EDUCATION CODE.

I, the undersigned parent, legal guardian or person acting as parent give permission for placement/service(s) as outlined on Page 1.

SIGNATURE OF PARENT, LEGAL GUARDIAN OR PERSON ACTING AS PARENT	DATE

OTHER AGENCY SERVICES ARE TO BE PROVIDED AS NOTED BELOW

SERVICES	DATE FROM	DATE TO	AGENCY	SIGNATURE OF AGENCY REPRESENTATIVE

COMMENTS REGARDING ABOVE SERVICE(S)

ATTACH TO I.E.P.
AS COMPLETED

OFFICE OF THE LOS ANGELES COUNTY SUPERINTENDENT OF SCHOOLS
DIVISION OF SPECIAL EDUCATION

SHORT TERM INSTRUCTIONAL ACTIVITIES

SCHOOL YEAR
19___ - 19___

Pupil _____ Birthdate _____ Grade/Level _____

Program _____ Site/District _____ Teacher/Specialist _____

Curriculum Content Area	IEP Goal/Obj. No.	Instructional Activities Designed to meet IEP Goals/Objectives	Assessment Criterion	Date of Report	Performance Level ANTICIPATED DATE OF COMPLETION
					Percentage / Baseline
					Percentage / Baseline ANTICIPATED DATE OF COMPLETION
					Percentage / Baseline ANTICIPATED DATE OF COMPLETION

SIGNATURES OF PARENT/PUPIL AS APPROPRIATE

SIGNATURE OF PARENT _____ DATE _____

SIGNATURE OF PUPIL _____ DATE _____

THE OFFICE OF THE LOS ANGELES COUNTY SUPERINTENDENT OF SCHOOLS
DIVISION OF SPECIAL EDUCATION

PRESENT LEVEL OF LANGUAGE-SPEECH PERFORMANCE
Remedial Language-Speech Program

Pupil: _____ Birthdate: _____ School: _____ District: _____

Case Selection Test Battery *

Columns: Auditory Association | Related Syllables | NSST-Receptive Syntax | Verbal Expression

Scaled Scores:
- +2 S.D. 48
- +1 S.D. 44, 42
- 40, 36
- −1 S.D. 30, 28
- −2 S.D. 26, 24

Years axis: 2–18

Percentile axis: 10–90

Test Dates:

Hearing Screening:
Pass ____ Fail ____ Referral Made ____

Articulation:

*L.A. County Norms

Additional Findings/Summary Statement:

_____   _____
Remedial Language-Speech Specialist   Date of IEP

Chapter 4

CONSULTATION

GERALD G. FREEMAN

The responsibilities of school speech-language pathologists (Ainsworth et al., 1964) include identification, evaluation, remediation, and consultation. Although these services are adaptable to various work environments, school clinicians frequently find it difficult to engage in effective consultation. It is the purpose of this chapter, therefore, to explore some of the ways in which clinicians may meet the challenges of consultative opportunities in the schools. While consultation is an interactive process, this discussion will emphasize the responsibilities and contributions of speech-language pathologists rather than those of other professional personnel.

THE NATURE OF CONSULTATION

The primary purpose of professional consultation is to seek the opinion of a person with particular knowledge, information, and skills. School speech-language pathologists, no less than others, should be prepared to fulfill this purpose. However, they must also recognize that the school environment requires the integration of consultation into all aspects of the speech-language program. Therefore, school-based clinicians must have a broader orientation to consultation than may be necessary in other settings.

Traditionally, professional consultation has been a culminating activity. Speech-language pathologists, therefore, have used consultation as the capstone of their other services—identification, evaluation, and remediation. That is, they have largely engaged in consultation, as a consequence of other services, to interpret their findings, impressions, and recommendations to professionals and parents. These practices, although legitimate, are too narrow to meet present consultative demands in schools.

Today, school speech-language pathologists must respond to the mandates of special education laws and the variable requirements of their profession. As a result of these influences (a) educators are placing greater emphasis on the relation between verbal skills and academic achievement, (b) more children with special needs, including speech and language, are being placed in regular classrooms, and (c) changes are occurring in the concept and implementation of school-based speech and language programs. All of these factors demand the greater involvement of professionals and parents, through consultation, in all aspects of school services. Consequently, effective consultation in the schools is an integral part of each of the speech-language pathologist's other responsibilities. It is a concurrent service—a dynamic process through which identification, evaluation, and remediation may be shaped. Consultation in schools is used to effect on-going exchanges of information as well as to provide culminating interpretations of clinical data.

The key to effective consultation is proficient clinical practice and the projection of a competent clinical attitude. Historically, school speech-language pathologists have found it difficult to achieve these objectives; schools, by nature of purpose and organization, are not clinical facilities in the usual sense of the term. Therefore, in many instances, school practitioners have had to be unusually resourceful in adapting clinical practices to their work environment.

Once again, recent special education legislation has substantially changed these circumstances. State and federal laws now mandate that handicapped students receive multidisciplinary evaluations, individualized educational plans, and placement in the least restrictive environment. These demands require a high level of clinical performance on the part of various school specialists, including speech-language pathologists. They also imply the need for school personnel to develop interpersonal relations that foster effective consultation.

To meet this challenge, speech-language pathologists must be fully knowledgeable of their discipline. They also need to feel confident in (a) their commitment to the profession, (b) their understanding of the relationship between verbal communication disorders and the educational process, and (c) their role as members of school teams. A brief discussion of each of these areas follows.

REQUISITES OF CONSULTATION

Commitment to the Profession

A number of circumstances have always seemed to confuse the professional identity of speech-language pathologists who work in the schools. (a) Many school practitioners have come into the profession from other fields; (b) for many years state laws have required speech-language pathologists to earn teaching credentials to qualify for school positions; (c) the public thinks of professionals working in schools as teachers; (d) school speech-language pathologists engage in remedial teaching; (e) school speech-language services are a part of special education; and (f) the speech-language-hearing profession, at large, has had a continuous problem defining itself. It is no wonder, then, that school clinicians have had trouble maintaining their professional identity.

Nevertheless, as Garbee (1964) states, the specific responsibilities, skills, and basic identity of school speech-language pathologists should remain the same as those of their collegues who work in other settings. Certainly, school clinicians, along with others in the field, must have an understanding of their environment so as to integrate their services into the broader framework. At the same time, however, it hardly seems possible for them to exercise effective consultative practices, as demanded in schools, unless they are viewed as specialists in speech and language development and its disorders.

There is no intent in this context to suggest that the term "specialist" implies any degree of superiority. School speech-language pathologists may or may not be superior persons. However, they are professional specialists in the same manner that they would be were they working in community agencies, hospitals, university clinics, or other settings.

Consequently, as consultants, school speech-language pathologists must earn the confidence of others through demonstration of specific competencies in the area of communication disorders. They must be committed to the speech-language-hearing profession and to the belief that the demands of their profession can be rewardingly fulfilled in the schools.

Communication Disorders and Education

The philosophy that public education should provide opportunities for individuals to develop to their fullest potential long has served as the foundation for clinical speech-language services in the schools. Further, Black (1964) suggests that the schools provide a logical means of reaching children with communication disorders in a natural setting where speech-language services are readily accepted. These services, therefore, have become an integral part of school programs.

The relationship between education and speech-language services also has been acknowledged by The American Speech-Language-Hearing Association. In 1974, this association endorsed the concept that school programs should provide a continuum of services (Healey, 1974) that recognizes the wide range of needs among children and accommodates each. As a result, school clinicians must use a variety of service and scheduling models designed to cover a span of functions from the prevention of speech and language problems to the remediation or alleviation of serious communication disorders. Concurrently, through consultation, they must variously involve other school professionals and parents along this continuum.

At the same time, the number and types of school programs and services for exceptional populations of children have expanded rapidly. Consequently, the speech-language pathologist is faced with ever larger numbers of children whose verbal communication disorders are one aspect and an integral part of broader educational problems. These children include those who are physically, mentally, visually, acoustically, emotionally, or otherwise handicapped and for whom speech-language services are essential components of their educational programs.

Finally, general and special educators are placing greater emphasis on the relationship between verbal communication skills and reading. They are recognizing that the development of auditory-verbal skills significantly relates to children's achievement in other language modes. In fact, the primary language skills are prerequisite to literacy; reading is dependent on language (Kavanaugh, 1968; Venezky, 1968). The development of auditory-verbal skills, therefore, has assumed a prominence in the curriculum that clearly places it within the responsibilities of speech-language pathologists, classroom teachers, and reading experts and requires the coordination of their various competencies.

Role of SLPs on School Teams

For many years speech-language pathologists considered the team approach highly desirable but found opportunities to engage in team efforts discouragingly limited (Knight et al., 1961). The schools, as an institution, failed to employ the range of professionals uniformly found in other work environments. Furthermore, interdisciplinary involvement tended to focus on the diagnostic process, excluding, as a priority, consultation related to program planning and implementation.

During the last decade this situation has changed dramatically. School resources have rapidly increased in number and sophistication in response to state and federal mandates. Consequently, speech-language pathologists now function, routinely, as part of formal multidisciplinary evaluation teams and educational teams. These teams may include administrators, teachers, other school specialists (psychologists, social workers, reading experts, counselors), medical personnel (physicians, nurses, occupational therapists, physical therapists), and parents. Furthermore, the combined responsibilities of the teams include evaluation, individualized program planning, and the implementation of programs.

Under these circumstances, speech-language pathologists have unparalleled opportunities to serve as vital educational resource consultants. As members of school multidisciplinary evaluation teams their role in planning for children's educational programs should include (a) providing a comprehensive summary of children's linguistic competencies, (b) identifying and interpreting relations between children's linguistic competencies and performances on psychological and educational assessments, (c) establishing correlations between children's observable motor, adaptive, and personal-social development and their speech-language behavior, and (d) formulating generalizations regarding children's learning patterns for speech-language as they relate to the academic environment of the classroom (Robertson and Freeman, 1974).

In addition, as members of educational teams, speech-language pathologists must engage in continuous consultation with the various professionals involved in providing children's individualized programs. The educational-team approach, by nature, involves the integration of each member's competencies into a unified management program; it matches children's needs to professionals' teaching-remedial strengths, regardless of preconceived territorial boundaries (Freeman, 1977). As members of educational teams, therefore, speech-language pathologists must determine the relationships between children's verbal communication disorders and learning, interpret these relationships to others, and consult with others about the role each is to play in the remediation of their common students' auditory-verbal problems.

CONSULTATION IN THE SCHOOLS

Speech-language pathologists earn the role of professional consultant through exemplary clinical behavior. Although the establishment of a full range of clinical practices in schools is not always easy, it is possible and essential to effective consultation. It begins with an understanding that the clinical approach in schools is active rather than nominal. That is, the clinical approach is a function of the committed clinical person.

The school environment tends to present a number of constraints to which clinical practices must be adapted. For example, despite mandatory special education, case loads in some school districts remain larger than they would be in other work environments, making it difficult or impossible for speech-language pathologists to provide intensive individual work to the extent that they would prefer. Also, the itinerant nature of most school-based jobs and that speech-language pathologists rarely work in the same building with others in the field may lead to a type of professional isolation uncommon in other settings.

Despite these constraints, clinically oriented school speech-language pathologists capably find ways to apply their discipline. They demonstrate concern about children and their behavior disorders, specifically disorders in verbal communication and their relation to the educational process. They engage each child in diagnostic teaching. They resist the use of superfluous time-saving activities and develop clinical methods to meet the needs of individual children within small groups. They are aware of their distinctive professional competencies, those of other professional workers, and areas in which these competencies overlap. In a word, through clinical practice they establish themselves as well-defined professional workers to whom others turn for consultation.

Types of Activities

Most of the consultations in which school speech-language pathologists engage are concerned with (a) specific children and their verbal communication disorders, (b) interpretation of the profession and its relation to the local school program, and (c) materials and techniques that may be used by others to support the remedial program. The nature and purpose of a given consultation determine the degree to which any of these areas may be emphasized.

The speech-language pathologist called upon to discuss a particular child, for example, inevitably becomes involved in interpreting the program in which the child is enrolled and recommending assistance for the child. Similarly, a session with teachers concerning the logistics of the program can hardly avoid some attention to a delineation of professional roles and responsibilities.

The ensuing discussion provides suggestions that relate to the core of a variety of actual consultative situations. The information, as provided, is specific for the sake of clarity. In practice, effective consultation usually would be broader and more overlapping in content than illustrated.

CONSULTING WITH SCHOOL SPECIALISTS

Administration

The Superintendent

The success of school speech-language pathologists in gaining the support of superintendents largely depends on the specialists' ability to interpret the relation between clinical speech-language practices and educational objectives. Consequently, speech-language clinicians should identify the commonalities among their concerns and those of other school personnel and clarify these commonalities with superintendents. Although school clinicians are workers in the speech-language-hearing profession, they need to indicate that their functions have an integral and necessary relation to the accomplishment of students' academic achievement, social-emotional well-being, and self-sufficiency. Speech-language pathologists who are able to make these clarifications and project them into consultations with their superintendents will foster understanding, respect, and support.

Boards of Education

The well-informed superintendent generally represents the speech-language pathologist's viewpoints to the school district's board of education. Periodically, however, clinicians may be called upon to present a summary of their programs to a board of education. As elected officials, one of the chief concerns of board members is the appropriate expenditure of funds. Therefore, it behooves speech-language pathologists to consult with board members regarding the educational significance of clinical speech-language practices and the relationship between auditory-verbal skills and educational goals.

Directors of Special Education

Many school speech-language pathologists are responsible to directors of special education. In these cases, clinicians should keep their directors informed about all aspects of the communication disorders program. In regard to the consultative component, specifically, clinicians should assure that their directors are aware of the role of speech-language pathologists, as described above, and the nature and purpose of their various consultative contacts, which will be described later.

Aside from this administrative type of consultation, speech-language clinicians are often called upon to consult with directors of special education about specific cases, particularly as participants on multidisciplinary evaluation teams and educational teams. Clinicians must recognize that special education directors are responsible for the identification, evaluation, placement, and educational goals of handicapped students. The directors must coordinate the findings and impressions of various team members and transform these data into educational practices. Therefore, speech-language pathologists assist directors most effectively when they are able to (a) interpret their findings in educationally significant terms, (b) design speech-language programs to meet students' individual needs, and (c) identify ways in which their data should be applied to the communication disorders program, the classroom, or other school services.

Principals

Principals are the chief administrators in their schools. They are responsible for their staffs and the educational programs and services provided in their buildings. Although most speech-language pathologists conduct itinerant programs, they are bona fide staff members in each building in which they practice. Therefore, they are as directly responsible to their several principals as are other personnel in these schools. Their professional management of children with speech-language disorders is under the principal's jurisdiction. They are expected to appreciate principals' concerns about the educational needs of each child and the programs provided to meet these needs, including speech-language services.

Most principals are eager to provide speech-language services in their schools. However, each principal has a different perspective of these services and the problems connected with providing them. Further, from one building to another, principals establish different educational philosophies; they have variable expectations based on the needs of their student populations. It is essential, therefore, that speech-language pathologists consult with each of their principals about ways in which the communication disorders program may be positively or adversely affected by circumstances within the building.

In consultative contacts with principals, speech-language pathologists must differentiate practices and programmatic adaptations which should be professionally determined from policies that are rightly determined by the school administration. The goal should be to enable principals to gain an appreciation of clinical speech-language practices that will lead to administrative policies which support the communication disorders program. To this end, clinicians must provide principals with information, opinions, and judgments in a capable, tactful, intuitive manner. They must demonstrate skill in presenting the objectives and policies of the program; they should keep their principals informed through conferences and written reports (Powers, 1956).

It is impossible to enumerate all of the areas in which speech-language clinicians might serve as consultants to principals. However, past experiences indicate that principals frequently need information or clarification about (a) the professional framework within which speech-language clinicians function, (b) service and scheduling models, (c) referral procedures, (d) speech-language consultations with parents and other personnel and (e) the case load.

First, the practices of speech-language pathologists are governed by state and federal laws and local administrative policies; they are further influenced by the code of ethics of the American Speech-Language-Hearing Association. School principals usually are well acquainted with local policies. However, they frequently are less familiar with state and federal special education requirements and, most often, know very little about standards and guidelines developed by the ASHA. They need information on how these influences affect speech-language services in relation to their own demands and expectations. With a better understanding of the constraints within which programs must be adapted, principals can be more appreciative and supportive of clinicians' needs to establish priorities and to strive for more idealistic goals.

Second, principals need to understand that speech-language pathologists must use a variety of service and scheduling models. Clinicians who are committed to delivering services along a continuum recognize the need for (a) ensuring communicative competence for all children, (b) providing direct or indirect service to children who demonstrate mild or transitory deviations, and (c) working intensively with children whose communication disorders interfere with academic achievement and/or social adjustment (Freeman, 1977). The traditional itinerant model—working with small groups of children on a biweekly basis—does not provide the flexibility and diversification necessary to meet the range of children's needs. Principals need to be willing to accept changes in service and scheduling models and the initial inconveniences created by them.

Third, SLPs should consult with principals about the process for referring children to other specialists. In schools, as elsewhere, referrals are expedited more efficiently when appropriate channels have been established. Frequently, the principal serves as a referral clearing house to avoid duplication of services and to prevent several staff members from simultaneously sending children and their parents in two directions. In other instances, principals conduct weekly multidisciplinary staff meetings—building team sessions—at which referrals are coordinated. Speech-language pathologists should serve as consultants to principals by indicating the needs for referrals, providing them with pertinent written information, participating in referral procedures, and when necessary, working with them to improve these procedures.

Fourth, clinicians should keep principals informed of their consultations with parents and other school personnel. Speech-language pathologists frequently interview parents with whom principals have had little or no contact or no reason to conduct an extensive interview. The information obtained by clinicians in these meetings, including physical, social, and emotional data, may be as pertinent to a child's total educational program as it is to speech-language behavior. Therefore, the clinician should consult with other personnel about these implications and share all information with the principal.

Finally, as a consultant, the speech-language clinician should supply principals with lists of children in the case load. These lists should be kept current. They should enable principals, at a glance, to know the number, distribution, and names of children being served. In addition, clinicians would be wise to provide principals with an annual written summary report of current services and projected program needs. Specialists who provide and discuss these types of reports with principals are assured of more accurate representation at administrative council meetings.

Consultation is the process through which clinicians may help principals support the provision of the best possible speech-language services in their schools. The task is not easy, since the differences in characteristics of schools prevent the use of a uniform consultative model. On the one hand, it may involve basic groundwork in a school where speech-language services are treated as peripheral to essential school functions. On the other, it may involve a slight alteration of a scheduling procedure where the speech-language program is established and integrated into the school curriculum. In any event, the need for improvements in any school is probable; well-informed principals make these improvements possible.

Teaching Personnel

Classroom Teachers

Successful speech-language services in the schools must include the participation of classroom teachers. Although the concept of interdisciplinary cooperation between teachers and speech-language specialists is not new, frequently these professionals have failed to interact effectively to achieve their common goals. Some teachers have viewed auditory-verbal skills as circumscribed behaviors that have little to do with academic achievement; they have been satisfied to delegate the total responsibility for children's verbal communication needs to speech-language pathologists. Similarly, some clinicians have failed to establish that their roles and functions are significant, even essential, to the academic program. They have conducted their services surrounded by an aura of specialization.

As mentioned above, current educational philosophy has emphasized the importance of varied interdisciplinary programs to meet the different individual needs of children. However, the success of such programs is largely dependent upon the ability of the participating professionals to establish compatible working relations. The most significant of these relations are those of speech-language specialists and classroom teachers. These professionals, aside from their own areas of expertise and competence, must share a common body of knowledge and concepts. They must appreciate each other's professional capabilities and limitations so they may complement and supplement each others' efforts.

To this end, school clinicians should consult with teachers, as one professional to another, about the nature and implications of speech-language services. They must engage teachers in dialogues and experiences that enable each professional to assess the other's unique and overlapping contributions. They must establish working relations designed to achieve the educational goals common to both professions.

Classroom teachers can play significant roles in the identification, evaluation, and remediation of children's communication disorders. To do so, they need to understand the speech-language program and ways in which they may become an integral part of each of its components. It is the responsibility of speech-language pathologists to consult with teachers about the specific processes involved in the communication disorders program and ways in which teachers' contributions to these processes will lead to coordinated efforts in behalf of mutual students.

Identification

The usual methods of identifying children with communication problems are (a) screening and (b) teacher referrals. By nature, screening procedures are subject to a certain amount of error. They may fail to identify some children and misidentify others. Consequently, the role of classroom teachers in verifying the presence or absence of speech-language problems is extremely important. Clinicians must inform teachers that they rely on them to observe and assess children's daily verbal behavior in various academic and social contexts. The specialists should consult with teachers about the kinds of data needed to substantiate or refute the suspicion of a bona fide problem.

Some speech-language pathologists depend totally on teachers to identify and refer children with possible or actual communication problems. This circumstance places even greater responsibility on clinicians to consult with teachers about the nature of speech-language development and its disorders. Clinicians should ensure that the teachers' level of familiarity with this information enables them to identify children in need of further evaluation.

Evaluation

Although speech-language pathologists assume the major responsibility for evaluating children's auditory-verbal communication skills, classroom teachers have an important role in each aspect of the process. Comprehensive speech-language evaluations require the collection and coordination of data obtained through (a) case histories, (b) specialized standardized tests and procedures, and (c) observations of behavior. Speech-language pathologists should consult with teachers about ways in which their participation in data collection augments the evaluative process.

Case Histories

Speech-language clinicians should ask teachers to share historical information that may be critical to understanding the nature of specific children and their problems. For example, teachers frequently can be very helpful when clinicians are concerned about parents' attitudes toward their children's communication problems. Because of their contact and regular interactions with parents, teachers may know a great deal about family situations and parental insights and feelings about the difficulties. They also may be able to identify environmental factors that contribute to communication disorders and to assess the parents' willingness and ability to become involved in the remedial process. These impressions are critical to the clinician's program of parent counseling.

In addition, teachers are an important source of information regarding the children's feelings about and attitudes towards their communication problems and the effects of these problems on their school lives. Clinicians should consult with teachers about the importance of sharing these impressions and jointly implementing management techniques found to be successful in the classroom.

Tests

It is essential that speech-language clinicians provide classroom teachers with information about the nature, value, and limitations of standardized speech and language tests within an appropriate educational perspective. Too often, school personnel become preoccupied with children's test scores and use these scores exclusively for educational decisions. Clinicians, at the same time, behave as if the tests they administer are preferred or beyond the grasp of those outside the field. In fact, they should consult with teachers about children's specific behavioral responses to test items, as well as their scores.

Scores, per se, often provide teachers with little more than confirmation of their previous impressions—those impressions which initially motivated them to refer a child for evaluation. Scores do not convert into educational programs. Descriptions of behaviors, however, are clear to teachers and clinicians alike. They may be discussed as focal points for jointly planned teaching or remedial strategies.

Observations

A valid speech-language evaluation considers recorded observations of children's spontaneous communication in natural environments. Furthermore, observations of children's motor, adaptive, and personal-social behaviors and their intercorrelations with speech and language are necessary considerations in planning remedial programs. Speech-language pathologists, therefore, should consult with classroom teachers about the need for sharing the responsibility of collecting observational data. The specialists also should interpret these data to teachers from their own perspective to add a dimension to program planning.

Interpreting the Problem

In interpreting the nature of speech-language problems to teachers, SLPs should strive to foster insight and action. Teachers generally want to know about the nature of communication disorders and the pedigogical implications of these problems. They want to learn what they can do to help. Speech-language pathologists, therefore, should provide teachers with straightforward, understandable information that reflects current knowledge as well as the state of the art.

One of the most effective ways to interpret speech-language problems to teachers is through description rather than classification. This approach deliberately eliminates excessive use of professional jargon, a vernacular that often is an enigma even to those in the field. It focuses on the behavioral aspects of the communication disorder. The approach is based on the premise that an analysis of what children do is more meaningful, in this context, than categorical pronouncements about them. In other words, in the perspective of school life, what children *do* is more significant than what they *are*.

There are several advantages to this orientation. First, it promotes a child-centered conference rather than a discussion that focuses on the labels used to designate speech-language disorders. It encourages specialists and teachers to exchange ideas about observed behaviors that are understood by both, rather than spending valuable time in clarifying the meanings of classifications. As a result, teachers and clinicians, together, may identify students' auditory-verbal capabilities and weaknesses. They may direct their attention to a commonly understood body of information.

Second, speech-language pathologists' descriptive analyses usually are not startling findings to astute classroom teachers. In fact, these analyses often corroborate teachers' impressions. If so, the analyses serve to establish a comfortable environment in which specialists and teachers may (a) discuss children's speech-language patterns, and (b) relate these patterns to other aspects of behavior and school adjustment. Jointly, the professionals may share observations and identify factors in the classroom that precipitate or perpetuate undesirable behaviors. They may relate auditory-verbal tendencies to children's learning processes and styles.

Third, a behavioristic approach lends itself to a planning structure with which most educators are familiar. The clinician's goal — enabling children to learn appropriate speech-language patterns —

in many ways resembles the teacher's daily goals for other skills. Both are concerned about the individual characteristics of children and the application of appropriate principles and theories of learning to meet the needs.

Finally, the establishment of this commonality of efforts among teachers and specialists highlights the interrelations between the educational process and the speech-language remedial process. SLPs should enable teachers to view speech-language behavior in its complex relations to other behavioral modes. Descriptive analyses lead to this end and, at the same time, lay the groundwork for consultations regarding ways in which specialists and teachers may share the responsibility for speech-language objectives.

The Remedial Program

The main purpose of speech-language programs is to enable children to modify their verbal communication behavior. Since each child's communication problem is different, however, clinicians must organize and implement individualized programs to meet the range of needs and to identify specific target behaviors for modification. The range may extend from indirect environmental support for children with normal maturational speech-language differences to very intensive, direct speech-language remediation for children with severe communication problems.

As a result of this range, comprehensive speech-language programs are organized along a continuum (Healey, 1974). The key points of this continuum are (a) a communication development component at one end, (b) a communication deviations component in the middle, and (c) a communication disorders component at the other end. The continuum accommodates the needs of all children in a district. Furthermore, the delivery of services along the continuum requires the cooperation and active participation of classroom teachers.

Communication Development

The communication development component of speech-language services is a preventive program. In the past, this component, known as speech improvement (Pendergast, 1963), created confusion in school programs. Speech-language specialists felt that communication deviations within the normal range were the responsibility of classroom teachers. The American Speech and Hearing Association (Ainsworth et al., 1964) stated that the clinician's role in speech improvement should be one of consultative help in the development of procedures directed toward supplementing the efforts of teaching personnel.

Today, speech-language pathologists recognize that the development of auditory-verbal skills is basic to the academic achievement of all children. Further, the improvement of children's primary language skills prevents the development of communication disorders. Although the primary responsibility for communication development remains with classroom teachers, among school staffs, speech-language specialists usually have had the most training and experience in this area. Therefore, clinicians should participate as active consultants in a district's communication development program.

Speech-language specialists should consult with teachers, particularly those at the early elementary level, about the need to include listening-speaking activities in the curriculum. They should work with teachers to organize and present sequenced curricular activities that address the needs of their students. If necessary, the specialists may provide periodic demonstration lessons or introduce new units, as consultative support.

In addition, speech-language pathologists should consult with early elementary teachers about techniques that promote the prevention of auditory-verbal problems through positive environmental support. These techniques include (a) modeling and expanding children's utterances, (b) limiting the length of directions to accord with children's maturational level, (c) permitting children to talk and listening to them without interruption, thereby encouraging them to listen, (d) offering children verbal choices, and (e) accepting maturational errors (Freeman, 1977).

Although communication development is not legally mandated, speech-language pathologists have a vested interest in the prevention of auditory-verbal problems. Furthermore, communication development programs provide school clinicians with opportunities, as consultants, to establish credibility as members of the educational team who are concerned about the development of basic academic skills — primary speech-language skills — as well as remedial procedures.

Communication Deviations

The communication deviations component of a speech-language program is designed to meet the needs of children with mild to moderate auditory-verbal differences. These children require more than the indirect approach of a preventive program although less than the intensive contact demanded for severe communication disorders. Speech-language clinicians have the primary responsibility for this component, but classroom teachers have an important supportive role in fulfilling its goals.

In particular, teachers are an essential part of the carry-over process. SLPs, therefore, should consult with teachers about the importance of carry-over in the classroom, as a sequential step to children's integrating new verbal patterns into their daily speech-language behavior. They should advise teachers about ways to promote carry-over, including (a) being aware of children's new habit patterns to reinforce and reward their spontaneous use, (b) providing indirect correction through modeling, (c) offering reminders to the children to use their new skills, and (d) capitalizing on routine classroom activities as opportunities for children to practice specific verbal skills.

Past experiences have indicated that school speech-language pathologists at times have been unrealistic in their expectations of classroom teachers to participate in the carry-over process. Consequently, teachers have felt that their responsibilities for carry-over have exceeded their level of training and have been too demanding for the available time. Therefore, SLPs should provide teachers with well-defined carry-over activities that can be readily adapted to daily classroom activities.

Speech-language pathologists in their earnest zeal often provide teachers with elaborate schemes for promoting carry-over in the classroom. They sometimes supply teachers with a portfolio of sounds and words that should be reinforced for each child. Despite their concern for children, teachers may rightfully resist involvement in too many extracurricular functions. They have little inclination to study or remember exhaustive lists of specific speech-language modifications to be made by each student enrolled in a remedial program. Again, these situations are best resolved through consultation that emphasizes logically structured, skill-by-skill reinforcement, adaptable to regular classroom procedures.

Along these lines, speech-language pathologists have been inclined to coordinate the vocabulary of remedial speech-language activities with that used in classroom materials. This method is intended to enable teachers to work on carry-over during reading, spelling, or other lessons that require verbal responses. However, the approach has proven unsatisfactory, since the teacher's chief concern at these times is subject matter rather than improved verbal communication.

An effective, well-defined, and relatively effortless method of coping with this problem is the coordination of vocabulary used in remedial activities with that applicable to classroom procedures instead of curricular materials. The teacher, in this instance, structures specific procedures to enable given children to use and practice meaningful speech-language responses that they have mastered.

For example, the clinician should advise the classroom teacher when a given child uses the /k/ sound appropriately in such phrases as "come up" or "take one." The teacher, in turn, may reinforce the child's spontaneous use of these types of responses and may also capitalize on more direct, yet natural, opportunities to strengthen the patterns. How many times, for instance, are papers or materials distributed to class members? If chosen to distribute these items, a given child could practice "take one" a number of times and receive the praise and acknowledgment of teachers and peers. Or, during dismissal, often a table-by-table or row-by-row procedure, the child in question could be asked to assist—"Come up row two."

The opportunities for structured classroom carry-over activities are boundless and seem to be a logical intermediate step between remediation and spontaneous usage. They permit classroom teachers to become involved in the remedial process without feeling the stress of additional responsibility, the need for more time, or concern about lesson interference. The speech-language pathologist who consults with teachers about this approach demonstrates understanding of teachers' responsibilities and a willingness to adapt techniques to the school environment.

Communication Disorders

The communication disorders component of the speech-language program provides intensive service to children with severe auditory-verbal deficits. Frequently, these children's linguistic handicaps are complicated by physical, intellectual, or emotional factors. Therefore, they require the coordinated remedial efforts of several educational team members.

As the mainstay of children's education, classroom teachers are the keystone to the educational team's plans. SLPs, therefore, have the responsibility to provide teachers with adaptive materials for students with communication handicaps and to consult with them about techniques that meet these students' auditory-verbal needs. The specialists should support teachers in integrating the students into classroom programs.

Clinicians and teachers should share information about their mutual students' learning patterns and the extent to which communication disorders seem to be affecting reactions to learning. The professionals should plan joint strategies that increase these children's learning probabilities. For example, some children with auditory-verbal deficits have difficulty comprehending or following verbal directions. They require shortened instructions, simplified vocabulary, or visual cues. When teachers are aware of these circumstances, they are able to modify their strategies and enhance the children's possibilities for success.

Similarly, speech-language pathologists should know about the various types of achievement tests and educational instruments that teachers routinely use. These assessment tools, most often, are verbally weighted and place children with communication disorders at a decided disadvantage. Clinicians, therefore, should help teachers develop adaptive methods of measuring the progress made by children with speech-language disorders.

In the case of children with severe language deficits, SLPs also must attend to curriculum. They should work with teachers to organize, present, and coordinate sequenced curricular activities that address these children's specific needs. For example, some of the students require classroom work that stresses concept development, while others need emphasis on syntax. Speech-language specialists should identify these needs and provide teachers with supportive materials and techniques that respond to them.

Finally, speech-language clinicians should consult with teachers about ways to augment the remedial program of students with severe speech-language problems. In many instances, the carry-over techniques as described previously are as applicable to these students as to those with communication deviations. However, students with severe problems also may need coordinated counseling to gain insight into their problems and to enable them to set realistic goals for changing their verbal behavior. Clinicians, therefore, should consult with teachers about the role each professional should play in counseling efforts.

Interpreting The Program

Classroom teachers must understand the speech-language pathologist's program if it is to be integrated into the educational framework. Although case conferences about given children or problems provide numerous opportunities to interpret specific aspects of the program, they frequently fail to address clearly the broader educational issues that are the foundation of school speech-language services. SLPs, therefore, should seek ways of providing teachers with this information through in-service training programs, including participation in workshops, conferences, and building meetings.

A major objective of this type of consultation is to encourage teachers to recognize that auditory-verbal skills are basic educational skills. On the one hand, teachers tend to view oral communication as one aspect of the language arts program. On the other, they place little curricular emphasis on the development of verbal skills. As a result, clinicians must make the point that primary language skills—listening and speaking—deserve the same curricular considerations as reading and writing. Further, children with primary language deficits cannot be expected to respond well to the standard language arts curriculum; they require modified approaches.

School clinicians should make every effort to inform classroom teachers, particularly at the elementary level, about the development of speech and language and its disorders. Teachers need this background if they are to assume some of the responsibility for referrals, carry-over, communication development programs, and remedial support. In addition, informed teachers appreciate the reasons for providing a continuum of services, the resulting variances in scheduling required to meet individual needs, and the factors that determine why, how, and to whom services are provided. They are willing to become involved in the speech-language program.

Special Education Teachers

Many of the students enrolled in categorical special education programs demonstrate speech-language problems as one aspect of their primary educational handicap. These students, as a group, require classroom instruction in the development of speech-language skills. At the same time, some students in a class may also need clinical speech-language services. It is essential, therefore, that speech-language pathologists and special education teachers cooperate in designing and implementing classroom-clinical programs that meet each student's unique circumstances.

Speech-language pathologists should assist special education teachers in (a) evaluating the general auditory-verbal needs of their classes, (b) developing sequential curricular objectives that respond to these needs, and (c) organizing activities and materials for classroom use. They should consult with teachers about ways in which the curriculum may provide opportunities for the entire class to learn new speech-language patterns as well as ways to promote carry-over for students enrolled in the clinical speech program.

Clinicians have the responsibility to decide which aspects of the students' auditory-verbal skills are managed best in the classroom and which demand the more specific attention of the speech-language pathologist. They should evaluate all children in special education classes to determine the degree to which the presenting speech-language problems are fairly typical of and attributable to the primary educational handicap (Freeman and Lukens, 1962). In atypical cases, SLPs and teachers should consider the students' need for a clinical program in addition to the classroom-based communication skills program.

The nature of speech-language disorders among otherwise handicapped children requires that clinicians become involved in planning educational procedures. They should establish themselves, therefore, as curricular consultants to special education programs. At the same time, they must maintain their clinical responsibilities to children who require specialized services. In this regard SLPs should provide special education teachers with the same consultative support available to regular classroom teachers. The combination—curricular and clinical consultation—enables special education teachers and speech-language pathologists to meet the auditory-verbal needs of handicapped students.

Other School Personnel

As members of multidisciplinary evaluation and planning teams, school speech-language pathologists have the opportunity to contribute significantly to the educational management of children with communication disorders. They should be able to integrate their findings, impressions and recommendations into children's total educational plans. They must be prepared, therefore, to consult with other team members—psychologists, social workers, reading specialists, and similar personnel—about ways in which auditory-verbal problems affect children's learning.

In this process speech-language pathologists alternately seek and provide information. They depend on other specialists to contribute to the broad base of data necessary for the evaluation and management of children with communication disorders. At the same time, the nature of clinicians' requests of others tends to reflect their own functions and concerns. Therefore, during consultative interaction they inform others about communication disorders, increase sensitivity to their informational needs, and provide the means for coordinating speech-language services with other aspects of educational programs.

Psychologists

Speech-language specialists require psychological data to gain increased insights about ways in which mental and emotional factors may be affecting children's auditory-verbal behavior. Therefore, it is important for clinicians to consult with psychologists about (a) the relations between psychological test findings and speech-language evaluative data, (b) psychological factors that relate to a child's learning patterns, and (c) information pertinent to behavior management techniques that may enhance a child's remedial speech-language program.

While seeking these data, SLPs have a chance to provide psychologists with insights about the effects of children's speech-language problems on psychological test performances. Since many psychological tests and subtests are language weighted, clinicians must point out the ramifications that communication disorders may have on children's (a) ability to comprehend and interpret test directions, (b) responses to specific verbal test items, (c) tendency to demonstrate discrepant responses to verbal and performance items, and (d) test scores.

This type of dialogue permits speech-language clinicians to inform psychologists about communication disorders as well as to request psychological information. It enables both specialists to direct their attention to interrelated concerns for children with speech-language disorders.

Social Workers

Social workers are adept interviewers. They frequently take detailed case histories from parents of handicapped students, including those with communication disorders. Therefore, they can provide speech-language pathologists with (a) developmental information, (b) analyses of family and environmental factors which relate to the precipitation or perpetuation of auditory-verbal problems, and (c) advice regarding counseling approaches.

Most social workers, however, must be made aware of ways in

which they can contribute to the communication disorders program. As a start, therefore, SLPs should inform social workers about (a) the landmarks of speech-language development, (b) the relations between environmental factors and speech-language development and its disorders, (c) the need to coordinate counseling programs, and (d) the speech-language pathologist's need for guidance in the use of counseling techniques.

With this information and orientation, social workers should be called upon to augment the communication disorders program by (a) collecting data regarding speech-language development as part of the routine case history, (b) identifying environmental factors that adversely affect speech-language, (c) selecting adverse environmental factors that are likely to be responsive to manipulation, (d) sharing counseling methods directed toward facilitating environmental changes, and (e) indicating ways in which speech-language clinicians may support the social work program. The two professionals, speech-language pathologist and social worker, should coordinate efforts into a unidirectional remedial program.

Reading Specialists

In recent years speech-language pathologists and reading specialists have recognized overlapping areas of roles and responsibilities in the delivery of services to children who have difficulty learning to read. Since the primary linguistic skills—verbal comprehension and verbal expression—are prerequisite to literacy, some cases of reading failure actually reflect inadequate mastery of aural-oral skills (Rees, 1974; Stark, 1975). Consequently, the remedial programs for these children should stress the development of auditory-verbal skills prior to reading. This task requires a combination of professional competencies.

In general, speech-language pathologists should assess the primary linguistic skills of children who demonstrate reading failure. They should consult with reading specialists about evaluative findings, the consequences of identified language problems on the reading process, and the necessary steps that should be taken, from their viewpoint, to implement a remedial program.

Since the background and experience of individual speech-language pathologists and reading experts vary considerably, their general expectations of each other's professional skills may prove inadequate in specific situations. Therefore, through consultation, these team members should reveal their strengths and weaknesses and use each other as resources.

For example, some speech-language pathologists view themselves as specialists only in the area of auditory-verbal skills, despite peripheral knowledge about reading and writing. Others have had extensive background in all aspects of language. Similarly, reading specialists may have variable knowledge of primary linguistic disorders and their remediation.

Even when speech-language clinicians and reading specialists clearly define and divide their responsibilities, there remain overlapping areas of concern. Therefore, each should rely on the other as a resource for personal continuing education. After all, the distinctions between professional roles are less important than the common goal of providing the best available program to children with language problems.

Other Speech-Language Pathologists

Many speech-language problems are complex, involve a large number of variables, and are difficult to resolve. Therefore, speech-language clinicians welcome the opportunity of consulting with others in the profession about puzzling clients. These consultations contribute to professional growth and enable clinicians to provide improved services.

Unfortunately, speech-language pathologists frequently fail to serve as consultants to each other. Due to their relative inaccessibility, many do not make the extra effort required to arrange and to participate in regular procedures for sharing knowledge and experiences. This situation detracts from their clinical effectiveness and the clinical nature of their programs. Therefore, although it is not easy, speech-language pathologists should actively pursue the consultation of their colleagues.

One of the most valuable consultative experiences is to observe another speech-language clinician interacting with a difficult case. This activity provides the regular clinician with new perspectives. It serves to stimulate discussions of diverse observations and opinions. The SLPs benefit from the exchange of information and viewpoints; their cases benefit from modifications in programs effected through clinicians' increased objectivity and new insights.

Another method of using the skills and knowledge of other speech-language clinicians is through regular staff meetings. In districts that employ only one or two clinicians these meetings may be arranged on a regional basis. The meetings should provide opportunities to discuss clinical problems, innovative practices, and developments in the field. They also may include case presentations and demonstrations followed by group discussion and case planning. They should result in practical in-service training designed to keep SLPs current and stimulated by the challenges of their profession.

CONSULTANT TO THE COMMUNITY

Speech-language clinicians can provide a variety of consultative services to members of the community. These include (a) participating in programs designed to educate and inform parents and other interested adults, (b) serving as a liaison between the schools and community agencies, and (c) consulting with members of related professions.

Educating the Community

Most communities have a number of child-centered organizations whose members are concerned about speech and language. Some of these are closely allied with the schools and are the logical means for informing parents about speech-language development and its disorders and the school program. The groups include parent-teacher associations and various organizations of parents whose children have specific handicaps—parents of retarded children, hearing-impaired children, learning disabled children, and so on.

In addition, speech-language pathologists should provide continual consultative services to child study groups and parents of children in preprimary schools or programs. These groups should be encouraged to practice measures that promote communication development and prevent speech-language problems. For example, in today's child-pressuring society, it is important that speech-language pathologists continuously emphasize that many early speech deviations are maturational and normal. Premature and undue pressure to correct these errors may lead to negative feelings about communication, personal or social maladjustment, or other attendant school and home problems. Adults need guidance in providing young children with positive, age-appropriate speech-language stimulation.

Community service clubs also should receive the attention of school speech-language clinicians. These groups frequently offer financial assistance, transportation, or other services to children with special needs. SLPs should provide club members with background information about speech-language disorders and concomitant problems. A well-informed group appreciates the needs for its services and is willing to participate when called upon to do so.

Agency Contacts

In given cases it is necessary for speech-language clinicians to work closely with child guidance clinics, family service agencies, and other social service organizations. In fact, clinicians are in an optimum position to serve as a liaison between these agencies and the schools. Their background and experience provide an appreciation of both environments, enabling them to interpret the viewpoints of each to the other.

Through consultation, SLPs may use this position to promote greater understanding between schools and community agencies in behalf of specific cases as well as with general reference to programs, services, and facilities. When this type of consultation is successful, the recommendations of agencies to schools become more practical, the referrals from schools to agencies become more appropriate, and the mutual expectations of schools and agencies become more realistic.

Related Professions

Speech-language pathologists sometimes are called upon to coordinate evaluative and remedial plans with professional members of the community—physicians, occupational and physical therapists, dentists, and others. This situation usually occurs when school-based multidisciplinary teams recommend a referral, or parents of a student, independently, wish to seek additional advice. Under these circumstances, school speech-language pathologists become members of a community resource team.

Community resource teams, unlike school teams, may never meet face to face to evaluate and discuss a case. Therefore, it is necessary for team members to exchange written case material. Speech-language pathologists, in doing so, should remember that methods used to seek information and the types of information requested can serve consultative ends. They reflect on the clinician's professional capacity and competency. Communications with other professionals, therefore, should ask specific questions and clearly state the relevance of answers to future school management practices.

Whenever possible, speech-language pathologists should take advantage of opportunities to address specific professional groups. These presentations should attempt to clarify roles as well as interrelate them. Speech-language pathologists should establish the scope and limitations of their professional responsibilities. They should indicate their appreciation of the contributions and limitations of others and elicit the same treatment in return.

SUMMARY

The schools present many opportunities for speech-language pathologists to engage in consultations of the highest professional order. As in the case of all clinical functions, the success of consultative services depends on practitioners' ability to adapt to the needs of their work environment. When school speech-language clinicians orient their specialized roles to the broader educational framework, their consultative responsibilities increase in number, scope, and depth. On the one hand, consultation is the means through which all professional functions may be integrated into school programs; on the other, it is an intrinsic part of daily clinical speech-language procedures that can be practiced successfully in schools.

STUDY ACTIVITIES

1. What factors enhance the school speech-language pathologist's opportunities to function as a consultant? What factors mitigate against consultation? How may they be changed?
2. What is the "clinical approach in the schools"? How does it relate to consultation?
3. On what matters should principals be particularly consulted?
4. What are several ways in which consultation with classroom teachers can fail? How can these failures be avoided?
5. How does the "continuum of services" affect consultation?
6. Who has the responsibility for the speech-language programs of otherwise handicapped children? What role does consultation play in their programs?
7. What are the major objectives of consultation with other school specialists?

REFERENCES

Ainsworth, S. et al. The Speech Clinician's Role in the Public School. *Asha,* 6, 189-191, 1964.

Black, M. *Speech Correction in the Schools,* Englewood Cliffs, Prentice-Hall 1964.

Freeman, G. G. The Assessment of Oral Language as a Precursor of Reading. In W. Otto, N. A. Peters, and C. W. Peters (Eds.), *Reading Problems: A Multidisciplinary Perspective.* Reading, Mass.: Addison-Wesley, 121-135, 1977.

Freeman, G. G. *Speech and Language Services and the Classroom Teacher.* Minneapolis: CEC, 1977.

Freeman, G. G. and Lukens, J. A Speech and Language Program for Educable Mentally Handicapped Children. *The Journal of Speech and Hearing Disorders,* 27, 285-287, 1962.

Garbee, F. E. The California Program for Speech and Hearing Handicapped School Children. *Bulletin California State Department of Education,* 23, 1964.

Healey, W. C. *Standards and Guidelines for Comprehensive Language, Speech and Hearing Programs in the Schools.* Washington: American Speech and Hearing Association, 1974.

Kavanaugh, J. F. (Ed.). *Communicating by Language: The Reading Process.* Washington: U.S. Govt. Print. Office, 1968.

Knight, H. et al. The Public School Clinician, V Professional Definition and Relationships. *The Journal of Speech and Hearing Disorders, Monograph Supplement 8,* 10-21, 1961.

Pendergast, K. Speech Improvement and Speech Therapy in the Elementary

School. *Asha,* 5, 548–549, 1963.
Powers, M. H. What Makes an Effective Public School Speech Therapist. *The Journal of Speech and Hearing Disorders,* 21, 461–467, 1956.
Rees, N. S. The Speech Pathologist and the Reading Process. *Asha,* 16, 255–258, 1974.
Robertson, M. L. and Freeman, G. G. Applying Diagnostic Information to Decisions about Placement and Treatment. *Language Speech and Hearing Services in Schools,* 5, 187–193, 1974.
Stark, J. S. Reading Failure: A Language-Based Problem, *Asha,* 17, 832–834, 1975.
Venezky, R. L. Spelling-to-Sound Correspondences. In J. Kavanaugh (Ed.), *Communicating By Language: The Reading Process.* Washington: U.S. Govt. Print. Office, 1968.

Chapter 5

SUPERVISION

Lee I. Fisher

Quality supervision is recognized as an important aspect of all areas of education. There is considerable justification for the provision of supervision of speech-language pathologists and audiologists in the schools. Leadership is needed to develop and implement programs for children; to assure the provision of appropriate, effective, and efficient services; to supervise speech-language-hearing personnel working in the schools; to insure equality of opportunity for students; and to evaluate programs and personnel. The supervisor has multiple responsibilities and should be viewed both as a leader who is an advocate for students with communication problems and as an advocate for speech and hearing personnel working in the program. The supervisor often serves as a catalyst in the process of generating and expanding new ideas, planning program changes, and implementing them effectively. The supervisor is a facilitator who is responsible for helping to make good things happen.

Major improvements have occurred in both regular and special education during the past decade. These continuing changes have affected all students but especially have had an impact upon services to the handicapped. Speech-language pathologists and audiologists are two of the many vital and important special education personnel provided to the educational system. Speech-language pathology and audiology have their own relevance and importance in the schools and are a part of the larger, total regular and special educational system. As such, speech-language-hearing personnel, whether serving as supervisors or specialists being supervised, must realize that we no longer work independently but must relate to the needs of the total child and the total educational system. Speech-language pathologists and audiologists working in the schools continue to represent the largest percentage of the members of our profession working in a given setting. Given quality supervision, most professionals are excited about the challenges and rewards resulting from working in an educational setting with children who have communication problems. On the other hand, poor supervision can result in dissatisfaction and less desirable programming. To be sure, there is considerable variability in the manner in which speech-language pathologists and audiologists provide services in both special education and regular education in many school districts. Our profession has begun to document the need for the provision of supervised services to assist children in overcoming their communication problems and to help them reach their educational potential.

The American Speech-Language-Hearing Association appointed a task force in 1970 to study the need for supervision of speech-language-hearing programs in the schools. The task force suggested that many school administrators are interested in having a comprehensive speech-language-hearing program that would provide not only diagnostic and remedial services but would include such other activities as preventive services, preschool language development programs, specialist involvement in curriculum development, publications and consultation for regular classroom teachers, and public relations activities.

To ask an administrator—one who has not been trained in the field and who has other administrative duties—to establish procedures and goals for speech-language-hearing programs, to determine goal achievement, and to evaluate effectiveness of the speech-language pathologists and the clinical process is unrealistic. It is also unrealistic to expect that school speech-language-hearing programs can have maximum effectiveness when several staff members are attempting to provide quality services with limited or no coordination of activities, with high turnover disrupting continuity, and with no speech-language pathologist authorized to serve as consultant when specific problems arise. Unfortunately, these conditions exist too frequently. School programs greatly need to employ supervisors with specialized competencies who will provide administrative, consultative, program development, and evaluative services.

Since school districts vary so much in size and complexity as well as philosophy regarding the provision of supervisory and consultant services, a supervisor-to-clinician ratio applicable to all schools is difficult to estimate. Every speech-language pathologist and audiologist should have access to a supervisor trained in the field. It is recommended that one supervisor be assigned to every ten to twelve speech-language pathologists. Any time a school district employs at least two speech-language pathologists, the more competent person should be given the authority and responsibility for coordinating the daily activities unless the immediate superior is trained in the field of speech pathology and audiology.

Supervisors may be employed on a full- or part-time basis. Small school districts might wish to share a supervisor. Districts near universities can often use university personnel on a part-time cooperative basis. Many speech-language-hearing programs are so large that one supervisor cannot perform all the administrative, consultative, and program development activities necessary for efficient program maintenance and evaluation. In such cases, the supervisory responsibilities should be divided. One speech-language pathologist or audiologist should be responsible for administration and program development, and additional supervisory personnel should be employed using the recommended ratio as a guideline.

The recommended supervisor-staff ratio is essential if the major responsibilities of the supervisor are to be accomplished. Evaluating the speech-language pathologists in the clinical process has top priority and is possible only if the supervisor-pathologist or audiologist ratio is low enough to provide time for this vital responsibility. Effective supervision can increase competency and services.

The supervisor should hold the ASHA Certificate of Clinical Competence in the area in which the supervision will be done. He should have a minimum of three years of experience working in the schools and should hold appropriate certification from the state in which he plans to supervise, according to Healey et al. (1972).

Nearly a decade later there are still many school speech-language-hearing programs without adequate supervision. Some programs do not have a supervisor, others are supervised by personnel who are not trained in our profession, and many large city systems have one supervisor for 100 or more staff without assistance in the supervisory process. As a profession we need to continue to work together for the goal of adequate supervision for every school speech-language-hearing program in the future. This can be done effectively by developing rationale and justification for local programs and should be done tactfully, working with the special education director and other administrators.

There are many facets to the supervisory process for both those who are supervising as well as those who are being supervised. Hundreds of volumes have been written on endless aspects of supervision and management of personnel. More of this writing has occurred in business and industry than in education.

Anderson, of Indiana University, continues to be an excellent advocate for quality supervision of speech-language-hearing programs in the schools. In 1974 Anderson described some important aspects of the emerging role of supervision in the schools as follows:

> The position of supervisor or coordinator of speech, hearing, and language programs in the schools, although it has existed in limited numbers for some years, is rapidly developing as a major component of the profession. As this role emerges, it is imperative that the profession of speech pathology and audiology assume the following responsibilities:
>
> 1. Support the need for supervision of school programs for communicatively handicapped children and communicate to school administrators the contribution a supervisor can make to such programs.
> 2. Take the initiative in defining the role of the supervisor of speech, hearing, and language programs in the schools.
> 3. Identify the components of the supervisory process and the competencies of supervisors, particularly those who work in the schools.
> 4. Establish training programs for supervisors with special emphasis on leadership in school programs.
>
> Assumption of these responsibilities by the profession would require a recognition of the large numbers of communicatively handicapped children who are served in the schools and the large numbers of clinicians employed there. It would imply a commitment to the clinical process and the supervisory process and to research directed toward these areas.
> Supervisors of school programs have traditionally been selected on the

basis of seniority, proven expertise, and interest or willingness to serve, and not on the basis of specific preparation for the role. In a 1972 survey of 211 supervisors of speech, hearing, and language programs in the schools, only 10% reported having had a course in supervising speech, hearing, and language programs. However, 92% of the full-time supervisors and 81% of the part-time supervisors in the survey said that supervisors of such programs should have special training. (Pp. 7-9)

Formal training programs are still not readily available for speech-language-hearing supervisory personnel. Consequently, the majority of supervisors serving in the schools learn most of their supervisory skills on the job without the benefit of graduate training in supervision or management of personnel and/or programs. University training programs are increasing in this area, but training in supervision is still not available in approximately 50 percent of the training programs. This unmet need offers a real challenge to the training programs, as leadership is essential in the schools as well as in all other employment settings. Consequently, most school supervisors must resort to ongoing training from three primary sources: (a) district and agency management in-service training programs; (b) state department of instruction supervisory meetings, seminars, and sharing sessions; and (c) personal growth and development: reading supervisory and managerial literature, and attending conventions.

The school district or area service agency has a great deal of responsibility in determining how programs and personnel are supervised. There is wide variability in the supervisory process, ranging from minimal supervision to superb leadership. The administration and the board of education of the district or agency are ultimately responsible for the quality of the supervisory leadership. Even though massive special education programs have developed in the United States as a result of Public Law 94-142, there is little guidance in this legislation for standards of supervision of specific programs. Consequently, school personnel are caught in a dilemma between the conservative educational establishment and the need for professional freedom in establishing a broad continuum of efficient and effective quality services. The supervisor often has the responsibility of working through this dilemma.

This chapter will deal with supervision of programs and of

personnel. These two factors are separable, but *inseparable* in many ways. The first section will include information on organizational structure and programming, program planning and implementation, critical work activities and job descriptions, goals and objectives, leadership, the negotiated contract, collective negotiations, politics in education, budget considerations, interaction with other specialists, and supervisory decisions based on severity rating data. The second part of the chapter will deal with supervision of personnel and will include sections on the principles of supervision, communication, motivating staff, and evaluation of personnel. The final section of the chapter will deal with supervision of student speech-language pathologists and audiologists and will include responsibilities of the training program, the supervisor, and the student.

ORGANIZATIONAL STRUCTURE AND PROGRAMMING

School districts and intermediate service agencies develop organizational structures to meet their needs as described in Chapter 3. The organizational structure varies in complexity and is usually diagrammed with a district or agency flow chart with the Board of Education being ultimately responsible for all programming and personnel. The organizational chart often combines line-staff responsibility and program responsibility. At times there is a separate organizational chart for programs. The administrator or superintendent is directly responsible to the Board of Education with the assistant or associate superintendent(s) and/or director(s) being responsible to the chief administrator. The director of special education reports to the administrator and is responsible for all special education programming in the district or agency. All programming is carried out in keeping with district or agency policies and procedures and with state and federal regulations. The special education program supervisors are responsible to the associate director or director, and the speech-language-hearing personnel are responsible to the supervisor of the service in most special education units. Following the "chain of command" from the Board of Education down through the staff ranks is generally expected. Likewise, speech-language pathologists and audiologists should communicate with the program supervisor as the first line of communication. In the event that an issue cannot be resolved at this level it is appropriate to go to a higher level to seek resolution. Bypassing the supervisor or other management levels is not advisable. Should this be necessary, it should be with the knowledge of the immediate supervisor.

Organization is the key to success in the managerial process. Effective organizational skills are essential in supervising programs and personnel. If one analyzes *effective* special education organizations, certainly highly organized structure and organized supervisory and managerial personnel will be found. There is a definite need for personal organization for both the supervisor and the speech-language pathologists and audiologists being supervised. We cannot expect to provide effective and efficient services without a considerable degree of organizational skills on the part of everyone. The challenge is to improve the organization of the program and to motivate the staff to carry out the program in a highly organized manner. Within every organization there is a need for structure. The Board of Education, administrator, director(s) and supervisors assume the responsibility for setting the tone of the organization and organizing the structure of the educational unit so the intended program goals can be accomplished. Ideally the staff also have input in this planning process.

Written program descriptions spell out the general and specific details of each program. A program description should exist for communication services and should include all the components of speech-language-hearing services. The program should be carefully described in writing and constantly updated in keeping with ongoing program changes and developments. Developing and updating the program descriptions is a great asset to program organization. The program should be organized to accomplish the long-range and short-range program goals and objectives. The program should be organized to use the skills of key staff members with special skills, those with leadership potential, and all staff members in selected activities.

In a large district or service agency the speech-language and/or hearing staff is often too large to meet together to accomplish work tasks. Supervisors frequently use committees and task forces to deal with a specific problem or to develop a certain aspect of the program. This provides incentive to become involved in a special project, encourages participative input, uses skills effectively, and provides numerous growth opportunities. The committees or task forces are often asked to report to the entire group when a business or in-service meeting is held. In smaller districts and intermediate agencies, all speech-language-hearing personnel may be able to work together on a given project. In either case, the supervisor gives careful consideration to the selection of the committee chairperson.

When new staff members join the service organization, it is important for the supervisor to clarify organizational matters for them. This can be done through a program description book, staff handbooks, policy books, slide-tape presentations, and/or personal orientation on individual matters. This orientation is especially important in a large organization so new staff members are properly informed about all aspects of the organization and program. In the event that this information is not provided by the supervisor, the staff should be encouraged to seek out information whenever they have a question. The supervisor should be in a position to answer the majority of questions, but if an answer cannot be provided immediately, he should take the initiative to obtain the information and get back to the staff member.

The supervisor should organize each day on a regular basis. This can be done in one of several ways. One suggestion is to make a list of things to be accomplished for the day and then list priorities. Another method is to develop a list showing the persons the supervisor wants to communicate with on a given day and the issues to be worked on or resolved. When planning a day, time should be considered for phone calls, dictation, meetings, visitations, communications, committee meetings, planning, in-service, and a multitude of other activities. If the day is not planned, the supervisor is likely to become bogged down in trivia. Considerable planning and organization can also occur during the summer months so that information is ready to provide to staff to implement new program plans when school begins.

PROGRAM PLANNING AND IMPLEMENTATION

Quality supervision depends upon the supervisor's ability to plan and implement programming effectively. The supervisor must always be alert to ways and means to improve the provision of services. Many major changes have occurred in our profession during the past two decades. Frequently these changes originated in the schools as a result of effective planning. Trends in our profession are often established in the schools as a result of planning. The management team, including the administrator, director, and supervisory personnel, has the major responsibility for developing short-range and long-range plans. Short-range plans should include anticipated changes and activities for the current year. Long-range plans should be projected for three to five years in the future. There is a constant need to plan for the future. Supervisors and speech-language-hearing personnel need to be highly imaginative and bold in planning changes because we live in a constant state of change. One should never underestimate the importance and value of involving the staff in the planning process. For example, in the speech-language-hearing programs this writer has supervised for the past fifteen years, the staff has met annually for a full day at the end of the school year to plan for the future. The basic question is, "How can we improve services for the future?" As a result of the ideas generated by those providing the service, we have frequently implemented major improvements during the following year. Each year numerous minor and major changes occur as a result of this activity. After the ideas are generated, they are discussed, and priorities are established. The supervisor has the responsibility to review these ideas and select changes that are desirable and practical. At times the supervisor and/or administration must reject an idea, but this is the exception. The best feature of this activity is that the staff has had input—they have an investment in their program. As a result, they are often knowledgeable of changes and, more important, are highly motivated to implement the changes under the guidance of the supervisor. Whenever a change is being considered, the supervisor needs to give thought to the impact the change will create. Will this change result in greater effectiveness? Will this change result in greater efficiency?

Another way to approach planning is to analyze the program and identify aspects of the program that are weak or that need to be expanded or upgraded to be in compliance with local, state, or federal guidelines and legislation. During such an activity the following questions need to be answered: Are the critical needs being met? How *well* are they being met? Which needs are not being met? After this exploration it is important to plan what changes are needed and to consider alternative ways to improve service. There are nearly always alternative ways to resolve an issue. The alternatives should be listed, and the best alternative should be selected. This can be done effectively by a task analysis and by seeking input and alternative solutions not only from the staff but from school administrators, teachers, parents, and the students themselves.

Whenever major changes are being considered, the supervisor needs to discuss the proposed ideas with the associate director and/or director to determine if the concept(s) fit into the overall goals and plans of the educational organization. If the supervisor seeks support from the appropriate administrative level(s) and from the staff for a given change, the change will likely occur smoothly. However, there is always someone who may resist change for one or more specific reasons. If this becomes a problem for the supervisor or the staff member, the logical step is to sit down and discuss the change and to seek understanding and resolution. Occasionally there may be some justifiable reason(s) why change cannot occur.

One of the greatest challenges facing all areas of special education at this point is planning and implementing programs in keeping with energy shortages, declining enrollments, and inflationary costs of programming. Costs are increasing rapidly because of increased operating expenses, rising salaries, greater fringe benefits, and new and expanded programming. In the future, supervisors will constantly be confronted with the questions, "How can we provide the most effective service with the budget we have? Are there better ways to serve children with communication disorders without increasing costs?"

CRITICAL WORK ACTIVITIES AND JOB DESCRIPTIONS

School districts and intermediate educational service agencies should identify critical work activities and should have written job descriptions for their supervisors and speech-language-hearing personnel. This is just as important for a small, individual district as it is for large agencies serving a large city or a multitude of districts or counties. Identification of critical work activities and written job descriptions serve a multitude of needs for the school district, educational agency, special education program, and speech-language and/or hearing personnel employed in the schools.

The critical work activities should be identified and listed separately for both the supervisor and the speech-language-hearing personnel providing the service. If the critical work activities have not been listed, the supervisor should be responsible for developing a list of all the tasks that need to be accomplished. There should be one list for the supervisor and one list for the staff. These lists should be reviewed at least annually and changed and updated to be consistent with ongoing program changes. The list of critical work activities includes all activities that are important to accomplishing the goals and objectives that will be described in the next section. Stated simply, this is a list of tasks and activities that must be done to provide an effective program and to be in compliance with local, area, state, and federal guidelines.

Following is a sample listing of the critical work activities for supervisors of speech-language pathology services in the schools.

Critical Work Activities

Supervisor, Speech-Language Pathology Services

1. Plan and implement new programs based on perceived needs.
2. Assist in recruitment of speech-language pathologists.
3. Assign personnel and plan overall schedule of service in cooperation with local school districts.
4. Be responsible for orientation and regularly scheduled staff meetings.
5. Promote positive attitudes and be supportive to staff.

6. Develop and insure implementation of annual program goals and objectives.
7. Provide direct supervision for speech-language pathologists.
8. Serve as supervisor/consultant for hearing conservation and education program if audiologists are not employed in the schools.
9. Evaluate staff in keeping with division and negotiation agreement policies.
10. Evaluate speech-language programs annually and plan future improvements.
11. Facilitate communication and serve as liaison between staff and groups such as parents' associations, diagnostic centers, physicians, ear doctors, etc.
12. Initiate and/or support meaningful research activities.
13. Keep abreast of professional change and development.
14. Facilitate staff and program development.
15. Be involved in student conferences and staffings on occasion.
16. Perform division and agency responsibilities as assigned.
17. Serve public relations role in all activities with a positive approach.
18. Maintain a high standard of professional ethics.
19. Be responsible for establishment and maintenance of speech-language pathology records and reports.
20. Support purchase of adequate materials.
21. Promote the philosophy and goals of the division, district, or agency.
22. Develop and monitor budget.
23. Prepare written program description, policies, and procedures.
24. Support practicum experiences for students in training.
25. Establish and maintain open and effective lines of communication.
26. Comply with local, state, and federal guidelines and mandates.

The school district or educational service agency also needs written job descriptions at the supervisory level and for the speech-language pathologlists and audiologists employed in the schools. In essence, the job description organizes, categorizes, and places priorities on the critical work activities. Furthermore, the job description provides insight as to who is responsible for accomplishing the critical work activities and how they are to be accomplished. Stated simply, the job description spells out the specific responsibilities of the speech-language-hearing personnel that are expected by the employing agency. To be sure, there is considerable variability in job descriptions from program to program, and there may be vast differences. However, with the advent of Public Law 94-142, there is likely to be considerable similarity in many aspects of the job description from one program to another.

The job descriptions are important not only for supervisors but also for speech-language pathologists and audiologists working in the schools. Everyone who is seeking employment in a given district or agency should ask to see a written job description. The job description should be carefully reviewed before accepting a job and signing a contract. Once employed, the speech-language pathologist and audiologist should keep abreast of the changes in the job description, since many educational agencies are now developing evaluation procedures based upon the job descriptions.

Following are sample job descriptions for supervisors of speech-language services and educational audiology services in the schools. Job descriptions for speech-language pathologists and audiologists working in the schools are considerably different from supervisory job descriptions.

Supervisor Job Description

Professional Responsibilities: Speech and Language Services

1. The supervisor assesses the overall needs of the local schools concerning programs and services for communicatively handicapped students.
2. The supervisor plans and implements new and expanded programs based on perceived needs.
3. The supervisor works with the personnel department and assists in recruiting, interviewing, and recommending personnel for employment.
4. The supervisor is responsible for formulating short-range and long-range goals and measurable program objectives.

5. The supervisor works with the management staff in planning, implementing, and carrying out the program budget.
6. The supervisor is responsible for assigning speech-language pathologists to schools and for developing their annual calendars.
7. The supervisor provides direct supervision for speech-language pathologists on the staff and for associate supervisor(s).
8. The supervisor is responsible for planning and conducting regularly scheduled staff meetings.
9. The supervisor is responsible for planning and implementing an ongoing in-service education program based upon expressed needs of the staff.
10. The supervisor evaluates the speech-language programs and personnel in keeping with division, district, and agency policies and negotiated agreement(s).
11. The supervisor provides a positive image for the program and staff and promotes this concept for all staff members.
12. The supervisor develops a written program description including policies and procedures for all phases of the speech-language program.
13. The supervisor participates in department, division, district, and agency meetings.
14. The supervisor serves as a consultant to the staff, other professionals, local schools, and other agencies.
15. The supervisor analyzes and disseminates appropriate statistical information regarding current programming and uses this information as a basis for expanded programming.
16. The supervisor supports participation in relevant research in keeping with division, district, and agency policy.
17. The supervisor works with the staff in developing and using appropriate records and reports.
18. The supervisor works with training programs in providing beneficial school practicum experience for student speech-language pathologists.
19. The supervisor cooperates with the supervisors of other programs in a concerted effort to meet the needs of children with communication problems.
20. The supervisor establishes and maintains effective communi-

cation for the staff and program(s).
21. The supervisor works with the staff on being in compliance with local, state, and federal guidelines and regulations.
22. The supervisor makes sincere efforts to be supportive to staff on a regular basis.
23. The supervisor may be responsible for the hearing conservation and education program in some districts.
24. The supervisor develops a program for personal professional development in leadership and clinical expertise.
25. The supervisor performs division and district or agency responsibilities as directed and promotes the goals of the program, division, and agency.
26. The supervisor promotes the need for adequate facilities, materials, and equipment.
27. The supervisor maintains a high standard of professional ethics at all times.
28. The supervisor provides supervision for personnel seeking certification from the American Speech-Language-Hearing Association.

Following is one example of a job description for a speech-language pathologist in the schools. Note the significant differences between the responsibilities of the supervisor and the speech-language pathologists working in the schools. Also note the many different responsibilities a supervisor has in supervising staff with these diverse tasks.

Job Description
TITLE: *Speech-Language Pathologist* REPORTS TO: Supervisor, Clinical Speech-Language Services

Position Overview:
The speech-language pathologist provides efficient and effective service to communicatively handicapped students within the parameters of the Rules of Special Education. This is accomplished through assessment, remediation, consultation, referral, staff development, compliance procedures, and research.

Position Responsibilities:
  I. Assessment
     A. Screening
        The speech-language pathologist identifies students in need of communication assessment included in the areas of articulation, voice, language, fluency, and auditory processing by:
        Using systematic screening procedures for specific populations dependent upon the needs of the school population.
     B. Evaluation
        The speech-language pathologist assesses identified and referred students with possible communication handicaps in the areas of articulation, language, fluency, voice, and auditory processing for possible referral, educational recommendations, and/or remediation by:
        1. Administering an appropriate diagnostic battery for evaluation of these areas.
        2. Using informal observation and assessment procedures, as appropriate.
 II. Referral
     The speech-language pathologist refers students in need of additional services to appropriate internal or external agencies, programs, or individuals for supplementary services based upon information derived from screening procedures, testing, remedial services, and observations or other professional contacts.

     The speech-language pathologist participates in staffings of children for whom speech and language deficits may contribute significantly to their educational needs.
III. Remediation
     The speech-language pathologist provides remedial services to the communicatively handicapped student. The services will be provided in individual and/or group speech-language therapy and may be provided via classroom settings, on a consultative basis, or in a school program by:
     A. Enrolling children based upon the judgments of sever-

ity, potential for improvement, availability of other public school services, and scheduling considerations.
B. Developing an individualized education program (I.E.P.) for each student in the clinical speech-language case load.
C. Adapting and using materials and remediation techniques that meet the communication needs of each student.
D. Distributing to parents, teachers, or appropriate individuals information relative to remediation.
E. Maintaining formal and informal interaction with teachers, parents, and other personnel in implementing the program developed for each student.
F. Maintaining systematic records regarding each student's progress.

IV. Consultation

The speech-language pathologist disseminates information relative to the communication process to teachers, parents, and local district or agency professional groups by:
A. Providing written and/or oral consultation with parents and appropriate school personnel and other professionals regarding speech-language services.
B. Providing opportunities for clinical observations to parents.
C. Participating in in-service presentations to classroom teachers, administrators, and interested school personnel regarding the role of the speech-language pathologist in the schools.

V. Compliance

The speech-language pathologist complies with discipline, division, state, and federal regulations relative to the provision of clinical speech-language services by:
A. Securing parental consent for assessment, placement, and remediation.
B. Preparing and reviewing individual educational plans.
C. Compliance with requirements regarding completion of annual reports, severity ratings, and state enrollment counts.
D. Compliance with all local, state, and federal require-

ments pertaining to speech-language services.
VI. Staff Development
The speech-language pathologist participates in organization, division, staff, group, and committee assignments.
A. Facilitate professional interaction.
B. Promote program development and expansion.
C. Increase the effectiveness of the clinical services provided.
VII. Research
The speech-language pathologist collects, analyzes, and reports information and data relative to students with communication problems when appropriate and approved by the management staff.

EVALUATION:
Performance of this job will be evaluated in accordance with provisions of the master contract and the Board's evaluation criteria as specified in this job description.

Many school districts are now beginning to employ audiologists. In large school districts or intermediate agencies an audiologist should be employed to supervise the hearing conservation and education program. Following is a job description for educational audiology services in the schools.

Supervisor Job Description
Professional Responsibilities
Educational Audiology Services

I. The supervisor assists in the recruitment and employment of all hearing staff members.
A. Works with the personnel department in recruiting and recommending employment of audiologists, audiometrists, and itinerant teachers.
B. Works in cooperation with the local education agencies (LEA) in recruiting and recommending employment of teachers of the hearing impaired.
II. The supervisor assigns hearing personnel and plans overall schedule of services.
A. Develops annual staff calendars.
B. Assigns audiologists and audiometrists to specific schools, districts, or regions.
C. Assigns specific responsibilities to audiologists, audi-

ometrists, and itinerant teachers.
- D. Assigns itinerant teachers to specific schools, districts, or regions.
- E. Recommends best utilization of hearing education teachers employed by the LEAs.
- F. Plans schedule for preschool program in cooperation with supervisor of early childhood program.

III. The supervisor is responsible for planning and scheduling fall orientation and regularly scheduled staff meetings.
- A. Plans and conducts annual fall orientation meeting for new staff members.
- B. Plans agenda and conducts regularly scheduled staff meetings.

IV. The supervisor develops and insures implementation of annual program goals and objectives.
- A. Works with the director, associate director, and staff in developing program goals and objectives.
- B. Reviews progress on a regular basis.
- C. Prepares annual evaluation reports.

V. The supervisor provides direct supervision for all staff members.
- A. Provides positive feedback on a regular basis and is supportive to staff members in the daily conduct of the program.
- B. Provides direct and indirect daily, monthly, and periodic supervision of the audiologists, audiometrists, and itinerant teachers of the hearing impaired.
- C. Supervises the secretary assigned to the program.

VI. The supervisor serves as the supervisor-consultant for the hearing education teachers employed by the LEAs.
- A. Serves as a supervisor-consultant for the teachers at all levels from preschool through high school.
- B. Works with building principals where classes are located on all aspects of programming.
- C. Provides materials and assists classroom teachers with consulting needs.
- D. Plans in-service program for instructional staff.

VII. The supervisor evaluates the staff in keeping with agency, division, and negotiation policy.

A. Evaluates all hearing staff members in keeping with the language of the negotiated agreement, division, and agency policy.
B. Works with the building principals who are responsible for evaluating hearing education teachers.

VIII. The supervisor evaluates hearing conservation and education programs annually and plans future improvements.
A. Meets with the hearing conservation staff each spring to evaluate the program and develop recommended changes for improvements.
B. Meets with the itinerant teachers and hearing education teachers each spring to evaluate the program and make recommendations for changes and improvements.

IX. The supervisor assists in the development of a comprehensive program for evaluating and serving students with auditory processing problems.
A. Provides active leadership in developing policy with regard to evaluation strategies and treatment plans for students with auditory processing disorders.
B. Serves as a primary resource for the Division of Special Education in the area of auditory processing.
C. Trains audiologists in the administration of specific auditory processing tests.
D. Plans remediation strategies for students with auditory processing problems.

X. The supervisor facilitates communication and serves as a liaison between staff and lay groups.
A. Communicates effectively with the hearing staff, division personnel, management personnel, LEA personnel, and parents.
B. Serves as a liaison with individuals and groups such as the state hearing consultant, parents association, diagnostic centers, physicians, hearing aid distributors, etc.

XI. The supervisor initiates and/or supports meaningful research activities.
A. Initiates meaningful research activities.
B. Supports meaningful research activities when participation is requested and the research is supported by the administration.

XII. The supervisor keeps abreast of professional development.
   A. Reads current professional literature on a regular basis.
   B. Attends a minimum of three professional meetings and/or conventions annually.
   C. Takes an active role in providing leadership for the State Speech and Hearing Association and the American Speech-Language-Hearing Association.
XIII. The supervisor facilitates staff and program development plans.
   A. Seeks ways and means and plans appropriate staff development in-service in keeping with changing staff and program needs.
   B. Plans appropriate program changes and development in keeping with professional, division, and agency changes.
XIV. The supervisor is involved in student staffings, conferences, individualized educational plans, and three-year reevaluation reviews.
   A. Participates in staffings of students recommended for a hearing education program.
   B. Attends parent-teacher conferences whenever special problems arise.
   C. Participates in I.E.P. Conference, annual reviews, and three-year reevaluation conferences.
XV. The supervisor performs division of special education responsibilities as assigned.
   A. Participates in division, district, and agency staff meetings.
   B. Performs division and agency responsibilities as assigned.
XVI. The supervisor promotes public relations to further public understanding of programs and services.
XVII. The supervisor maintains a high standard of professional ethics.
XVIII. The supervisor is responsible for the establishment and maintenance of records and reports.
   A. Assumes responsibility for the planning, development, establishment, and maintenance of all hearing conservation and education records and reports.
   B. Assumes responsibility for the development and sub-

mission of records and reports requested by the director and administrator.
XIX. The supervisor assigns and monitors the function of personnel and group amplification devices.
XX. The supervisor promotes the philosophy and goals of the division, districts, and the agency.
   A. Promotes the philosophy and goals of the division, districts, and agency in the provision of the hearing program.
   B. Assesses the ongoing hearing conservation and education needs of the local schools.
   C. Seeks ways and means to improve the effectiveness and efficiency of hearing programs and services on an ongoing basis.

GOALS AND OBJECTIVES

Supervisors are currently struggling with the ramifications of the age of accountability. This is included in the information provided in Chapter 6. In the future, accountability will become even more important in view of the vast numbers of children with unmet communication needs, rising costs of special education services, and energy shortages. Simply stated, effective planning is preestablishing a course of action in writing. Program planning includes, "Who will do what by when and at what cost?" The supervisor, working both with management and the staff, is primarily responsible for the development of short- and long-range goals and objectives. These goals and objectives may be viewed as a road map, a plan where you are going, and how you are going to get there. This planning is vital to the provision of quality services based upon actual and perceived needs and the production of effective results. Accountability includes the development of performance standards, measurement, and evaluation leading to performance improvement.

Dublinske (1970) has been a leader in our profession in advocating program planning and evaluation through the development of goals and objectives. Dublinske has indicated that one of the most important roles of the supervisor of the speech-language-hearing programs in the schools is accountability. All of us are aware of the push by taxpayers for accountability in the educational process. They are concerned with the amount of money placed in the educational coffers and are demanding that it be spent in terms of the following:

1. Efficiency: "Am I getting the most learning experience for my child in the least amount of time for the least amount of money?"
2. Effectiveness: "Is the money I put into learning experience programs used to develop effective procedures to achieve educational objectives?"
3. Economy: "Are there alternative methods of programming and administering that are less expensive than the present methods?"

All supervisors and speech-language pathologists and audiologists must get involved in the "Three Es" actively and soon. In the schools specialists are called upon to justify their positions more and more frequently. In many areas special service personnel are considered a "frill" and are the first to go when a large budget cut must be made. The "frill" element becomes quite evident when staff takes a look at the commitment the schools have made to speech-language-hearing services. Do they get the best possible rooms in which to work? Are they allowed to schedule cases on a basis similar to other educational services and activities? Do they get the quieter rooms for hearing testing? Do they get full cooperation from administrators and teachers? Unfortunately, in many cases the answer to these questions is no. If speech-language pathologists and audiologists are going to insure that their services become an integral part of the educational system, they must develop a system of accountability that will generate data that show they do provide a valuable service related to the total educational process.

One of the problems in discussing accountability with specialists is that when the concept of measurable objectives or performance criteria is mentioned, it brings to the surface the "can'tbedoneism syndrome." For some unknown reason, many speech-language pathologists and audiologists feel they cannot measure the job they are doing in terms of effectiveness or be held accountable for the job they are not doing. As professionals, speech-language pathologists and audiologists must develop their own program goals and objectives and set their own performance criteria before others do it for them.

Just what is accountability? Accountability is defined simply as knowing (1) what you are going to do, (2) when it is going to be done, (3) how you will know when you are there, and (4) the cost involved in getting there.

One system used to achieve accountability is called "Program Planning and Evaluation." Many systems have been developed to achieve management by objectives, and all include identifying needs, developing goals, writing measurable objectives, and putting a cost on achieving the various goals. Each state or local education agency may have its own term for the planning system it uses. Following are the ten steps of the Program Planning–Evaluation procedure.

1. Collecting Perceived Needs and Program Ideas
   All staff develop a list of (1) actions that have been part of previous service that should be maintained, (2) problems that need attention, and/or (3) perceived concerns about services or program activities. In developing this list, draw upon ideas from agency personnel as well as consumers such as teachers, administrators, students, clients, parents, and professionals in other disciplines.
2. Identifying Priorities for Action by Verifying Needs
   Typically, staff will identify more concerns that need attention than will be possible to complete within a year. This forces staff to determine priorities and decide where to spend their time and resources. Verifying needs involves seeing how many people are involved or affected by the problem. Use of questionnaires, review of records, and interviews can be used.
3. Getting Staff Needs Together
   Discuss what needs individual staff members within each section have and see how their verified needs group together. Combine the needs, where possible, with other professionals who have the same concerns. By pooling the needs, the staff will identify areas of major concern.
4. Writing Goal Statements for Areas of Major Concern or Special Efforts
   Goals for each section of the agency are defined in a clear

statement that will convey to others the major efforts of the agency for the year. Goal statements should indicate (1) WHAT is going to be done, (2) WHEN it will be done, and (3) the CRITERION for success.

5. Reviewing Goal Statements
The director, administrator, supervisor, and/or board review the goals developed by the staff and indicate approval, or return the goals for further consideration.

6. Writing Program Objectives for Specific Activities
All staff write program objectives for all activities they want to complete during the year. Staff should have objectives that account for 90 percent of their time, leaving 10 percent open for unanticipated activities that will need attention. Specifically, an objective must indicate WHAT is going to be done, TO WHOM it is going to be done, WHO is going to do it, WHEN it is going to be done, CRITERION that will indicate success, and the EVALUATION method that will be used to show the objective was accomplished. Objectives should be coded according to universal program functions necessary for comprehensive services.

7. Reviewing Program Plans for Each Section
The supervisor reviews the program objectives (program plans) for each staff member and approves the plan or requests modifications.

8. Reviewing Program Plans for the Entire Agency
The Board of Education reviews program plans for all sections and personnel in the agency and approves or requests modifications.

9. Implementing Plans and Making Changes as Needed
After all program plans have been approved, they are ready to be implemented. If changes are needed in the objectives, staff members and supervisors jointly work through modifications.

10. Keeping Others Informed of Progress
Periodically, staff and supervisors share information regarding accomplishment of goals and objectives with the director, administrator, board, and community.

The program plan is developed using a set of universal program functions such as (1) identification, (2) remediation, (3) referral, (4) consultation, (5) administration, and (6) research development. By writing program objectives specific to the program functions, specialists can indicate how many hours of service a child gets, how many parent conferences may be held, how many cases may be seen, how many cases may be dismissed, how many professional meetings may be attended, how many research projects may be developed, and how much planning time may be needed. To measure the effectiveness of the specialist-child relationship, which is really what accountability is all about, speech-language pathologists and audiologists must develop instructional objectives that tell how much progress the child should make in a specified time period, the criteria for determining success, and the evaluation procedures used to measure effectiveness, according to Dublinske (pp. 121-124 revised).

A goal may be defined as a broad general statement regarding a desired outcome of a perceived need. Goals may be short-range or long-range or may vary from general to specific. A perceived need may be described with a goal that may involve the program, supervisor, staff, students, school personnel, and/or parents. The supervisor contributes to the general philosophy of service, assesses the needs and expectations, develops short–and long-range goals, sets priorities for the attainment of specific goals, and defines precisely what must be done to reach each program goal.

Objectives are specific statements that relate to obtainable ends. There are four components to an objective. An objective should meet all of the following four standards: (a) identify the task to be performed; (b) identify who is to perform the task; (c) describe the conditions of the task—where, when, and what resources; and (d) identify the criteria for measurement and the desired degree of proficiency to be achieved. Written objectives should be realistic, compatible with established policies and procedures, state expected results, be quantifiable and measurable, identify the present condition, be achievable, include completion date, and be evaluated. The purpose of this chapter is not to detail how to write specific goals and objectives, as there are a number of excellent references existing for this purpose. Mager's book, *Preparing Instructional Objectives* (1962), is widely used for this purpose.

The pressures of accountability have resulted from state and federal compliance mandates, the need for expanded programming, and budget limitations. For example, Public Law 94-142 has resulted in the development of many new and expanded programs and has identified many requirements that were not in existence in the past. Consequently, throughout the country we are beginning to struggle with identifying the compliance issues, trying to determine what they mean, assessing where a given district or agency is in relation to meeting these compliance issues, and developing a plan of action to be in compliance with state and federal legislation by a given point in time. In the future, the supervisor and the staff of each district or agency will need to clarify their goals and objectives, document progress, and produce results if programs are to survive and expand.

LEADERSHIP

Staying on the Cutting Edge

The quality of speech-language-hearing programs depends, to a significant degree, upon the leadership of the supervisor. One of the major responsibilities of the supervisor is to provide leadership for the program and the staff. In the past when a program was well established, the supervisor was often content to repeat the same program year after year. Special education programming has changed drastically, and currently, programs are constantly being upgraded and improved. Consequently, the supervisor not only provides leadership for current programming but also spends considerable time and energy planning for the future.

Anderson (1970) identified several aspects of the leadership role of the supervisor in innovative programming as follows:

> One of the functions of the supervisor of a speech, language, and hearing program is to promote and develop innovative programs in the schools that will better meet the needs of children. This role may be facilitated by the following procedures:
>
> 1. Have an awareness of trends in general education, including interpretations at the local level.
> 2. Provide information and expertise to those involved in making educational decisions.
> 3. Apply problem solving techniques to implement innovative programs.

4. Secure commitment of staff members by utilizing committees (a) to study the problems, (b) to show needs, (c) to give evidence of inadequacies in the current program, and (d) to suggest changes and implementations.
5. Utilize resources outside the speech, language and hearing area in the school setting—classroom teachers, psychological service personnel, social workers, reading specialists, health service personnel, and others—to meet the total needs of children.
6. Obtain supplementary professional support for necessary innovations by making use of resources outside the school setting—state and local speech and hearing associations, state universities, and state departments of education.
7. Continue an innovative program long enough to develop valid evaluative criteria, to evaluate its effectiveness, and to retain that which is found useful.
8. Make known the results of innovative programs to the staff of the speech, language and hearing program, administrators, the local community, and interested professional personnel. (P. 154)

The supervisor, associate director, and director are all responsible for developing new ideas, implementing them, and evaluating them. Whenever implementing change, it is important to consider the degree of change, how the change should occur, when the change should occur, and how the change should be approached.

There are a number of characteristics that contribute to quality supervision. Two of these are likely more important than others. First, the ability to work effectively with people is an extremely important component of the supervisory process. The abilities to listen to, support, motivate, work with, build trust in, and evaluate staff are all important aspects of this component. Other personal qualities, such as flexibility, creativity, sensitivity, and dependability are important supervisory characteristics. Second, the supervisor needs to be knowledgeable, highly skilled, and up to date in the area he or she is supervising. At times there may be individual staff members who are more knowledgeable than the supervisor in a specific area, such as cleft palate or stuttering. These staff members can and should assist the supervisor in developing improvements in their area of expertise. The supervisor needs to be an advocate for the students, staff, and program and to speak out on new and

*Planning Processes**:
Thinking
Determining objectives
Developing procedures

Scheduling
Forecasting
Programming

Organizing Processes:
Establishing standards
Resource allocating
Establishing relationships
Distributing functions

Coordinating
Delegating
Designing organization structure
Developing policies

Leading Processes:
Decision-making
Selecting people
Stimulating
Initiating
Demonstrating

Advising
Communicating
Encouraging
Suggesting

Innovating
Motivating
Facilitating
Illustrating

Controlling Processes:
Directing
Expediting
Applying sanctions

Taking corrective
action
Dismissing people

Reprimanding
Regulating

Assessing Processes:
Judging performance

Measuring performance

Researching

*Processes are rather complex patterns of behavior. They permeate much of the behavior of task-oriented people and tend to be employed regardless of the nature of the task. All of these processes and activities are important in supervising speech-language and hearing programs.

Figure 5-1. Processes and activities involved in Supervision. From B. Harris, *Supervisory Behavior in Education,* ©1963. Reprinted by permission of Prentice-Hall, Inc., Englewood Cliffs, N.J.

better ways to improve service (Fig. 5–1).

A new trend in education is to provide leadership training for management staff. This is becoming increasingly important in view of the complex issues of special and regular education. This is also important in view of collective negotiations and the negotiated contract. Many supervisors learn through experience on the job with little or no formal training. However, school districts and educational agencies are currently encouraging and supporting leadership training at district and agency levels through attendance at state supervisor meetings and attendance at national conventions. In addition, supervisors can keep up with new trends by attending conferences, by taking courses, and by reading current management literature. There is great value in good state leadership. In Iowa, as in many states, quality leadership exists at the state level in speech-language pathology and in audiology. Two or three state supervisor meetings dealing with numerous aspects of supervision and programming are held each year. This has been a real asset to the State of Iowa and has resulted in program development and improvement in the area education agency, district, clinician, and child levels.

There are two excellent ways to improve services. The first is to upgrade quality through continuing education of the supervisors and staff. Educational units are generally supportive of continuing in-service plans and programs for their professional personnel. The supervisor should be an advocate for continuing education and responsible for selecting topics, inviting national leaders, designing specific goals and objectives for each in-service, and carrying through with implementation and evaluation. Viewed in this manner, in-service is a process, with effective change being the ultimate goal.

The second major way to improve service is through recruiting new staff members. An entire chapter could be written about recruitment of speech and hearing personnel. As a result of experience, this supervisor has learned the value and importance of recruiting exceptional staff members. The first and most important requisite, this supervisor feels, is hiring a positive person who can work and relate effectively with children, parents, school personnel, and the supervisor. One negative, complaining staff member may not only create problems for the supervisor but may also adversely affect other staff members or the entire program. The supervisor needs to review carefully the training, experience, and references of a potential staff member. References are frequently checked by telephone to verify written recommendations and to obtain additional information about an applicant. Personality characteristics are often given consideration during the interview process. Consideration must also be given to the importance of recruiting new staff from a variety of training programs to generate and implement new ideas. Carefully selected new staff members can be a great asset to the program. There is no substitute for hiring the very best candidate(s) available.

THE NEGOTIATED CONTRACT

The majority of school districts and area education agencies have established negotiated contracts as a result of collective negotiation legislation. There are still some school districts that do not have a negotiated agreement between the Board of Education and the professional employees of the district. In essence, the contract spells out the rights of the employing agency and management versus the rights of the staff. The negotiated contract is the most important agreement between the Board of Education and the employees on work conditions, hours, responsibilities, salaries, and fringe benefits. Nearly every negotiated contract has ramifications that are far reaching in nature. Therefore, it is essential for both the supervisor and the staff to be highly knowledgeable about the contents of the negotiated agreement.

The items contained in a contract vary from one employment setting to another. Following is a list of items that are frequently included in detail:

Recognition
Procedure for negotiations
Dues
Grievance procedure
Complaint procedure
Job classification
Evaluation procedures
Hours
Employee work year
Health provisions
Safety provisions
Transfer procedures
Travel procedures
Reduction of staff
Leave provisions and notices
    Association-Union
    Personal/disability
    Emergency
    Bereavement
    Family illness

Personal
  Professional
  Extended leaves of absence
  Military
Insurance provisions and notices
  Health and medical
  Long-term disability
  Life
  Travel accident
  Workmen's compensation
Salary
  Salary schedule
  Salary placement schedule
  Supplemental pay
  Compliance clause and duration

An attempt will not be made to cite examples of contract language because of the variability in the language and because the details of every contract are different. The supervisor and the staff should be aware of the policies and procedures that describe, clarify, support, and reinforce items in the contract. Frequently there is direct relationship between an employee's job description, the negotiated contract, and the personnel evaluation procedures. For example, job classifications are often identified in the language of the contract. The job classifications are defined in written job descriptions that are district or agency policy. The employees are evaluated on their performance in relationship to their job description.

Two important aspects of most contracts are the complaint and grievance procedures. Certainly there should always be clear communication between the supervisor and the staff he is supervising. However, from time to time issues ranging from insignificant to highly significant become concerns and issues between the staff member and the supervisor. Whenever the supervisor or staff member has a concern about an issue, the concern should be discussed and hopefully be resolved. If the concern is not resolved through this communication process, the staff member may file a complaint or grievance. It is extremely important that both the supervisor and the employee be well informed of the complaint and grievance procedures that are usually in the negotiated contract. If the supervisor cannot answer a staff member's question or needs advice in responding to a complaint or a grievance, the supervisor should listen to the concern(s) and take detailed written notes of the conversation. The concern(s) should be discussed with the next higher level of authority, and an appropriate written response should be given to the staff member as soon as possible. If the concern is still not resolved, the staff member may take the grievance to the next higher level until the issue is resolved or all levels have been exhausted. Whenever the complaint and/or grievance procedures are used, there is a need for written documentation on the part of the supervisor and the employee. There is no substitute for written dated documentation when handling unresolved issues. Following all details of the grievance procedure is critical if the process is to be effective.

Collective Negotiations

As a result of legislation that has been passed during the past decade, public employees in at least thirty states currently have the right to negotiate the details of their work contract. Collective negotiation is another area where legislation has had a major impact on the educational process—that of employee benefits and working conditions. The employees of a given district or educational agency have a right to band together to improve their benefits and working conditions. Employees have an opportunity or, in some cases, an obligation to join an association or a union that represents them in the negotiations process. In many larger cities both a teachers' association and a union exist, but legally the Board of Education will recognize only one negotiation unit.

The process of negotiations is political and emotional but follows a legal plan of action. During this process, the Board of Education and the management staff are often pitted against the employees. This can result in negative side effects in some situations. However, in other districts, this process improves communications. During the negotiation process, the expectations of the employing agency and the expectations of the staff are reviewed, discussed, and if necessary, changed. In reality, there are numerous benefits to be derived from collective negotiations, since the negotiated contract clarifies issues, upgrades working conditions, provides for fairness and equality, and often results in written policies and procedures to refine the details of the contract.

In numerous states collective negotiation is regulated by state legislation, and a given period of time is permitted for open and/or closed discussion between the "district or agency" and the "association or union" in an effort to reach agreement on the stipulations of the contract. The employees who are members of the association or union select a negotiation team to represent them, and the board selects a negotiation team to represent the board and management. Each team generally will have one chief negotiator employed for this purpose. Chief negotiators are often attorneys, labor relations personnel, or professional negotiators. Usually only the chief negotiator speaks "at the table" for either side. The team may be comprised of a variety of members, and the supervisor and speech-language-hearing personnel may be asked to serve on the respective teams. Collective negotiation takes considerable time and energy and is a "give and take" situation. There are often detailed strategies involved in "getting the most or giving up the least." The tendency for the board is to begin by making a minimal offer and for the association or union to exaggerate its requests and demands. After many hours of deliberating, the two teams sort out the issues, discuss them in detail, and provide supportive evidence for their arguments. The end result is often a compromise on salaries, benefits, and other contract items. However, a given side may stand firm from beginning to end on one or more issues.

There is a sequence of basic steps involved in the negotiation process. During the first step, there is an initial exchange of proposals followed by bargaining between the two parties in an effort to resolve the issues. State legislation and policy governing collective negotiation define timelines for the entire process. In the event that the two parties do not reach agreement by the specified date, an impasse is declared, and this is the beginning of step two. The first phase of step two is mediation. During this period a "neutral" nonpublic employee trained by the federal or state government tries to bring the two parties together through reasoning and compromise. The results of this step are nonbinding unless a compromise is reached and approved by both parties.

In some states, fact finding is the second phase of step two. A trained, nonpublic, neutral person appointed by a regulating board conducts a public formal hearing where arguments and exhibits are presented and exchanged. The fact finder may support management and the board of education, may support the union or association, or may develop a third proposal. The fact finding process is advisory and not binding. In this process a recommendation is made for each contract item on which the parties disagree. The states that do not have fact finding in their procedures go directly from mediation to arbitration.

The final step in the negotiations process is binding arbitration. This process is similar to mediation and fact finding, but there are two basic differences. First, the "arbitrator" cannot develop a new position. The arbitrator studies the arguments, hears supporting evidence and defends the board's position, the union or association's position, or the compromise position resulting from mediation and/or fact finding. The second difference is that the arbitration decision is binding. Binding arbitration is occurring more and more frequently in the public sector as an alternative to a strike. In the event that the two parties cannot reach agreement during the initial bargaining, they generally may continue to negotiate in an effort to reach settlement throughout this entire process up to the point when the arbitrator renders the binding arbitration decision. The end result of all of this activity is a negotiated contract between the board of education and the employees, usually for a one- or two-year term. At the expiration of this term, the negotiation process begins again.

POLITICS

Politics—simply defined as looking out for one's own interests—is very real in education today. Some political maneuvering is subtle and occurs behind the scenes in quiet strategic sessions, while other politicking is very obvious, open, and spoken loud and clear to an individual or to a group at meetings or in written memorandums. Politics is often associated with power to accomplish personal, program, division, district, or agency goals. One form of this power is expressed in control of budget, programs, and/or staff use. The staff may exert political influence on the supervisor in an effort to accomplish a given objective.

There are many political lines in an educational setting. Only two individuals or factions of the organization may be involved in a given issue, while at other times the entire organization may be involved in a political issue. The political lines include the board to the administrator; the administrator to the director; the director to the associate director(s); the associate director(s) to the supervisors; and the supervisors to the staff. These lines can also occur from an agency to a district or a group of districts or may occur within or across groups. There is tremendous variability in the political atmosphere from agency to agency, district to district, building to building, teacher to teacher, child to child, and parent to parent. Consequently, supervisors and staff must work with most of these political atmospheres all of the time. The manner in which the supervisor and staff approach a situation and conduct themselves will set the tone and determine how a given person will adapt to different political situations. It is important for the supervisor and the staff to learn what the political system is and to work within the system.

The political implication(s) of an issue may range from highly positive, to neutral, to negative. Supervisors should be good listeners, not display favoritism, and communicate openly and honestly. Professionals at all levels should be able to express their feelings on issues, but this should be done through the proper channels, with good timing, and with clear, concise communication. Personal emotions should be minimized—the discussion should be on the issue and not on the person or personalities involved. If the supervisor does not keep in tune with political issues, she is likely to be caught "in the middle" between top management and the staff.

BUDGETARY CONSIDERATIONS

The supervisor's involvement in the budgetary process varies greatly from program to program. The continuum ranges from no responsibility to total responsibility for the speech-language and/or hearing services budget(s). The majority of supervisors do have some responsibility for budget development and expenditures. The development of the budget is primarily a managerial responsibility and often involves not only the administrative level but the supervisory level as well. In reality, the staff working in the schools have little input in the budget process. The budget process also varies from district to district, agency to agency, and from one state to another. Generally speaking, the budget is developed during the fiscal year prior to the implementation of the budget. The board of education and/or administrator have a timetable for budget development. During the initial planning stages, the supervisors, associate director(s), and director review the current budget and begin to plan for the forthcoming year. One or more advisory committees are often involved in the planning process, especially if program expansion is to be considered. The total agency budget consists of all of the divisions in the district or agency. The special education budget and, in particular, the specific program budgets, are integral components of the total budget. Once the budget is developed, it is often reviewed by one or more budget review committees and is presented to the board of education for information. A public hearing and state review are often completed before the board of education takes final action on approval.

It is important for the supervisor and the speech-language-hearing personnel to understand basically where the dollars come from and how they are spent. Funding sources include local property taxes, county and/or state aid, federal funding, such as that provided by Public Law 94–142 and/or federal grants, and miscellaneous revenue sources. The income is proportioned on a needs basis to the various programs and services provided by the district or agency. Within a given program, funds are basically expended for salaries and fringe benefits, contracted services, travel, and materials and supplies.

Following is a list of general items the supervisor and management consider in the budget process. This is not a complete listing, but the items in this list are commonly found in speech-language-hearing program budgets. The list is as follows:

Salaries for supervisory and administrative staff

Salaries for speech-language pathologists and audiologists
Salaries for speech aides and/or audiometrists
Salaries for secretarial help
Social security
State withholding
Workmen's compensation
Unemployment compensation
Life insurance
Liability insurance
Travel insurance
Disability insurance
Travel — within area
Travel — within state
Travel — out of state
Instructional supplies
Office supplies
Postage
Telephone service
Production
Computer charges
Prorated administrative costs
Repair of equipment
Contracted services

As can be seen, the majority of budget items are fixed expenditures. Often there is little manipulation of funds, as most of the expenditures are for salaries and fringe benefits, and only a small percent of the budget consists of variable expenses.

After approval by the director and/or administrator the expenditures are subject to approval by the board of education on a regular basis. Often a business manager, accountant, or comptroller heads the business office and develops business practices for the entire district or agency. Supervisors and speech-language-hearing personnel are wise to acquaint themselves with the budgetary process. The requisition-voucher process and administrative approval procedures must be clearly understood and followed by the supervisor and staff.

Is the cost of supervision justifiable? The answer to this question should be positive and viewed from the standpoint of the need for supervision and management of the allocated investment. For example, special education has become big business. The budget for many educational agencies now runs into millions of dollars annually. The budget for speech-language services may exceed a million dollars each year. The cost of supervisory and managerial expenditures is justifiable on the basis of the amount of public expenditure for educational services and the need for direct supervision of staff and program. Unfortunately, there are no data to indicate that supervision makes a difference in the effectiveness of speech-language pathologists at any level of training or in the employment setting. Research on the values of supervision is needed desparately in this age of accountability. While the budget is often controlled by the board, administrator, and/or directors, the staff should be knowledgeable of the total cost of speech-language-hearing services, the cost per staff member, and a general idea of cost accountability. For example, what is the approximate cost of a two-hour evaluation? What is the cost of a one-half hour therapy session? What is the cost of a hearing screening and threshold test? Some cost accountability studies have been done in speech and language. These cost accountability studies are often initiated with a time study. Omans (1972) conducted a service accountability study of the time allocated to various aspects of the speech-language program in the Spokane Public Schools. Following are the program functions and the percentage of time spent on each function: Travel, 7 percent; Identification, 4 percent; Diagnosis, 8 percent; Program scheduling, 3 percent; Therapy, 31 percent; Planning and preparation, 10 percent; Administration, 13 percent; Consultive service, 9 percent; Supervision of auxiliary personnel, 7 percent; and Meetings, 8 percent. The actual cost of each aspect of the program was computed and evaluated.

As accountability becomes a greater issue in the future in the schools, supervisors and staff providing services will become more cost conscious and will analyze costs more carefully. For example, the majority of speech-language pathologists in the schools work on an itinerant basis and travel from school to school. In the past travel was a minor expenditure. However, in view of our current and future energy problems, the cost of transportation is rising in dollars and time to go from school to school. This is a very real factor in view of the itinerant nature of speech-language-hearing services.

The federal government has passed numerous federal mandates for special education, including Public Law 94–142. On the pretext of compliance with the federal legislation, the local education agency (LEA) and the state education agency (SEA) receive additional funding. If these agencies do not comply with the legislation, their funds may be reduced or terminated. There are two serious problems in this respect. First, the federal legislation is often dependent on the establishment of adequate state funding. Some states do and some do not provide adequate special education support funds; there is great variability in state funding. Some states are more dependent upon federal funding than other states. Second, the federal government is not appropriating the amount of funds that were allocated in keeping with the increasing share of the federal government in supporting Public Law 94–142 and other legislation. These budget limitations have contributed to the budgetary problems resulting from declining enrollment and have been complicated by rising special education costs and the need for new and expanded programming. Supervisors can expect to be confronted with increasingly complex budgetary issues in the future.

INTERACTING WITH OTHER SPECIALISTS

Speech-language-hearing supervisors are team members with other supervisors of a wide variety of special education services. There is frequent interchange of information regarding children and programs. This interchange is healthy and should occur not only at the supervisory level but at the staff level as well. All special education and regular education programs have equal importance in the total educational program even though there is considerable difference in the way various programs are organized and the manner in which services are provided. Speech-language-hearing supervisors and personnel working in the schools are unique in that we have knowledge and skills regarding aural and oral communication skills and abilities that affect all learning. As such, there is a greater need for interdisciplinary communication in serving children. The majority of special education programs are currently set up on an interdisciplinary service approach. As communication specialists, we provide vital contributions to both regular and special education. We must also be cognizant and supportive of the contributions of other specialists. We are past the age when the "speech teacher" or "speech therapist" walked in the back door, went directly to the broom closet, met with the children, and left, without talking with anyone else. Considerable change results not only from the direct service but also the interdisciplinary communication and united front of a number of people working together to create positive child change.

Speech-language-hearing supervisors should encourage interdisciplinary communication, consultations, evaluations, staffings, and development of student service plans. In reality, there are many different professionals who are directly or indirectly involved with the child's total educational program. Speech-language-hearing supervisors and staff need to relate to a host of regular education personnel and special education personnel. For example, in the school speech-language pathologists and audiologists work with the superintendent, principal, teachers, special teachers, special education teachers, counselor, nurse, and others. Likewise, in special education there is a need to communicate with the special education director and/or assistant director, supervisors, and staff of a variety of special education services, such as psychologists, social workers, vision personnel, occupational therapists, physical therapists, early childhood staff, and staff members for the emotionally disturbed. In addition, speech-language pathologists and audiologists may work with regular and special education consultants and coordinators. There is no substitute for effective interdisciplinary communication at the supervisory and staff levels. When additional information is needed, or when some other specialist may be more effective in evaluating or serving a given child, a referral is initiated to the appropriate service.

One excellent example of a variety of regular and special education personnel working together for a common goal is the staffing process. Public Law 94–142 now requires a multidisciplinary staffing prior to the placement of any child in a special education program(s). The staffings are usually conducted by a principal, a coordinator, or a counselor, or this responsibility is assigned to one of the staff members. In any event, speech-language-hearing personnel should be members of the staffing process whenever a communication problem is being considered. At times the supervisor is involved in this activity, especially in small programs or in special cases. The staffing process is one of the most effective avenues of child advocacy, which should be strongly supported by the supervisor.

In-service programming is another area where interaction should occur with other specialists. At least three to five workdays should be used each year for in-service programs in addition to release time to attend state and national meetings. In developing in-service plans, the speech-language and/or hearing supervisor should consider at least three components of the in-service program: First, in-service for continuing education designed to meet the identified needs of the speech-language and/or hearing personnel; second, the supervisor should plan joint in-service meetings with other specialists having common interests and goals; third, the supervisor should encourage speech-language-hearing personnel to conduct continuing education meetings for other disciplines. For example, interpreting an audiogram is a relatively simple task for an audiologist, as we know the effects of various degrees of hearing loss, but a social worker who is counseling a child for social-emotional problems may not possess our knowledge. Likewise, speech-language pathologists need to in-service classroom teachers on speech and language problems and how they can assist in the clinical process in the classroom. We often assume that everyone knows what we know, but such is not the case. This is only one example of an in-service that might be provided for members of another discipline. In any event, the supervisor should set the example for the staff and interact and communicate effectively with other specialists.

Supervisory Decisions Based on Severity Rating Data

Severity rating systems for the communication handicapped are being used in public school programs in several states. Freilinger et al. (1978) reported on the development of the *Iowa Severity Rating Scale for Communication Disabilities.* Other such scales are reported in Chapter 8. When using this rating scale, a severity rating may be assigned for each of four categories: articulation, language, voice, and fluency. The severity rating is based upon objective measures of communication behavior. Traditionally, the information obtained from a severity rating scale has been used for case load selection and making scheduling decisions by individual speech-language pathologists. Beste and Aller (1980) suggest that severity rating data may also be used as a basis for planning the total speech-language program for a district or intermediate agency and for making a number of important management decisions.

The majority of speech-language pathologists and audiologists employed in the schools are employed for 180, 185, or 190 days. Nearly all school districts operate on a calendar of 180 actual days of school per year. School personnel are generally expected to work an eight-hour day, but the students are rarely, if ever, in attendance for more than six hours per day. Consequently, there is a maximum of 1,080 hours of prime student contact time during a given school year. Conservatively, at least eighty hours of this time are used for in-service meetings, conference days, inclement weather, personal illness, personal days, and a myriad of other activities. In essence, there are only approximately 1,000 hours of prime student contact time per year. In this age of accountability, supervisors must assume the responsibility for effective and efficient scheduling of staff. Speech-language pathologists and audiologists, in turn, must assume the responsibility for effective and efficient scheduling of students to maximize the impact of speech-language-hearing services in the schools.

Beste and Aller have developed a system for using severity rating information in determining personnel needs, case load distribution, and making assignments to rural and urban school districts, taking the concept of prime contact hours into consideration. Severity rating data may also be used for public relations activities, determination of staff development needs, participation in the development of individual educational plan (I.E.P.) conferences, and child service audits.

The *Iowa Severity Rating Scale for Communication Disabilities* was used to rate approximately 3,000 students served by sixty speech-language pathologists in a large intermediate educational agency. As a part of the evaluation procedures, the speech-language pathologists completed a severity rating sheet for each student. Each speech-language pathologist also submitted a rating tally sheet for each facility. The data were analyzed according to type of problem, grade level, severity, and treatment strategies. The data were combined for each assignment and included with information concerning mileage and special program enrollment. Assignments were evaluated by using the following formula: $H \div I + G + 1\ FTE$.

The specifics of the formula are as follows:

Hours $(H) = 27$ prime contact hours (6 hours per day $\times$ 4½ days per week with ½ day per week reserved for coordination responsibilities)

Individual $(I) = 10$ individual sessions allotments

Group $(G) = 12$ group session allotments

FTE = full time equivalency

This formula permits scheduling an average case load of fifty students. Ten students rated as four or more (disorder) are scheduled for three individual therapy sessions per week, and forty students rated as two or three (deviations) are scheduled for group therapy. Three or four students are scheduled per group, and sessions are scheduled twice a week. All sessions are based on thirty-minute time periods in this particular formula.

Driving time to and from the schools is included in the eight-hour workday. In the majority of cases, the driving time does not interfere with prime student contact time. However, occasionally, additional driving time to a given school and/or additional cases in the disordered category may further reduce the case load and/or increase group size. Actual clinical use of the twenty-seven prime contact hours is determined by the individual speech-language pathologist.

The data may also be used to analyze incidence figures by type of problem, special population, and school district. This information may be used for evaluating treatment strategies by comparing changes in ratings as indicated by a records audit. Information may also be used in the budgetary process for planning staff expansion, staff development, public relations activities, and justifying assignments to local districts and intermediate agency administrators. Beste and Aller conclude there is considerable merit in using severity rating data as baseline data to assist in making a number of important supervisory decisions regarding assignment and use of staff.

SUPERVISION OF PERSONNEL

Most of the information presented thus far in this chapter has dealt with administrative and program supervisory responsibilities. The remainder of the chapter will address the supervision of personnel. Supervision of the staff is a major responsibility of the supervisor. This responsibility requires a multitude of skills in human interaction, motivation, and leadership of developing professionals. The role of a supervisor is vastly different from the role of a speech-language pathologist or an audiologist in this respect. In essence, when a person becomes a supervisor, this person changes professions. Supervising a group of professionals is much different from supervising a clinical program for a group of children.

In 1978 the Committee on Supervision of Speech Pathology and Audiology of the American Speech-Language-Hearing Association indicated that the supervisory process is the interaction that takes place between the supervisor and the speech-language pathologist or audiologist and may be related to the behavior of the professional or to the child(ren) or to the program in which the supervisor and staff member are employed. The tasks a supervisor may perform are divided into two categories—clinical teaching and program management. Clinical teaching may be defined as the interaction between supervisor/supervisee in any setting that furthers the development of clinical skills of students in training or practicing speech-language pathologists or audiologists as related to changes in child behavior.

Among the summary statements at the conclusion of a conference on supervision in the schools, according to Anderson and

Kirtley (1966), was the following:

"Although the supervisor of speech and hearing may function both as an administrator and supervisor, he is chiefly a leader of professional personnel and, as such, must be responsible for the development of common philosophies and beliefs about the therapy program and its goals" (p. 9).

Ideally all speech-language pathologists and audiologists are supervised in the schools by a certified speech-language pathologist or audiologist in their own area of expertise. Iowa has been a national leader in this respect and provides supervision in both areas of expertise through the Area Education Agencies. However, adequate supervision is still minimal or nonexistent in some states. In small programs speech-language pathologists and audiologists supervise their own personal program or a colleague is assigned supervisory responsibility on a part-time basis. Supervision for the majority of local district speech-language and hearing programs is still provided by a professional with only one level of certification—generally speech-language pathology.

There are various management styles that are used in the supervisory process. While each supervisor has an individual, personal style, the supervisory style tends to fall into one of three categories. The first style is an autocratic form of leadership. An autocratic supervisor sets herself apart from the staff and has a tendency to be a highly subjective, program-oriented person. The autocratic leader views herself as being more knowledgeable and skillful than the staff members. The majority of decisions are "personal" ones. Using this style of leadership, the supervisor may listen to the staff but have little regard for their feelings or ideas and insist upon doing it "my way" without regard for the outcome. The autocratic leader is usually a strong-willed person, often has difficulty relating to people, and is obsessed with the power of the supervisor's position.

The second style is a democratic form of leadership. Following this style, the supervisor provides some personal leadership but obtains input from both management and staff. The feelings and ideas of the staff are considered, and the majority rules. Issues are often brought to a vote, and the supervisor may be put in a position of supporting and implementing a concept that he or she cannot really believe in or support. On the surface this supervisory style has many advantages, but a closer analysis may reveal that the supervisor who primarily follows a democratic approach may be a "weak" leader and is often confronted with problems resulting from dealing with the effects of democratic decisions.

The third supervisory style is participative management. This style requires an open-minded, flexible, mature person. In participative supervision, all staff members have not only the opportunity but also the responsibility for input. Instead of saying "Do it my way" or taking a vote on an issue, the participative manager shares the supervisory responsibility with staff. When an issue is at hand, the supervisor takes the issue to the staff, listens to the input, develops alternative ways to solve the problem or develop an idea, considers the pros and cons of each alternative solution, and provides staff with an opportunity to assist in making the decision. In this management style, the supervisor retains the right and responsibility to make the final decision on a given issue. However, as a result of the participative input, the staff contribute to charting their own course. Program changes resulting from this style of leadership are often implemented more easily and smoothly, since staff are knowledgeable of the decision and how it was reached.

While there are variations on these three supervisory management styles, supervisors will generally fall into one of these three categories. There are pros and cons to each supervisory style, but the participative management style has the most merit for developing quality programming and for relating most effectively to the staff. The management style may be determined, in part, by the program administrator and/or director, and the supervisor may be caught in a quandary between the requirements of top management versus personal choice of management style. The supervisor is generally more effective if the supervisory style is consistent with and/or supported by the administrator and director.

Supervision Concepts

There are a number of supervisory concepts which are important to any management style. Each concept implies the need for developing competencies, many of which deal with human interaction. These concepts and principles pertain to all supervisory positions and are identified as follows:

1. The concept of leadership: The supervisor must assume a strong leadership role by providing direct and indirect supervision for all professional staff members. This concept requires numerous competencies for providing the supervision each staff member might need.
2. The concept of planning: The supervisor assumes the responsibility for assisting each staff member in the process of developing effective plans to carry out the staff member's job description responsibilities in keeping with the overall program plans. This principle requires competencies in planning a program, developing goals and objectives, and supporting individual variations in accomplishing a given task.
3. The concept of effective communications: The supervisor has major responsibilities for effective oral and written communications. In view of the significance of these competencies, a section of this chapter will address this topic.
4. The concept of staff and student advocacy: One important responsibility of the supervisor is to serve as an advocate for staff and students. There is a paramount need to be supportive to the staff members and to the students they serve. This concept suggests a need for supervisory competencies in advocacy, in tolerance for individual differences, and in being supportive.
5. The concept of being positive: The supervisor has the responsibility to set the tone of the program by being a positive example. This principle is demonstrated by being a positive person, fostering positive relationships, providing genuine positive feedback to staff, hiring positive staff, and providing frequent rewards of a positive nature.

6. The concept of effective listening: The supervisor needs to develop the ability to listen to the needs and feelings of the staff, take time to listen, get to know specific situations, and build relationships of acceptance and trust.
7. The concept of objectivity: The supervisor should establish and maintain an attitude of being open minded and objective on issues and relationships. This principle elicits competencies in understanding different points of view, being objective in dealing with issues rather than being subjective or emotional, and in using objective measures in self-ratings and evaluation of the staff.
8. The concept of motivation: The supervisor has a responsibility to serve as a catalyst in motivating staff to provide quality services and produce highly effective results. A supervisor can motivate staff most effectively by being encouraging and supportive, by stimulating their thinking, and by reinforcing them with a variety of rewards on a regular basis.
9. The concept of flexibility: The supervisor develops competencies in adapting supervision to the individual needs of each staff member, depending upon her/his training, experience, abilities, and different professional viewpoints. This principle implies that the supervisor provides different strokes for different folks.
10. The concept of being considerate: This principle solicits the supervisor's consideration of all staff members—their views, their methods, their efforts. A given task may be performed many ways, and often there is more than one *right* way to accomplish something. Staff members should be treated with respect.
11. The concept of evaluation: The supervisor has the responsibility to evaluate the performance of each staff member, generally in relation to the agency job expectations and job description. A segment of this chapter will deal with this concept in view of the importance of evaluation.

Staying in Touch

Supervisors of speech-language-hearing programs often spend in excess of 50 percent of their time communicating with their staff. As communication specialists, we are naturally interested in a constant interchange of information between supervisor and staff. Communication is of paramount importance to developing and maintaining effective relationships. It is of utmost importance that all staff members be encouraged to communicate freely with the supervisor. The supervisor should have contacts ranging from highly informal to formal communication with each staff member. An informal communication may be a phone call, a letter, or a chat at a meeting, whereas a formal communication might include such things as a planning meeting or a personal conference for a specific reason.

There are a wide variety of reasons for the supervisor to communicate with staff and the staff to communicate with the supervisor on a regular basis. The purpose of the communication will often dictate how important, urgent, and personal the communication is. The supervisor is encouraged to make personal contact and to take sufficient time when a really critical issue is at hand. In reality, then, the importance of the communication will dictate whether the communication should occur during a personal visit or conference, through a personal letter, a note, or a group announcement. The supervisor is encouraged to have an "open door" policy, which enables staff to talk with the supervisor when the staff feels a need to do so. Likewise, it is important to have a degree of privacy for some sessions. Activities should be carefully planned and concepts clearly communicated to the staff. There is a great variability in the frequency of communication from one supervisor to another. A supervisor with a small staff of only a few people can spend a great deal of individual time with each staff member. However, supervisors of speech-language programs may supervise 100 or more persons in a large city system. This is not an adequate supervisor-to-staff ratio. At the beginning of this chapter a supervisor-to-staff ratio of 1:10 was reported as recommended by the American Speech-Language-Hearing Association. This ratio may be somewhat idealistic. In the opinion of this writer, a full-time supervisor can adequately supervise a staff of twenty-five speech-language pathologists. If an assistant is employed to help the supervisor, it is often possible for one person to supervise twenty-five to fifty speech–language–hearing personnel.

Obviously, the larger the program, the less time the supervisor will have to communicate with each staff member individually. One caution suggested for supervisors of large city programs is that they should not isolate themselves from the staff but should stay in communication with individual staff members as much as possible. This writer can recall employing a speech-language pathologist from a large city system who related that she received a memo in the fall that stated she should come to the central office to receive her assignment and pick up the keys. At the end of that academic year she received a second memo from the supervisor indicating that she should return the keys to the central office. At no point during that year did the supervisor make any attempt to contact her. On the other hand, she did initiate contact with the central office on several occasions. Obviously, this is an extreme example. The antithesis of this is the supervisor who constantly looks over the speech-language pathologists' shoulders and makes the majority of decisions about programming. Speech-language pathologists are expected to have at least adequate training and skills when employed. Some need more help than others. Staff should be encouraged to contact the supervisor when they need assistance. The supervisor should not view this need as a weakness on the part of the staff member.

The length of the communication, whether it is a memo, a letter, or a personal conference, depends on the need for the communication. When a staff member comes to the supervisor with a concern or an issue, the supervisor should take sufficient time to listen, to discuss the issue, and to resolve the issue with the staff member at that time if at all possible. Some issues take only a few minutes to resolve—others may take months and perhaps years.

The most effective way to convey the information or to carry out the communication should be considered. For example, if information can be clearly communicated in writing, this may be the most effective method. On the other hand, some items are best communicated in person. Some items can best be communicated in a group meeting so everyone is informed simultaneously.

It has been said that the tone of a presentation, whether it be in writing or in person, conveys as much of the intent of the message as do the words. Consequently, the supervisor should always be aware of the tone of her voice in communicating the intent of the message. In a similar way, the language of a message carries important content about the message itself. The supervisor can also obtain important information about the seriousness of an issue by listening to the tone of the speaker's voice and the language being used. Some thought needs to be given to whether each communication should be documented or not. Oral communication is generally not documented. However, if the issue is significant, a supervisor should take the initiative to keep dated notes for future reference. In the area of written communication, a copy should always be kept in the supervisor's file, and copies should be sent to the appropriate persons.

Motivation

One important responsibility of the speech-language-hearing supervisor is motivating staff members to improve the effectiveness and efficiency of services. The supervisor needs to develop a relationship of trust with each staff member so motivational techniques can be used successfully. This relationship is essential before one can motivate a person effectively. A relationship of trust can be established by accepting a person as he is and by recognizing individual differences. The staff needs to know from the beginning that the supervisor will attempt to treat each staff member fairly and deal with issues openly, honestly, and humanely. If the supervisor expects the staff to respect her leadership, the supervisor should respect each staff member for his knowledge, feelings, and skills. A supervisor can stimulate and motivate staff more effectively if a relationship of trust is well established. The supervisor should take sufficient time to become acquainted with each person and to observe his performance not only in the supervisor's office but in the field as well. After the relationship of trust is established, it can be developed and strengthened into a viable motivational force on an ongoing basis.

Once a relationship of trust has been established with a staff member, the supervisor can use a number of motivational skills and techniques. The supervisor should display a personal interest in each staff member. This can be done best by taking time to listen to the person and by providing opportunities for the person to express his views, needs, and feelings. The supervisor should be attentive while the individual is talking and should take an interest in what he is saying and try to understand the person's ideas and feelings. Kagan (1970) suggested the importance of dealing with the affective elements of communication in the supervising process. When a staff member comes to the supervisor with a concern, the supervisor should resist putting the person down, or putting the issue off, and should work with the staff member in placing the problem in perspective and resolving the concern. This will motivate the staff to bring their problems to the supervisor and, in most cases, the problem will be brought to the supervisor's attention before it becomes a major personal or program problem.

Another way to stimulate and motivate staff is to demonstrate to staff members that you care about them, their work, and their results. This implies that the supervisor is considerate of each staff member as each day passes. One of the best ways to foster a caring attitude is to help the staff members feel they are vitally important. As indicated earlier, the supervisor should present a positive personal image and should promote a positive approach for all staff. Unfortunately, in reality there are always negative feelings, concerns, and viewpoints, but these can be minimized through a positive approach. Staff should be encouraged rather than discouraged to express new ideas and suggestions for changes that have merit for improving performance. Another way to motivate staff is to stimulate them to produce effective and efficient results. The supervisor can motivate staff by emphasizing the importance of their results in relation to the children they serve, to the children's parents, and to school personnel. Likewise, this stimulation is equally important for their own motivation and makes a significant contribution to the success of the total program. Teaching staff to observe changes in each child is an extremely rewarding motivator. If one were to analyze the effectiveness of services to individual children in the schools, one would find vast differences in the effectiveness of progress and results. As supervisors, we need to be concerned with the end product—communication change in children resulting from the provision of services. One of the greatest rewards a speech-language pathologist can experience is to observe a child correcting an articulation error or using an improved language structure or to see the smile on a child's face as he understands a language concept.

The supervisor should generate confidence in staff members— especially in new staff members. Staff should be encouraged to try new ideas, to create an atmosphere in which it is permissible to make a mistake, and to create an understanding that one learns through this process. The supervisor generates confidence in staff by supporting persons when they are "up" and when they are "down." The supervisor should spend more time with new staff during their first year than with experienced staff. This is important so that the supervisor can assist new staff in building skills, can reassure their efforts, and can build confidence that will continually motivate them to improve their progress.

The most important way to motivate staff is by rewarding them. Educational systems are continually upgrading their salary and benefit packages as tangible rewards for people who dedicate their time and energy to education. Salary and fringe benefits are improving. The major rewards in special education have no specified monetary value; the major rewards in our profession result from the personal satisfaction derived from the provision of human services and improved communication skills. Each staff member needs to be reinforced through the supervisory process. The supervisor can reward her staff in a variety of ways. This should be done in sincerity and with sufficient frequency to be satisfying to the staff member. Speech-language pathologists and audiologists may be rewarded by individual verbal praise from the supervisor, by group recognition, through letters of appreciation, and through public media. Everyone needs positive feedback for the results of his efforts. New and innovative techniques should be recognized. A school district can also reward staff members by encouraging them to share some of the exciting things they are doing through participation in state and national conventions and by writing articles for professional journals. There are many ways to challenge, stimulate, and motivate staff members to continue to strive for improvement in performance and excellence in programming.

Evaluation of Personnel

Evaluation of the work of speech-language pathologists and audiologists is a major responsibility of the supervisor. The supervisor uses a wide variety of skills during the evaluation process. For example, the supervisor needs to remain current in her knowledge of speech, language, and hearing problems and must keep abreast of the latest therapeutic techniques; must be skillful in observing human interaction and child change; must be a keen observer; must be able to record significant events accurately during the evaluation process; and must communicate clearly with the speech-language pathologist and/or audiologist when reviewing the evaluation.

Anderson (1974) indicated that

> It is not enough for a supervisor to be a public relations person; it is not enough for him to be a program developer—although these are important activities. If children are to receive higher quality services as a result of the supervisor's presence in a program, then that supervisor must not only be a competent clinician himself, he must also have some special skills in working with clinicians. He must have a thorough understanding of the clinical process. He must develop infinite skills in behavioral observation. He must be an expert in the communication of feedback. He must understand the modification of adult behavior. He must understand his own strengths and weaknesses as a clinician and as a person. He must be able to evaluate, encourage, reinforce, coordinate, facilitate, and moderate." (P. 10)

Basically, there are two purposes for evaluation. The first purpose is to evaluate the performance of the staff members in relation to what is expected in the general job description, personalized job description, and goals and objectives of the person and program. In reality, this process provides the most objective way to evaluate a person and to have an evaluation base for comparison purposes. The second purpose for evaluation is for improvement of performance. The second responsibility really involves teaching skills. This is often done by analyzing therapy techniques, offering suggestions for change, and by demonstrating alternative methods.

Evaluation of personnel should be viewed as a challenge and as an ongoing process. Evaluation systems vary considerably from informal, lax, and almost nonexistent systems to highly developed, intensive observations, personal conferences, and written procedures. In small or relatively new programs the supervisor may need to take the initiative to design and implement a personnel evaluation system. These procedures are well established in large school systems and in programs that have been in existence for several years.

There are three components to the evaluation process. The first component is a direct observation of the speech-language pathologist or audiologist working with children. In addition, other observations may be made, such as in the case of parent and/or teacher conferences. During the observation the supervisor should write an objective record of the observation, which should be reviewed as soon as possible with the staff member. The second component of the evaluation process is to compare the individual's performance with a job description and specific goals and objectives. This may be done in relation to both direct observation and indirect knowledge of the person's performance during the course of a given year. This evaluation should also be recorded in writing. The third component of the evaluation process is a personal conference between the supervisor and the staff member. During this conference the supervisor should review the observations and comments for the first two components of the evaluation and should have an opportunity to discuss the person's performance with her in detail. This process may occur once or several times during the course of a year and may be carried out with the combination of informal and formal procedures. During the evaluation conference the supervisor should provide positive feedback for the staff member, should discuss any problems or concerns arising from the evaluation process, and should offer suggestions for change and improvement. The evaluation process should be kept confidential and should be performed primarily by the supervisor rather than a building principal. Peer review certainly has some merit but, in the opinion of this writer, personal evaluation of the staff should not be done by fellow staff members but should be the responsibility of the program supervisor.

SUPERVISION OF STUDENT SPEECH-LANGUAGE PATHOLOGISTS AND AUDIOLOGISTS IN THE SCHOOLS

Public school programs provide a multitude of opportunities for practicum experiences for student speech-language pathologists and audiologists. Every student should complete practicum experience in the schools. This is important from the standpoint of becoming acquainted with programming in the schools and evaluating the setting as a possible work environment as well as for meeting certification requirements.

Directors and supervisors of the training programs are encouraged to develop good working relationships with the supervisors of school speech-language and hearing programs. It is mutually important for supervisors of training programs and supervisors of school programs to work closely together in providing quality opportunities for students in training. It should also be recognized that all professionals have a responsibility to assist in the education and training of future professionals. Speech-language pathologists and audiologists working in the schools often become the primary supervisor for students in training.

The purpose of this section is to describe some aspects of supervision of students in public school practicum experiences. There is an important common thread between supervisors in the schools and in the training program. The common thread is that supervision of students is a teaching process wherever experience and learning occur.

Goals for students in training should include the provision of a variety of training experiences, an opportunity for the students to do some in-depth planning, to gain confidence and skills through actual experience derived from working directly with children, to learn through the evaluative-teaching process and to improve and grow in knowledge and skill.

Anderson (1973) noted that the structure and methods of school practicum in speech pathology and audiology have closely followed the original model of student teaching as conducted in general education. There is an urgent need to investigate the efficiency and effectiveness of that model. If research determines that existing models are not productive, new models should be proposed, according to Anderson. All students should complete adequate course work before being assigned to student teaching practicum experience in the schools. Students should enter the practicum with sufficient background knowledge and skills as determined by professional standards and the training program.

Supervisors of school programs are encouraged to meet with the supervisor(s) of the training program(s) for the purpose of planning maximum opportunities for students in training. In many cases it will be necessary to have a series of planning meetings to develop a complete program for practicum experiences in the schools. It is advisable to include the special education director of the educational unit and the director of the speech-language and hearing clinic in these planning sessions for administrative understanding and support. The practicum plans should ultimately be approved by these administrative personnel. In addition to the series of planning meetings, it is envisioned that there will be ongoing communication between the supervisor of the school program and the supervisor of the training program after the procedures have been developed and put into practice.

There are a number of topics that need to be discussed and resolved during the initial planning process. These include the following:

1. List the different types of training experiences that are available in the schools.
2. Delineate responsibilities of the school supervisor, training supervisor, and student(s).
3. Develop procedures for student practicum experiences.
4. Assure appropriate level of professional certification of training program(s), school program, and supervisory personnel.
5. Develop communication strategies.
6. Determine plans for assignment of students.
7. Plan program for orientation of students.
8. Determine length and timing of practicum experience(s).
9. Develop cooperative plans for supervision of students.
10. Develop cooperative plans for evaluation of students.

The school supervisor also has the responsibility to assign students to staff members who are willing to accept this additional responsibility. These staff members are expected to establish a good working relationship with the student, provide him with a variety of professional experiences, allow the student to experiment within accepted limitations, provide frequent opportunities for observation, confer frequently with the student about plans, and provide ongoing evaluation of the student's progress.

The training program supervisor maintains a responsibility to work with the student in the school setting. There are a variety of practices in this regard. In some cases the training program supervisor assumes responsibility for on-site evaluations, conferences, and grading. In other cases the supervisor of the student in the schools assumes these duties. At times, supervision is done on a cooperative basis. In any event, practicum experience should be viewed as a learning opportunity and as a teaching process. The training program supervisor should not delegate all of the responsibility for this teaching process to the school personnel but should develop a working relationship with each student by maintaining frequent contact with him and his school supervisor during the practicum experience.

The student assumes a number of responsibilities in the practicum experience. The student should take the initiative to become acquainted with all aspects of the practicum experience, enter the experience with a willingness to learn, plan appropriate goals and objectives, prepare adequately on a regular basis, be objective, communicate clearly at all times, request help when needed, develop confidence in himself, and assume a positive attitude toward the evaluative-teaching-learning process.

Freilinger (1973), Consultant for Clinical Speech Services for the Iowa Department of Public Instruction, commissioned a task force to investigate problems of the practicum experience and to develop guidelines for a more systematic approach in providing a quality learning experience for student speech-language clinicians in the schools. The results of the task force were reported in a 1975 report of the Iowa State Department of Public Instruction. Baldes et al. (1977) summarized the information and recommendations of the task force.

> The qualifications and characteristics of the University Supervising Clinician and the School Supervising Clinician in the schools are *similar* in more respects than they are *different*. These personnel shall hold the Certificate of Clinical Competence from the American Speech and Hearing Association. The University Supervising Clinician should have experience as a public school clinician other than her/his own practicum experience and should have had courses in supervision and management at the graduate level. The School Supervising Clinician should have at least

two years of experience in the public schools and should have some training in supervision. The University Supervising Clinician shall be a faculty member of the Department of Speech Pathology and Audiology. Supervisors of Clinical Speech Programs in the schools should provide and assist speech clinicians in getting supervisory experience. More and more graduate programs are providing their outstanding graduate students with practical experience in supervising beginning speech-language clinicians.

The University Supervising Clinician and the School Supervising Clinician must possess leadership qualities which require the utmost consideration of human relations. The following suggestions are made for supervising clinicians in working with a student speech-language clinician.

1. Have a friendly, understanding attitude and acceptance of the student speech-language clinician as a colleague.
2. Be a model for students of conduct expected in professional life.
3. Have the ability to provide objective evaluation and recognition of success through assistance in planning and evaluation, instruction, and frequent conferences and guidance in self-analysis.
4. Be sensitive to the student-clinician's need for an orientation to school environment which includes the extent of the student-speech clinician's authority and responsibility, importance of records and reports, and the importance of maintaining good public relations.

In addition, the key to the student speech-language clinician's success, and the success of the University Supervising Clinician and the School Supervising Clinician, is that there be effective communication.

Two distinct differences between the University Supervising Clinician and the School Supervising Clinician are noted.

1. The responsibility for the well-being of the school program and the clients therein remains the prime concern of the School Supervising Clinician.
2. Should problems arise, the student speech-language clinician should attempt to resolve the matters with the School Supervising Clinician. If, however, either the student speech-language clinician or the School Supervising Clinician feels the matters need further discussion, one or both should contact the University Supervising Clinician.

The length of the practicum should be such that the student speech-language clinician has time to become involved in the varied experiences unique to the public school setting. Although the most desirable internship is for a full year, it must be recognized that this may not be feasible at this time. It is believed, however, that no practicum period should be less than eight weeks and that the full day be included, five days per week. It is felt that the student speech-language clinician should be exposed to full-time experience so as to better understand the real work environment of the speech-language clinician who works in the schools. It would seem that student speech-language clinicians would be better prepared for the comprehensive clinical practicum in the public school setting after they have completed their course work and their on-campus practicum. The case load in the public schools usually includes language, articulation, fluency and voice problems of varied etiology and severity. Thus, it is very important that the student speech-language clinician be thoroughly prepared in techniques of management for the variety of problems.

Evaluation criteria should be formulated as a cooperative endeavor of both the University Supervising Clinician and the School Supervising Clinician. These criteria should be formulated for each of the three evaluators: (1) the University Supervising Clinician, (2) the School Supervising Clinician, and (3) the student speech-language clinician. Since each of these individuals will be evaluating the student speech-language clinician during his/her school practicum, it is imperative that each person involved in the evaluation process understand the areas to be evaluated—methods, purposes, results— and how the evaluation information will be used.

The University Supervising Clinician should directly observe and confer with the student speech-language clinician, School Supervising Clinician or program supervisor at least every two weeks. The University Supervising Clinician should assume the responsibility for designing those areas which will be evaluated when making observations of the student speech-language clinician and should assume the responsibility for informing and explaining that evaluation process to both the student speech-language clinician and the School Supervising Clinician. It is highly possible that the University Supervising Clinician may continue to utilize evaluation methods and procedures which are employed within the particular university, or one may wish to design and utilize evaluation methods and procedures which are more "tailor-made" to the rather unique clinical environment found in the majority of public school programs.

The School Supervising Clinician along with the University Supervising Clinician should be responsible for designing and formulating the evaluation criteria to be utilized during the student speech-language clinician's school practicum. Separate written evaluations based on these criteria should be prepared by the University Supervising Clinician and School Supervising Clinician at least twice during the student speech-language clinician's assignment.

It is suggested that the student speech-language clinician evaluate his/her performance with the same instrument and as frequently as the School Supervising Clinician. In the long run, the evaluation that will lead to improvement in the student speech-language clinician will be the evaluation he/she makes of himself/herself. (Pp. 7–12)

Figure 5-2 includes the suggested parameters that should be used in an evaluation format for the school practicum experience(s). The format was suggested by the Iowa Committee for evaluation of the student speech-language clinician.

I. IDENTIFICATION
  A. Skill in screening for:
     1. language disorders
     2. voice disorders
     3. articulation disorders
     4. fluency disorders
     5. hearing screening (when applicable)
  B. Appropriate utilization of screening materials and equipment.
  C. Ability to follow standardized screening procedures.
  D. Accuracy in interpreting test results.
  E. Skill in interpreting and communicating screening results.
  F. Accuracy of screening records and reports.
  G. Based upon these criteria, a brief description about this student speech-language clinician is as follows:

II. DIAGNOSTIC EVALUATIONS
  A. Skill in diagnostic evaluations for:
     1. language disabilities
     2. voice disabilities
     3. articulation disabilities
     4. fluency disabilities
     5. acoustically handicapped
     6. mentally handicapped
     7. neurologically handicapped
  B. Appropriate selection of diagnostic instruments and procedures.
  C. Accuracy in interpreting diagnostic results.
  D. Skill in interpreting and communicating evaluation results with teachers, parents, administrators, and other staff members.
  E. Accuracy of evaluation records and reports.
  F. Effectiveness of processing and initiating referrals.
  G. Based upon these criteria, a brief description about this student speech-language clinician is as follows:

Figure 5-2. Suggested parameters for school practicum experience.

III. SCHEDULING

   A. Selection of case load
      1. Selection of case load is based upon case selection criteria.
      2. Grouping of children is consistent with speech and language needs of the individual child.
      3. Devises a workable service schedule which will adequately meet the child's communication needs.
      4. Clears service schedule through the appropriate school personnel.
   B. Initiates appropriate referrals.
   C. Plans indirect services for children not enrolled (if applicable)
   D. Based upon these criteria, a brief description about this student speech-language clinician is as follows:

_____

_____

_____

_____

IV. MANAGEMENT

   A. Management of a broad variety of communication disabilities.
   B. Appropriate selection of target behaviors.
   C. Appropriate selection and use of materials.
   D. Management in accord with diagnosed needs.
   E. Effectiveness of goals and objectives for each pupil.
   F. Demonstrates flexibility in modifying services in relation to results and evaluations.
   G. Consistently participates in ongoing evaluation and programming.
   H. Effectively assesses pupil progress.
   I. Directions given to pupils are clear and appropriate to the child's level of functioning.
   J. Maintains accurate records and reports for each pupil.
   K. Establishes effective rapport and liaison with pupils, parents, and allied professionals.
   L. Follows specific criteria of dismissal of pupils.
   M. Utilizes appropriate transfer and maintenance and follow-up procedures.
   N. Based upon these criteria, a brief description about this student speech-language clinician is as follows:

_____

_____

_____

_____

V. PROFESSIONAL AND FAMILY RELATIONSHIPS

   A. Is aware of referral criteria.

Figure 5-2-*Continued*

Supervision

B. Knows available materials and personal resources.
C. Seeks information from appropriate sources.
D. Makes use of available professional and supportive personnel and agencies.
E. Integrates the special program with the educational program.
F. Demonstrates ability to utilize appropriate resources.
G. Communicates effectively with supervisor, teachers, administrators and school patrons regarding goals, objectives, results and current status of pupils and the program.
H. Actively participates in local staff meetings and pupil-relations programs.
I. Based upon these criteria, a brief description about this student speech-language clinician is as follows:

_____
_____
_____
_____

VI. Which of your personal qualities and professional skills do you believe have helped you have a successful student experience?

VII. Which of your personal qualities and professional skills do you believe need to be improved?

VIII. Based upon this evaluation, goals are as follows:

SUMMARY:

EVALUATION FOR: _____
EVALUATION BY: _____
DATE: _____

Figure 5-2—*Continued*

SUMMARY

Quality supervision of speech-language and hearing programs in the schools is a necessity. There are many legitimate reasons to support this need. Program supervisors have a multitude of responsibilities. These responsibilities basically fall into two categories—supervision of the program and supervision of the speech-language-hearing personnel. Program supervisors are frequently selected from the staff and often have little training or expertise in program and/or personnel management. Training programs are encouraged to develop and provide more opportunities to learn supervisory skills.

The supervisor has a number of important responsibilities relating to management of the program. The supervisor is responsible to the director of special education. The district or area administrator and board of education assume the ultimate responsibility for programs and services. Organization is the key to success in the managerial process. Written program descriptions should be developed to spell out the general and specific details of each program.

Quality supervision depends upon the supervisor's ability to plan and implement programming effectively. Staff should be involved in the program planning process. It is important to determine if the needs are being met, the degree to which they are being met, and to identify existing needs. Alternative plans should be considered when planning program improvements. In the future, supervisors will be challenged to implement changes resulting from energy shortages and inflationary costs.

School districts and intermediate educational service agencies should identify critical work activities and should have written job descriptions for supervisors as well as for personnel. The critical work activities should be identified by listing the tasks and activities that must be accomplished to comply with local, area, state, and federal guidelines. The job description lists the major professional responsibilities for the program supervisor(s).

The supervisor contributes to the general philosophy of service, assesses needs and expectations, develops short– and long-range goals, sets priorities for the attainment of the specific goals and objectives, and defines what must be done to reach each major goal. In this age of accountability, the supervisor must provide leadership to clarify goals and objectives, document progress, and produce program results if we are to survive and expand. The quality of the program depends to a large degree upon the leadership of the supervisor. Among the characteristics that contribute to quality supervision are the ability to work effectively with people and to be highly knowledgeable and skillful in dealing with communication disorders.

Legislation permits collective negotiations and the development of a negotiated contract in many states. Management personnel must work within the limitations of the negotiated contract and district, agency, state, and federal policies, rules, and regulations. Many decisions in the supervisory process are no longer left up to the discretion of a given supervisor but are clarified in the negotiated contract and supporting policies, rules, and regulations. If a negotiated contract is in existence, it is essential for both the supervisor and the staff to be familiar with the contents of the master agreement. The supervisor may or may not be involved in the collective negotiation process.

Supervisors often become involved in the budgetary process. It is important for the supervisor and the speech and hearing personnel to understand sources of income and expenditures. Cost accountability studies can be completed in an effort to identify the cost for specific aspects of a program.

There is a wide diversity of special education programs in existence today. These range in size from small school districts and services for a few hundred children to complex programming for hundreds of thousands of students. As such, a supervisor may supervise anywhere from a few professionals to several hundred professionals. Every person should have a supervisor. The supervisor to staff ratio should not exceed 1:25 unless the supervisor has assistance. Speech-language-hearing supervisors should encourage interdisciplinary communication, consultation, evaluations, staffings, and development of student service plans.

There are a number of management styles employed in the schools. A participative management style is encouraged. This style implies frequent input and interaction with speech-language pathologists and audiologists as well as maintaining communication with upper levels of management. A number of supervisory concepts that relate to dealing with human interaction are identified in the chapter. Communication is of paramount importance in developing and maintaining effective relationships.

Evaluation of speech-language pathologists and audiologists is a major responsibility for the supervisor. Evaluation generally consists of one or more observations, an evaluation of the individual's performance in relationship to goals and objectives and his job description, and a personal evaluation conference.

There are a multitude of opportunities for student speech-language pathologists and audiologists to gain experience in the public school environment. The supervisor is encouraged to work closely with the supervisor of training programs in developing and providing these opportunities.

STUDY ACTIVITIES

1. Read the articles written by Jean Anderson listed in the Bibliography.
2. Evaluate yourself or a fellow student using the suggested format developed in Iowa for evaluation of the speech-language clinician.
3. Invite a school supervisor to talk to one of your classes about supervision of speech-language and hearing programs in your area.
4. Develop a list of situations or potential problems that could affect the relationship between a supervisor and a staff member. Role-play these situations and problems using problem-solving techniques and develop alternate ways to resolve a given issue.
5. Explore opportunities to visit and observe a supervisor of a school program.

REFERENCES

American Speech and Hearing Association. Program supervision. *Standards and Guidelines for Comprehensive Language, Speech and Hearing Programs in the*

Schools. Washington, D.C., American Speech and Hearing Association, 1973–74.
American Speech and Hearing Association. *Essentials of Program Planning, Development, Management and Evaluation.* Washington, D.C.: American Speech and Hearing Association, 1973.
American Speech and Hearing Association. Supervision in the Schools. Report of Task Force on Supervision. *Language, Speech, and Hearing Services in Schools, 3,* 4–10, 1972.
Anderson, J. Training of Supervisors in Speech-Language Pathology and Audiology. Unpublished paper presented at The American Speech and Hearing Convention, 1978.
Anderson, J. Supervision of School Speech, Hearing & Language Programs—an Emerging Role. *Asha, 16,* 7–10, 1974.
Anderson, J. Status of College and University Programs of Practicum in the Schools. *Asha, 15,* 60–68, 1973.
Anderson, J. Handbook for Supervisors of School Practicum in Speech, Hearing and Language. Unpublished. Bloomington, Indiana: Indiana University, 1972.
Anderson, J. Status of Supervision in Speech, Hearing and Language Programs in the Schools. *Language, Speech, and Hearing Services in Schools, 3,* 12–23, 1972.
Anderson, J. (Ed.). *Conference on Supervision of Speech and Hearing Programs in the Schools.* Bloomington, Indiana: Indiana University, 1970.
Baldes, R., Goings, R., Herbold, D., Jeffrey, R., Wheeler, G., and Freilinger, J. J. Supervision of Student Speech Clinicians, *Language, Speech and Hearing Services in Schools, 8(2),* 76–84, 1977.
Baldes, R., Freilinger, J. J., Goings, R., Herbold, D., Jeffrey, R., and Wheeler, G. *Report of the Task Force on Supervision of Student-Speech Clinicians.* Des Moines: Department of Public Instruction, 1975. Available from ERIC, ED 108482; EC 07–3083.
Beste, P. and Aller, K. Using Severity Rating Data in Public School Program Management. Unpublished paper submitted for 1980 American Speech-Language-Hearing Association Convention, Detroit, 1980.
Brown, J. and Freilinger, J. *Lecture Notes on Management and Supervision.* Des Moines: Department of Public Instruction, 1973.
Cramer, W. and Trent, R. *Performance Objectives.* Cincinnati,: Educational Horizons Publishers, 1972.
Culatta, R. and Seltzer, H. Content and Sequence Analysis of the Supervisory Session: A Report of Clinical Use. *Asha, 19,* 523–526, 1977.
Culatta, R. and Seltzer, H. Content and Sequence Analyses of the Supervisory Session. *Asha, 18,* 8–12, 1976.
Diedrich, W. and Crouch, Z. *Programmed Instructions for the Use of Charting in Speech Pathology.* Kansas City, Kansas: Hearing and Speech Department, University of Kansas Medical Center, 1972.
Dublinske, S. Program-Planning-Evaluation. In J. Anderson (20), *Conference on Supervision of Speech and Hearing Programs in the Schools.* Bloomington, Indiana: Indiana University, 1970.

Freilinger, J. J., Baldes, R., Barker, K., Jenkinson, P., and Wilson, K. *Iowa's Severity Rating Scale for Communication Disabilities.* Des Moines: Iowa Department of Public Instruction, 1978. Available from ERIC, ED 159–863, EC 112–291.

Harris, B. *Supervisory Behavior in Education.* New York: Prentice Hall, 1963.

Kagan, N. Human Relations in Supervision. In J. Anderson (Ed.), Conference on Supervision of Speech and Hearing Programs in the Schools. Bloomington, Indiana: Indiana University, 1970.

Kirtley, D. (Ed.). *Supervision of Student Teaching in Speech and Hearing Therapy.* Indianapolis, Indiana: Department of Public Instruction, 1967.

Mager, R. *Preparing Instructional Objectives.* Palo Alto, California: Fearon Publishers, Inc., 1962.

Mager, R. *Goal Analysis.* Palo Alto, California: Fearon Publishers, Inc., 1972.

Omans, M. Special Study Institute: Management and Supervision. Des Moines: Iowa Department of Public Instruction, 1973.

O'Toole, T. Supervision of the Clinical Trainee. *Language, Speech and Hearing Services in Schools, 4,* 132–139, 1973.

Chapter 6

SYSTEMS FOR PROGRAM PLANNING, MANAGEMENT, AND EVALUATION

William C. Healey

On the first day of employment in a school district, every speech-language pathologist, supervisor, and administrator in a program for children with communication disorders is confronted with the need to amass information and to begin answering the following questions:

What are the needs and problems?
What procedures can be used to verify the needs and problems?
What alternative strategies exist for meeting the needs and solving the problems that are verified?
What resources are available?
What constraints exist?
What instructional/program goals and objectives are needed immediately and over time?
What evaluation procedures should be used to document the achievement of goals and objectives?
What systems can be used to help conduct the role and responsibilities in an effective, efficient, and economical manner?

Acquiring the necessary information and taking the steps required to answer these questions can be accomplished most effectively, efficiently, and economically in school districts that have formal program planning, management, and evaluation systems.

The need for program administrators and practicing clinicians to understand the principles and practices of formal program planning, management, and evaluation has been reinforced, in part, by several recent, interrelated events: (a) the enactment of Public Law 94–142, which requires states and local school districts to have comprehensive plans and to offer a continuum of free, appropriate educational services; (b) the requirements in Public Law 94-142 that specify the development of an individual educational program (I.E.P.), which must be planned, implemented, and evaluated on an annual basis, and (c) the increasing need for special program professionals to provide the highest quality services for the greatest number of handicapped children in the least amount of time and with decreasing availability of adequate funding. Being knowledgable about the procedures for program planning and evaluation is as important to the direct service provider as it is to the program administrator or coordinator. Each should be familiar with such activities as needs assessment; goal and objective setting; methods and materials selection; program implementation monitoring; goal and objective attainment determination; and program revision procedures based on results of competent evaluation.

LEVELS OF PROGRAM PLANNING, MANAGEMENT, AND EVALUATION

Conceptually, three levels of program planning, management, and evaluation should be coordinated in any school district providing special education and related services for children with communication disorders. They include (a) the school district plan, which encompasses all departmental and individual programs and constitutes the organizational structure that will bear most responsibility for the service delivery system; (b) departmental program planning, which focuses on all special services provided directly and indirectly for children with speech-language-hearing disorders; and (c) individual program planning, which is geared to each child with a need for special instruction and related services and for whom the I.E.P. will be developed, implemented, and evaluated.

Although the principles of program planning and evaluation are similar at each level, the methods used tend to differ considerably. Figure 6-1 depicts the steps involved in program planning, development, management and evaluation (PDME) proposed by the American Speech-Language-Hearing Association (1974) for use in school districts. Implementing a PDME or related system is

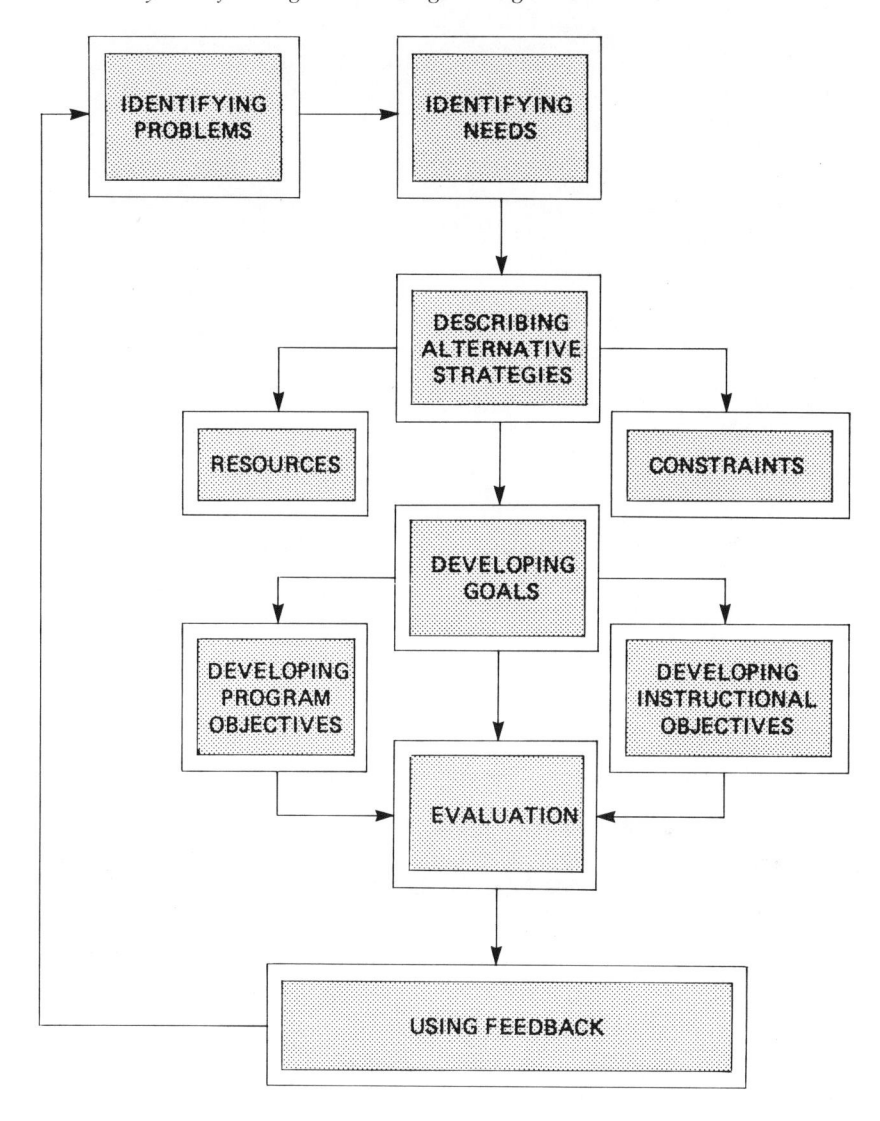

Figure 6-1. Program planning, development, management, and evaluation model.

essential for school speech-language-hearing programs as a means of (a) identifying and serving the needs of all handicapped children; (b) assuring efficient program management; (c) evaluating pupil progress; (d) evaluating personnel competence; (e) demonstrating accountability; and (f) determining costs. In general, formal systems serve as management devices that facilitate decision making and establish procedures for formulating goals, deriving measurable objectives, and managing programs that are consistent with the goals and objectives of the department and the school district. Establishing appropriate goals and objectives at the three levels of management requires comprehensive, cooperative planning.

Planning Systems

Planning, which is a formal process of establishing goals, objectives, and procedures, must be cooperative and should be complementary at each level of program and student management. For example, the superintendent will have a comprehensive plan for the school district; the director of special education will have a comprehensive program plan for serving all handicapped children; and the director of the speech-language-hearing program will work with each supervisor and direct service provider to develop a comprehensive plan that will meet the needs of the school district, the special education program, and the individual children and parents needing services.

Comprehensive planning is basic to the performance of every program within a school district. As seen in Figure 6-1 planning incorporates (1) the identification of key needs and problems; (2) the accumulation of accurate data about these needs and problems; (3) an analysis of interrelationships between existing services and the needs or problems identified; (4) the extrapolation of alternatives for the future that are derivatives of present conditions; (5) the assessment of potential consequences that could occur as new variables are introduced, choosing the more desirable alternatives to represent each program's basic goals; (6) developing a sequential plan for implementing objectives and procedures that will achieve the goals; and, (7) formulating a built-in feedback system that permits periodic reevaluation of the goals, objectives, and procedures used to achieve the goals and objectives. While each school district, program, and individual has a responsibility for planning, the scope of the responsibilities varies and so does the authority to implement the plans. In many school districts, for example, the appropriate implementation authority frequently is a matter of some controversy. Planning cannot succeed without a clear delineation of each person's authority and responsibility.

For the last two decades, education has been forced to address the issue of rapid growth. As a consequence, comprehensive plans have been directed primarily to the establishment of orderly and efficient accommodation procedures for enrollment increases, especially in serving children who are handicapped. The present and immediate future will require a different type of planning in which personnel must focus on the qualitative problems of maintaining and improving appropriate programs and services, probably without the extensive growth experienced during the last decade. The need for more detailed planning at both the state and local educational agency levels actually will be greater because the policy options are becoming more difficult and sensitive. An economic crisis pervades many school programs, and local districts are having to serve more handicapped children with fewer personnel, less equipment, and reduced capital outlay. In addition, laws such as Public Law 94-142 and Section 504 of the Rehabilitation Act of 1973, discussed in Chapter 3, have forced school personnel to serve a much broader population of handicapped children with more extensive needs than previously encountered in the schools. These changes require planning that assures the public, including legislators, that program policies are not arbitrary but are designed to meet the needs of constituents in an effective, efficient, and economically appropriate manner.

Program directors and individual providers of special services who commit considerable energy to planning are more likely to have a clear sense of the priorities governing the provision of comprehensive, qualitatively appropriate services. Using effective planning processes permits program managers to be cognizant of the concerns and aspirations of their internal and external constituencies. Planning addresses the fundamental questions of purpose, policy, and priority in a way that is considerably different from managerial functions, which tend to be more concerned with maintenance of appropriate daily and weekly responsibilities. Planning provides an opportunity for proposing innovations. Planning can provide a forum where long-term educational needs and societal needs become complementary through reconciliation, compromise, and consensus. For the individual program administrator or the service provider, planning should be viewed as one of the few opportunities, at least initially, to be totally creative. Program administrators should bring together people with the highest technical expertise and creative imagination. On the other hand, planning can be a threatening experience, a precarious process, and an exercise that results in futility. Planning is not a panacea, especially when it falls under the influence of parochial interests, is used to introduce greater rigidities instead of flexibility and responsiveness, or is abused by persons or groups who are not committed to the need for such activity. Failure to effect comprehensive planning, however, offers more dangers than the potential pitfalls mentioned above. When comprehensive planning is absent, program personnel ultimately experience lack of direction, expedient and short-term decision making, and political interference. Lack of planning makes longer term effectiveness improbable. Some changes in personnel, school population, and financial status are inevitable, and failure to identify the needs and problems that arise with such changes can result in the perpetuation of inadequate policies and procedures or the provision of inappropriate services.

Assessment of Needs and Problems

Some program planning, management, and evaluation systems refer to problem assessment as a process that is separate from needs assessment. In essence, they may be considered as a similar process. When program personnel identify an unsatisfactory state of affairs, they typically describe it as a problem that needs to be solved. Consequently, one can formulate any statement of problem as a statement of need. Statements of problems or needs are indicators that help is required. The system must, however, be able to determine whether or not the state of affairs as presented actually represents an unsatisfactory status and not the misperception of individual staff members, parents, or community representatives.

School programs tend to have common problems that can be stated as needs. These needs generally may be classified as follows:
- A. Economic: the need for continuing or increasing the present levels of financial support that are required for program survival or growth.
- B. Administrative: the need for revising or implementing new efficient and effective procedures that delineate each step required between initiating and terminating a management task.
- C. Clinical/Instructional: the need for assistance in the development, modification, or use of diagnostic and teaching methods or technology.
- D. Communicative: the need for establishing or improving lines of interpersonal relationships among staff who are working to achieve the programmatic goals and objectives.
- E. Political/Professional: the need to define roles and distribute the power of authority and responsibility among groups or individuals.
- F. Legal/Legislative: the need to assure rights of individuals or groups through due process or regulatory procedures.

A need may be characterized as a discrepancy between the current state of affairs and a desired state. A need exists when internal or external personnel can demonstrate that an issue is adversely affecting the behavioral, social, physical or organizational equilibrium or quality of the program. The purpose of needs assessment is to identify those actions that must be taken to increase the appropriateness of services to children and their parents and/or to improve the efficiency and effectiveness of program operations. This also is a form of *evaluation* which is discussed in more detail later in this chapter. The needs assessment process requires the use of various procedures for obtaining and assigning a priority to information in a way that will verify and lead to an exact specification of each need. Dublinske and Grimes (1971) cite several methods for obtaining information about needs, which include (1) standardized questionnaires; (2) standardized achievement tests; (3) district comparisons; (4) standard measures of characteristics, e.g. attitude, ability; (5) interviews; (6) observations; and (7) program records and data analyses. The following examples of

1. Questionnaire

This tool is one that allows contact with populations too large for direct interviews. It is not always necessary to question an entire population, e.g., all parents in a school district. A limited random sample is adequate. To be effective, however, the questions must be specific and non-ambiguous and the respondent must know what *yes* and *no* answers or rating scales actually mean. Otherwise, those responding will not necessarily share the same reference point. A limitation of questionnnaires is that respondents may be a select group – those with strong biases. Less concerned persons may not respond, thus distorting the broad view of the problem.

<u>example</u>

Speech-Language pathologist please rate: (in terms of importance)

District #3–Possible Goals of L–S–H Program	3	2	1
1. Provide expanded services so that the waiting list of 140 pupils with language disorders will be decreased.			
2. Increase the frequency of direct contact for language impaired pupils now seen on a twice weekly basis.			
3. Design criteria for identifying four year old children with language problems.			
4. Provide service to 80 language impaired trainable retarded pupils.			
5.			

Scale:

3–Very important, start immediately.	2–Fairly important, of concern for next year or after all 3s are solved.	1–Unimportant, of lowest priority or can be ignored.

2. Recording

All requests for service that go unfilled, all instances of having problems brought to your attention, and requests for consultations should be recorded. Collectively, they may underscore areas of need or indicate unrecognized needs.

example

Pupils Referred By West Hospital Speech and Audiology Center

Name	Address	Age	School	Reason for Referral
Jane Smith	10 East Avenue	4	to enter Gay Elem.	Language Disability
Gregg Barr	100 Scott Lane	5½	Stokes Elementary	Articulation Disorder

and

1981 Waiting List—Stokes Elementary School

Name	Grade	Problem	Severity	Date Assessed
Barr, G.	1	Articulation	Moderate	9/79
Brown, R.	3	Dysfluency	Moderate	11/79
Gold, S.	2	Language	Mild	10/79
Harris, M.	K	Language	Moderate	9/79
James, P.	2	Articulation	Mild	5/79
Klaus, H.	4	Voice	Mild-Moderate	3/80
Perry, L.	3	Articulation	Mild	9/79
Ralston, P.	K	Language	Mild-Moderate	9/79

3. Comparison

With this process you compare the services you offer to those provided by a comparable school district or service center; or you compare your service population with an appropriate research population. Large differences in either set of comparisons may indicate service needs.

example

	District Enrollment	Number of Speech-Lang. Paths.	Pupils Served in S-L-H Program
District #1	30,000	20	1,000
District #46	20,000	16	800
District #3	45,000	20	1,240

4. Interview

This process allows direct contact with others affected by or interested in the problem. This method of contact assures that responses will be made, and that ambiguity of both questions and responses will be minimized. A standard set of questions should be used to allow the results to be pooled as group information. Interviews should be held with a number of persons in the same environment, e.g., the principal and several teachers in a selected school.

example

> **Supervisor:** "Mrs. Harper (principal), the speech-language pathologist in this school has received ten referrals from kindergarten classroom teachers. Eight of the children who have been referred and tested have serious problems in either comprehending or using language. Do you think it is important for us to develop a special program for this group of preschool pupils?"

5. Data Analysis

You can also verify the magnitude or scope of problems by further analysis of program and case level information, such as numbers of pupils served; waiting lists; and/or test results.

example

> We have identified 75 pupils in 40 kindergarten classes who have mild to moderate language disorders.

several methods listed above are taken from the PDME Manual (Healey and Jones, 1973), which is available from the American Speech-Language-Hearing Association.

As a rule, opinion surveys should be designed around potential program goals, objectives, or outcomes. The person being surveyed indicates his opinion about the extent to which a goal, objective, or outcome is currently being achieved and the extent to which it should be achieved. Most of these needs assessment methods also may be used in program evaluation.

Ranking Needs by Priority

If numerous needs have been identified, a process of establishing priorities must be used before program planners and staff can determine appropriate plans of action that will meet the needs. Program planners typically attempt to achieve consensus pertaining to (a) the degree of importance or value of meeting each need; (b) the time requirement in meeting the need; and (c) the potential effects of failing to meet the need at all and within the time requirement as specified.

Achieving consensus frequently is difficult because individuals may approach the resolution of an issue from discrepant perceptions or have differing reasons for assigning a rank, weight, or time to meeting a particular need. In such instances, the perceptions and reasons of the participants must be discussed and evaluated. Following these discussions and evaluations, priority scales, i.e. nominal, rank order, or interval, may be used to achieve consensus. Another alternative is to postpone the process of establishing priorities until the potential strategies, resources, and constraints for meeting each need have been reviewed.

Reviewing Alternative Strategies

Alternative strategies may be defined as the identification of several possible solutions to a problem or various promising approaches to meeting a need. Each strategy proposed should relate directly to the verified need, lead to measurable outcomes, and offer a reasonable expectation that the discrepancy between the current and desired status will be reduced appreciably or eliminated. For example, the school district speech-language pathologists may conduct a summer diagnostic clinic for prekindergarten children and identify twenty five year olds who have severe language disorders. These children are scheduled for enrollment in their neighborhood kindergartens in the fall. The following strategies for meeting these children's needs appear to be feasible:

Strategy #1: instruct kindergarten teachers in the management of language disorders

Strategy #2: reserve time for these children in the schedules of speech-language pathologists serving these schools

Strategy #3: establish two special language development classes that will permit these children to have intensive, daily assistance by highly qualified specialists in the management of language disorders

Each of these alternatives may appear to be possible, but which ones are preferred and which are feasible? To answer these questions, it becomes necessary to review the school district's current and future constraints and resources.

Reviewing Constraints and Resources

Constraints are those variables which circumscribe the means that may be used in meeting a need or solving a problem. Constraints are the "minus" factors in the environment that mitigate against or limit the possibility of success in pursuing a given strategy. For example, a frequent strategy selected for improving a speech-language-hearing program is that of employing additional personnel. An equally frequent discovery is budget constraints, which will not provide for the allocation of new, salaried positions. Other constraints emanate from restrictions in state regulations that govern the types of services that can be provided, local school district policies, lack of space, and limited experience or skills among staff in the area of need. Constraints in budgeting generally affect the selection of strategies, while constraints in staff attitudes, knowledge, or skills tend to affect judgments of the prognosis for a specific strategy. For example, the strategy of teaching kindergarten teachers how to modify severe language disorders in five-year-old children may be considered both economical and an ideal management procedure from the program administrator's perspective. However, the speech-language pathologists may suggest that even if the teachers acquire the necessary knowledge and skills, they will not be able to schedule the time required to ensure appropriately individualized instruction. Consequently, the kindergarten teachers may not be selected as the primary resource in meeting the need to provide special services in their classes for language handicapped children.

Gallager et al. (1973) identify *resources* as those human, technological, and organizational "plus" factors that increase the probability that a particular strategy or set of strategies will be successful over time in meeting a need or solving a problem. In a formal program planning, management, and evaluation system, each strategy proposed should be accompanied by a list of constraints and resources.

Selecting and Implementing Strategies

Once a list of strategies, constraints, and resources has been developed, the selection and implementation processes require decisions that should involve the clinical/instructional staff. The first task is that of determining the *prime strategy.* This strategy can be defined as the choice that holds the highest probabiliy for resulting in a desired outcome within the least amount of time and at an anticipated cost that is both affordable and reasonable in relation to the potential benefits. The second task involves the development of an action plan that will answer the following questions: What must be done? How will it be done? Who will do it? When will it be done? Where will it be done? How will it be monitored? What evaluations should be done? From answering what will be done, the staff has taken a preliminary step toward the formulation of a program goal. By answering the questions of *how, when, where,* and *what,* the staff has begun to identify objectives that may be stated in terms that are measurable. The specific steps that will be required in meeting the objectives represent *procedures.* It becomes important at this point to: (a) formulate general goal statements; (b) develop measurable objectives; (c) structure the procedures that will be followed in meeting the objectives; (d) establish authority and responsibility for monitoring progress in meeting the objectives; and (e) set preliminary criteria that will be used in evaluating progress and ultimate success in achieving the goal and objectives.

Preparing Goals

The term *goal* refers to a major end result or product. Goals generally represent broad statements of an educational program's long-range purposes. An organization with no goals is without a plan for looking forward and could be judged as having no clear concept of its future. Goals provide standards and guidelines for immediate and futuristic decisions and actions. Speech-language-hearing personnel may establish *program goals* and *instructional goals.* The program or organizational goal articulates philosophy, ideology, and policy, which summarize the program's *raison d'être* and what can be expected of it. Instructional goals may be group or individually oriented and emphasize learning or positive behavioral change.

Goals should be measurable. Writing goals that are too global or timeless is a frequent error in planning. On the other hand, people with limited experience in planning or projecting into the future find it extremely difficult to envision goals that would be appropriate five to fifteen years from today. Educational systems are just beginning to emulate the long-range planning that has been a common practice of most large corporate entities such as General Motors (GM). GM designers already have a rather firm concept of society's transportation needs through the year 2000. The anticipated needs may have to be modified as a consequence of economic or other variables, but the long-term goals provide direction and bring together the assumptions, values, and hopes of the organization.

Educational organizations need short– and long-range goals as a prerequisite to the following:

A. Establishing fundamental policies
B. Facilitating decision making
C. Guiding additional planning
D. Determining the content of management information systems (as discussed later in the section on management)
E. Effecting evaluation systems (see section on evaluation)
F. Achieving accountability

Goals, to be measurable, must include the components of *When*, *What*, and *Criterion*. The *When* generally is the anticipated date for goal accomplishment. The *What* is the activity, and the *Criterion* is an indicator of how successful the program or provider of services expects to be in reaching the goal. The Criterion used in the goal statement generally is not as qualitative as the criteria that may be used in evaluating the appropriateness or success of each objective used to meet the goal. Examples of goals with all three components are presented:

> Example #1: By (date), two language development classes will be established to meet the needs of all kindergarten children diagnosed as having severe language disorders and requiring intensive special education

In this example, the *When* is a date, the *What* is two language development classes, and the *Criterion* is "all" kindergarten children with severe language disorders who need intensive special instruction. Program objectives must be written to delineate each major activity required for achieving the goal and to identify *Who* will be responsible.

>   Example #2: By September 1, 19••, 100 percent of the school district's speech-language pathologists and audiologists will have completed a workshop on procedures to be followed in using the new computerized program and client management data system..

Again, the *When* is a date, the *What* is a workshop, and the *Criterion* is 100 percent of the district's speech-language pathologists and audiologists.

>   Example #3: By December 1, 19••, 75 percent of the special language class kindergarten children will have increased their language performance by at least fifteen points on the verbal scale of the WIPPSI (Wechsler test for preschoolers).

This instructional goal uses a date to state *When;* a statement of performance to identify *What;* and a *Criterion* of 75 percent.

In developing goal statements, some experienced planners tend to become somewhat ethereal and write such goals as "facilitating learning through systematized educational management" or "creating knowledge through applied research and dissemination." Although these goals are considered primary in the educational establishment, they nearly defy measurement and fail to communicate any idea of when they might be reached or what outcomes can be anticipated in relation to major program or instructional concerns. After writing either the broad, high-order goals or those that may be considered more narrow or lower ordered, the next tasks are those of describing and scheduling the activities that will be needed to accomplish each goal. These activities are known as *objectives.*

Writing Objectives

Objectives are statements of specific activities or behaviors that are measurable and have a set time for completion. In a speech-language-hearing program, the *program objectives* are those sequentially scheduled actions which must be taken to reach a goal and generally relate to some aspect of providing comprehensive services for children with communication disorders, parents, instructional staff (such as in-service education), or the community. *Instructional objectives* refer to the clinician/client relationship and generally indicate those clinical/instructional behaviors that constitute the immediate and longer term performance steps that must be completed to achieve an instructional goal. Although the term "behavioral objective" occasionally is used in the literature, this author considers any appropriately written instructional objective to be behavioral.

Properly written objectives provide administrators, staff, parents, and other interested constituents with an in-depth understanding of the activities, time requirements, and personnel responsibilities involved in meeting the goals established.

Writing objectives is a process of planning each activity in advance and can be accomplished best when the following questions are answered:

A. WHEN is it going to be done?
B. WHO is going to do it?
C. WHAT is going to be done?
D. TO WHOM is it going to be done?
E. CRITERIA that will indicate success of the objective
F. EVALUATION that will be used to determine completion

One example of a program objective follows:

WHEN: By October 15, 19••
WHO: This speech-language pathologist in Future Elementary School #1.
WHAT: Will conduct comprehensive, standardized language assessments
TO WHOM: On kindergarten children failing to pass a speech-language screening examination
CRITERION: 100%
EVALUATION: Lists of children failing screening and assessment protocols submitted to the program director on October 17.

This program objective indicates that the speech-language pathologist will allot time until October 15 to conduct comprehensive language assessments of all kindergarten children who fail a speech-language screening test. The program director can anticipate receipt of the assessments and can use this information in identifying any kindergarten children who may need to be considered for placement in the new language development classes that represent a program goal already established and discussed earlier in this chapter.

An instructional objective uses the same components and may be written in the following manner:

WHEN: By the end of clinic session number five
WHO: The audiologist
WHAT: Will select an appropriate hearing aid
TO WHOM: For Billy Jones after determining
CRITERION: Best overall auditory performance on each of five aids using
EVALUATION: A record of correct and incorrect responses with each aid in four communication environments

This instructional objective indicates that the audiologist plans to select an appropriate hearing aid for Billy Jones after meeting with him in five clinical sessions. Since the objective is task-specific, it must be assumed that the audiologist has studied Billy's hearing loss and has selected five aids that potentially may be suitable for the type of auditory impairment that Billy is experiencing. Such assumptions would not be required if each of the audiologist's objectives for Billy could be presented. With a complete set of objectives, the activities leading up to the example should make it clear whether or not this objective is appropriate at this time.

Several additional points about writing objectives need to be understood.

A. Proficiency in writing objectives increases with practice and experience.
B. Writing clear objectives, ultimately, will prove to be a time-saving device for three very important reasons: (1) you will have identified those steps that will give your program direction; (2) many objectives involving routine activities such as screening, diagnostics, parent conferences, or preparing materials do not have to be rewritten completely each year; and, (3) well-sequenced and effective instructional

objectives can be used for many children who have the same disorder and level of performance.
C. New objectives must be written for every new goal, and the criteria used in the objectives must be consistent with and complement the criteria defined in the goal statement.
D. The format presented for writing objectives does not discuss one additional component that is critical to successful program management. For each objective, the person writing the objective should be prepared to describe how an objective will be met. These are the procedures that will be followed. For example, if the objective is one of developing and publishing a language development curriculum for five-year-old children, the procedures might be described as follows:

> The program director will select a writing team of two language specialists, two kindergarten teachers, one curriculum specialist, and one child development specialist who will be employed for eight weeks during the summer. The team will identify the instructional goals and objectives and will assemble the curriculum using commercial materials, staff generated materials, and language development guides. Permission to duplicate the commercial materials will be obtained from the publishers and authors. A draft of the curriculum will be submitted to the program director on or before July 15. At this point, at least two printers will be asked to meet with the director and writing team to discuss the requirements for publication of the material and to obtain estimates of printing costs. A final draft of the curriculum will be submitted to the printer that meets the time and production requirements, and five copies of the curriculum will be purchased for use in the special classes. The director will schedule meetings with the classroom specialists and the writing team as necessary throughout the school year to solve any problems that are encountered. Each member of the writing team, one principal, and two parents will use procedures developed in cooperation with the program director to evaluate the appropriateness of the new curriculum.

Although this description of potential procedures may not be exhaustive, it serves as an example of the *how* that frequently must accompany a stated objective.

Planning Procedures

The following checklist of planning procedures should be used in describing the basic, substantive components of a group or individual program.

Step 1: Review the statements of goals and objectives.
Step 2: Categorize the goal statements, including their objectives, as: (1) educational; (2) economic; (3) social; (4) group; and (5) individual. This process of categorization seems to help the planner quantify the goals and understand where each fits into the total program or pupil management system.
Step 3: Review and analyze the school district's enrollment, fiscal and physical resources, and programs that will complement the services needed and offered in the department of speech-language-hearing and in the SLP's individual pupil management program. For example, the administrator must have a comprehensive understanding of the pupils needing special services; the number-frequency-intensity of services needed versus those currently provided; the present and desired use of educational technologies; the opportunities for staff in-service and continuing education; and the geographic availability of personnel and services within the district, community, and state.
Step 4: Complete program projections for the next two to five years, which represent short-term planning. Follow this process by making projections for five to fifteen years, which can be considered as intermediate planning. For example:
  A. Analyze enrollment trends categorized by *level of programming* (preschool, elementary, secondary); *type of program*, i.e. self-contained special class, resource room, and itinerant; *types of disorders by severity*, e.g. language, speech, voice, hearing; and *continuum of services*. In studying enrollment for planning purposes, an overall prevalence figure of approximately 6 percent (Hull et al., 1976) of the total school population may be used if the goal is one of serving all handicapped children who manifest some form of communication disorder or deviation (*see* Fig. 6-2). If the goal includes the provision of speech-language and auditory development experiences for preschool and early elementary children, for instance, the number of children, classes, and contacts must be projected and added to the overall prevalence figure of 6 percent.

264   Speech-Language Programming in the Schools

	Communicative Disorders ----▶	Deviations ------------▶	Development
Population Served:	Pupils with severe language, voice, fluency, articulation, or hearing disorders	Pupils with mild to moderate developmental or nonmaturational deviations in language, voice, fluency, or articulation, and those with mild hearing loss requiring minimal oral rehabilitation procedures	All pupils in regular or special education classes
Program Goals:	Provide direct, intensive, and individualized clinical-educational services to effect positive changes in the communication behavior of pupils with handicapping disorders	Provide direct and/or indirect clinical-educational services to stimulate and/or improve pupils' communication skills and competencies	Provide prevention-oriented, sequenced curricular activities to help pupils develop communicative behaviors in appropriate social, educational, and cultural contexts

Figure 6-2. Continuum of communication needs. From W. Healey, Continuum of communication need, *Asha*, 1973. Courtesy of American Speech-Language-Hearing Association.

In reviewing the *types or levels of program models* that may be used, see Figure 6-3.

SEVERITY OF HANDICAP (MORE SEVERE → LESS SEVERE)

CASE MANAGEMENT STRATEGY (MOVE ONLY AS FAR AS NECESSARY / RETURN AS SOON AS POSSIBLE)

- HOSPITALS AND TREATMENT CENTERS
- HOSPITAL SCHOOL
- RESIDENTIAL SCHOOL
- SPECIAL DAY SCHOOL
- FULL-TIME SPECIAL CLASS
- PART-TIME SPECIAL CLASS
- REGULAR CLASSROOM PLUS RESOURCE ROOM SERVICE
- REGULAR CLASSROOM WITH SUPPLEMENTARY TEACHING OR TREATMENT
- REGULAR CLASSROOM WITH CONSULTATION
- MOST PROBLEMS HANDLED IN REGULAR CLASSROOM

◀—— NUMBER OF CASES ——▶

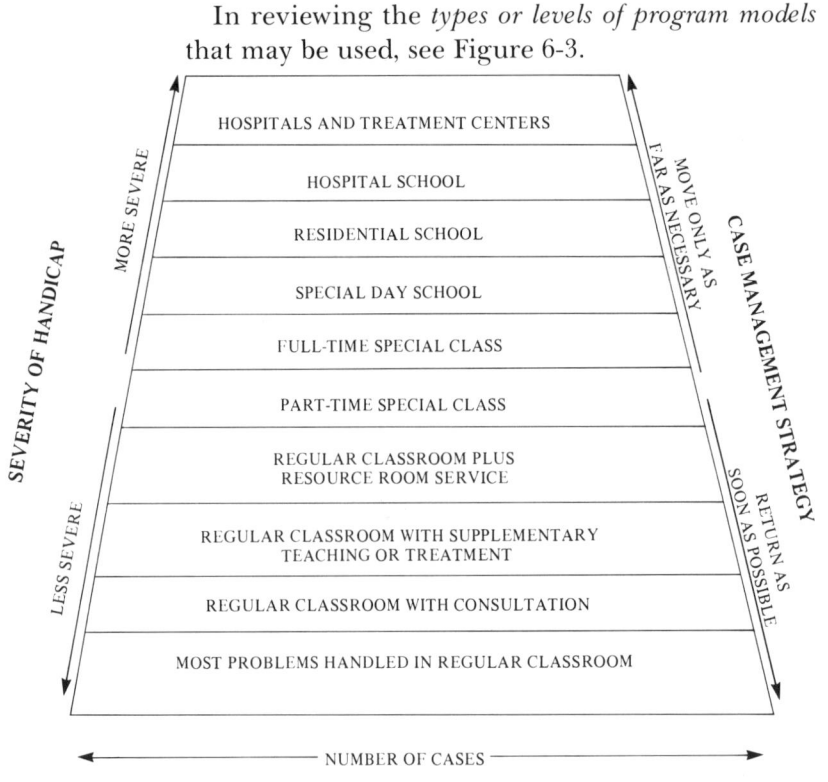

Figure 6-3. Conceptualization of administrative arrangements for serving handicapped children. From M. C. Reynolds, A Framework for Considering Some Issues in Special Education, *Exceptional Children*, 28:368, 1962. Courtesy of publisher and author.

Category of Exceptional Program	Prevalence Rate (%) Low/High
Educable Mentally Retarded	1.30 2.3
Trainable Mentally Retarded	0.24 0.50
Auditorily Handicapped	0.10 2.1
Visually Handicapped	0.05 0.1
Speech Handicapped	3.60 6.3
Physically Handicapped	0.21 0.7
Special Learning Disorder	1.12 3.0
Emotionally Disturbed	1.2 2.0
Homebound/Hospital/OHI	0.22 0.4
Multiply Handicapped	0.01 0.05

Figure 6-4. Prevalence of handicapping conditions.

Unpublished data collected in 1979 from 20 state and 143 local education agencies by the School Services Program of the American Speech-Language-Hearing Association.

Project the number of preschool, elementary, and secondary pupils that will require speech-language-hearing services in each model; by types of disorder or special need and by severity. A special consideration for planners may be helpful at this point. Among pupils being served by special education for physical, emotional, intellectual, sensory, and learning disabilities, at least 30 percent will need the services of speech-language pathologists and about 10 to 15 percent need audiologic services. Figure 6-4 summarizes the highest and lowest prevalence figures reported for pupils with each type of handicapping condition.

To project the *continuum of services,* determine which services from Figure 6-5 will be required to operate each program model in Figure 6-3 at each level of programming (preschool, elementary, secondary).

B. Projecting *personnel needs* is a somewhat complicated task. The administrator must follow each of

266 Systems for Program Planning, Management, and Evaluation

	CONTINUUM COMPONENTS		
Population Served	Severe ─────────────────────────────────────► Mild		
Program Goals	1. Provide prevention programs ───► 2. Provide direct intensive individualized and group lifetime services when necessary to effect maximum development 3. Provide information and assistance to all program participants		Provide necessary sequenced support activities to help develop appropriate behaviors in social, educational, and vocational contexts

Services Provided•	1. Identification ───►
	2. Comprehensive interdisciplinary ───────────────────────────────────────►
	   assessment (diagnostic evaluation)
	3. Referral (for additional services) ────────────────────────────────────►
	4. Parent or guardian counseling ───►
	   and instruction
	5. Client counseling and placement ───────────────────────────────────────►
	6. Staff counseling and in-service ───────────────────────────────────────►
	   orientation/instruction
	7. Direct management (medical, educational, vocational, social, recreational)
			Direct or Indirect Management

	8. Program evaluation ───► 9. Individual reassessment ───► Consultation (for individual client or groups) 10. Dismissal and follow-up ──► 11. Research ──► 12. Record and data maintenance ───►		
Program Types and Alternatives•	1. Diagnostic center placement ──► 2. Special-class educational placement	Special-class educational placement or resource room placement	Regular educational placement with supportive services or resource room services

	3. Vocational placement ───►
	   a. Prevocational services ──►
	   b. Work-study program (emphasis on individual work skills and attitudes) ─►
	   c. Sheltered workshops
	   d. Activity Centers
	   e. Community employment ──►
	4. Home or hospital services ──►
	5. Parent/infant instruction ──►
	6. Community and residential placement
	7. Organized recreation ───►
	8. Special living arrangements ──►		

Participants (most common)	Parents, teachers, administrators, aides, rehabilitation counselors, psychologists, physicians, psychiatrists, social workers, nurses, occupational therapists, physical therapists, dentists, audiologists, speech pathologists, recreational specialists, employers		

•Transportation-purchased services may be required to facilitate provision of a service continuum.

Figure 6-5. Continuum of services.

the procedures described above and establish a staff:pupil ratio for each program model that is anticipated and for each type of service to be offered, i.e. screening, diagnostics, consultation, etc. Next, the amount of time for each type of service per staff member should be estimated. Few guidelines in the literature are available to assist planners in ascertaining appropriate staff:pupil ratios or time allocations required for each component within the continuum of services. The determination of an appropriate case load or class size, for instance, is subject to many variables that must be studied, including the following:
1. The professional staff member's judgment or estimate of each pupil's needs and the frequency of contact required to effect the greatest positive change in communication skills in the shortest time period.
2. The types of program and scheduling models to be used.
3. Additional program responsibilities of staff (teacher consultation, parent services, record keeping, diagnostic staffing, screening, and so on).
4. The number of pupils needing help.
5. The geographic area to be served.
6. Socioeconomic nature of the community.
7. Availability of communication aides.
8. Number and availability of special education and pupil personnel staff.
9. Administrative, supervisory, and clerical support.

Historically, speech-language-hearing specialists too often have managed excessive staff:pupil ratios that resulted from inadequate numbers of trained specialists, inflated state and/or locally required case load maximums, and staff desire to provide some level of service for all pupils in need. Pupils with severe speech-language-hearing disorders affecting their social and learning behavior often failed to receive the quality of service required because of limited contact with the specialist. State departments of special education often have set a maximum case load requirement such as 60 or 90 pupils. These requirements have been arbitrary and, traditionally, have represented only the itinerant scheduling model. Other states have required at least one specialist for every 1000 nonhandicapped and handicapped pupils enrolled in a school district. This, too, has proven to be a short-sighted, ineffectual resolution of this continuing issue. Preferably, determinations of case load or class size should be established after the school district: (1) completes a needs assessment and identification program; (2) obtains diagnostic assessments of pupils with problems; and (3) establishes goals and objectives outlining all services to be provided (to each pupil, parent, teacher, and so on). Goals and objectives established in rural districts to meet pupils' needs may be considerably different from those in central city districts, and class or case load sizes should be tailored carefully to the needs and service models required. Obviously, new school districts or those without previous speech-language-hearing services need some guidelines for initiating programs. These districts can (1) contract with qualified outside agencies or personnel to conduct a needs assessment by completing an identification program and obtaining diagnostic assessments to determine the number, ages, and types of problems among pupils in the district and, then, make a determination of types of services and personnel required; or (2) employ staff using a fixed ratio (1:1000) to initiate the program. These staff can complete a needs assessment, determine the types of program models necessary for serving the pupils in need, and recommend appropriate staff:

pupil ratios. This author, in working with many school districts that truly wanted to meet all of their pupils' needs, found some specialists assigned to fewer than six pupils (preschool deaf or language-impaired class). The average case load for specialists providing quality support services for hearing-impaired pupils who are integrated full time into regular classes in some districts was twelve. Another specialist may provide speech-language-hearing services to twenty-five pupils with cerebral palsy. Some itinerant specialists with case loads composed of pupils having varying types and degrees of communication needs did not carry more than thirty pupils with moderate to severe disorders. The nature of service required and all other program variables should be evaluated carefully before staff:pupil ratios are determined. Within the continuum concept, the staff:pupil ratios will vary with each program component. In any component, for each staff member required to serve too many pupils, there will be several pupils who cannot compensate for the loss in service quality and, indeed, will not achieve to their fullest potential in school.

After completing the aforementioned processes, the number of personnel needed can be projected.

C. Estimate *resource requirements;* including physical facilities, materials and equipment, and operating and capital expenses. For budget planning purposes, one procedure may be of assistance. Determine the estimated average salary of all personnel for the program, calculate the total personnel budget (which generally will be about 85 percent of the total budget needed) and allot an additional 15 percent of the total personnel costs to equipment and materials; unless extraordinary costs are anticipated for the purchase of new, very expensive equipment such as an acoustic room for hearing assessments, or a mobile diagnostic and treatment van (Work et al., 1975).

School budget officers can be helpful in analyzing the needs for and costs of new or modified buildings and classrooms. For existing programs, standard forms for the request of materials and equipment (such as those used in the CASE Information System, ASHA, 1978) may be used to compute needs and costs. Rossmiller, Hale, and Frohreich (1970) completed a National Educational Finance Project in an attempt to identify the relative costs of programs for exceptional children. Their method incorporated the use of normative funding practices that, under usual circumstances, would not cause the cost index to vary significantly over time for a particular school district. However, any significant change in the district's staffing pattern, e.g. lower staff:pupil ratios, or aide employment, could result in major changes in the cost index. One technique used in the study for adjusting divergent resource allocations to special programs was to compute a mean (average) cost index; this statistic is relevant to a normally distributed population and, therefore, requires that a median cost index also be developed. For example, Rossmiller et al. (1970) found that a cost index for exceptional children generally was 1:81 when the regular education program average cost index for normal children was equal to 1:00. Figure 6-6 shows the per pupil cost indices established by Rossmiller et al., but several important points must be understood about the index in determining costs of programs for children with communicative disorders:

1. The cost index for "Speech Handicapped" was developed primarily on the itinerant model, and the average caseload in the districts that were studied is undetermined. Average case loads, nationally, at the time the study was conducted tended to be about eighty-five pupils per SLP. Lower average case loads would require adjust-

ment of the index to reflect a somewhat higher cost.
2. In programs having self-contained and resource rooms for children with speech-language disorders, the index established for "Special Learning Disorder" could be used.
3. An index needs to be determined for the cost of providing speech-language-hearing services for pupils classified as mentally retarded, physically handicapped, or emotionally disturbed if these case load numbers fall somewhere in between the numbers generally served in the resource room and the itinerant models.

Step 5: Review all local, state, and federal regulations governing the provision of services to pupils with special needs in speech-language-hearing and concomitant disorders.

Step 6: Establish management systems for each program process such as referral, screening, diagnostic assessment, and

Exceptionality	Mean	Median
Educable Mentally Retarded	1.92	1.87
Trainable Mentally Retarded	2.20	2.10
Auditorily Handicapped	3.15	2.99
Visually Handicapped	3.48	2.97
Speech Handicapped	1.25	1.18
Physically Hnadicapped	3.26	3.64
Special Learning Disorder	2.50	2.16
Emotionally Disturbed	3.70	2.83
Homebound/Hospitalized		1.42
Gifted	1.13	1.14
Multiple Handicapped	2.80	2.73

Figure 6-6. Per pupil cost indices.

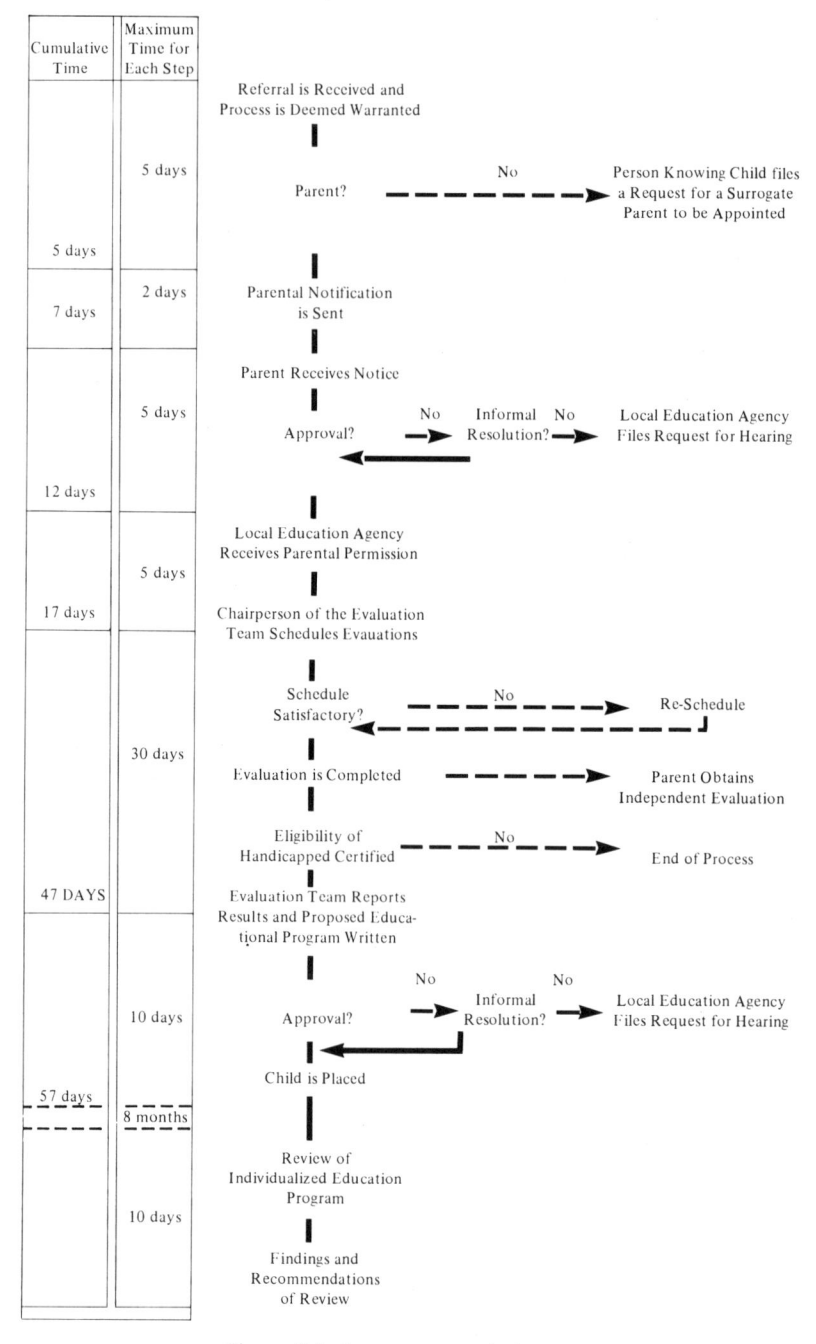

272 Speech-Language Programming in the Schools

Cumulative Time	Maximum Time for Each Step	Process
		Referral is Received and Process is Deemed Warranted
	5 days	Parent? — No → Person Knowing Child files a Request for a Surrogate Parent to be Appointed
5 days		
7 days	2 days	Parental Notification is Sent
		Parent Receives Notice
	5 days	Approval? — No → Informal Resolution? — No → Local Education Agency Files Request for Hearing
12 days		
17 days	5 days	Local Education Agency Receives Parental Permission
		Chairperson of the Evaluation Team Schedules Evauations
	30 days	Schedule Satisfactory? — No → Re-Schedule
		Evaluation is Completed — → Parent Obtains Independent Evaluation
		Eligibility of Handicapped Certified — No → End of Process
47 DAYS		Evaluation Team Reports Results and Proposed Educational Program Written
	10 days	Approval? — No → Informal Resolution? — No → Local Education Agency Files Request for Hearing
57 days		Child is Placed
	8 months	Review of Individualized Education Program
	10 days	Findings and Recommendations of Review

Figure 6-7. Assessment and placement.

Systems for Program Planning, Management, and Evaluation 273

placement. Figures 6-7 and 6-8 provide examples of outlines that might be used in establishing the timelines and procedures that are required in various program processes (*see* section on Management Systems).

Step 7: Review present and potential arrangements with other schools, agencies, hospitals, and physicians to maximize resources.

Step 8: Effect evaluation procedures as a method of analyzing the quality of existing programs and any proposals for expansion, reduction, or improvement.

Step 9: Analysis of the present degree of efficiency in the management and use of educational services currently available and proposals for increasing their efficiency.

Step 10: Determine public and private education relations, including present and projected state aid for both public and private agencies.

Step 11: Evaluate the adequacy of all complementary instructional and related services, including counseling for careers, vocational education, work-study, rehabilitation and rec-

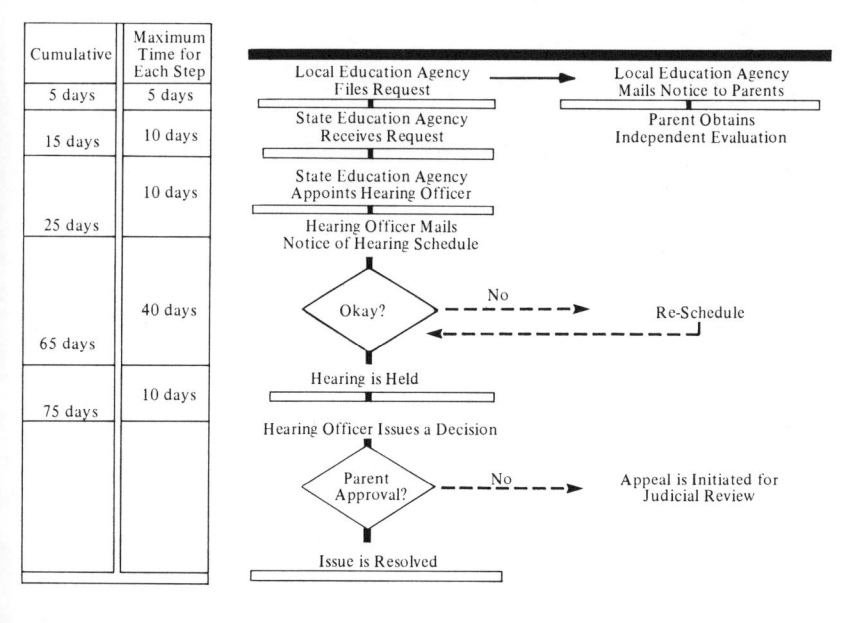

Cumulative	Maximum Time for Each Step
5 days	5 days
15 days	10 days
25 days	10 days
65 days	40 days
75 days	10 days

Local Education Agency Files Request → Local Education Agency Mails Notice to Parents

State Education Agency Receives Request — Parent Obtains Independent Evaluation

State Education Agency Appoints Hearing Officer

Hearing Officer Mails Notice of Hearing Schedule

Okay? --No--> Re-Schedule

Hearing is Held

Hearing Officer Issues a Decision

Parent Approval? --No--> Appeal is Initiated for Judicial Review

Issue is Resolved

Figure 6-8. Hearing process.

reational opportunities for the communication handicapped.

Kerr (1973) has indicated, "If change is inexorable and certain forms are more desirable than others, then change must be directed and managed rather than merely accepted and adapted to. . . . If we can no longer plan for an age of expansion, an age of building, we can and must turn our energies to planning for an age of creative refinement, . . . an age of intensive rather than extensive growth."

The following characteristics of planning are essential:

A. *Scope:* Planning works best when each of the persons responsible has a working knowledge of the goals and objectives for the total academic, remedial, and vocational education programs of the school district.

B. *Participation:* Planners must encourage participation from all external and internal constituencies, including the general public. Participation generally involves the use of informal consultation, public hearings, advisory committees, and questionnaires. Participation begins with the solicitation of representative opinions regarding the issues to be addressed, and it should include opportunities for reaction to preliminary findings, recommendations, or decisions.

C. *Implementation:* Persons having responsibility for implementation of each objective and procedure should be identified explicitly.

D. *Information:* The types of information that should be collected to monitor and evaluate the implementation process and success of any objectives within the plan should be specified, and the responsibility for data collection should be established.

E. *Amendment:* Specific procedures for revision of a plan should be incorporated within the plan.

F. *Reevaluation:* A specific time for systematic review of the plan should be established.

G. *Integration:* The relationship of the speech-language-hearing services plan to the planning efforts of the educational agency should be clear and, as possible, complementary.

H. *Assumption:* The principles and assumptions upon which

the plan is based should be articulated, including assumptions about societal trends, educational trends, and the learning process.

I. *Future agenda:* Issues that arise during the planning process but are not addressed in the plan should be listed with a time schedule for their consideration.

J. *Incentives:* Funding and administrative policies should be analyzed to assure that they do not constitute disincentives to implementation of the plan and, as possible, provide incentives for implementation.

In designing a plan to meet particular needs, the following caveats require consideration: (1) the course of action must be understandable to administrators and other personnel; (2) the plan must have enough detail and flexibility that consensus can be obtained; (3) the plan must be organized and communicated clearly to all interested constituents; (4) the plan must have a reasonable chance of being adopted and implemented.

The essence of planning is the attempt to assess the future and to formulate decisions for dealing with it. These activities are desirable in any program but are indispensible in planning for children and youth who are handicapped.

MANAGEMENT SYSTEMS

An anonymous writer once observed that the best kind of pride is that which compels a person to do the very best work, even when no one is watching. The promise of such pride is available to administrators, supervisors, and direct service providers who use program management systems as a means of conducting their activities in a manner that is highly organized, efficient, effective, and economically appropriate.

A *management system* incorporates an organized set of principles, procedures, and resources that are interdependent and interact to form a unified operational structure. A management system should facilitate getting the most work finished, in the shortest period of time, at the highest level of quality, for the least cost possible.

Management, then, is a process of working with individuals and groups to accomplish individual as well as organizational objectives and goals. Each of us is a manager of our professional and personal roles and responsibilities.

The processes involved in managing a case load, class, program, or school district include planning, organizing, motivating, controlling, and evaluating. The skills of a manager charged with the responsibility of providing comprehensive instructional/clinical services for pupils with communication disorders might be classified and defined as follows:

A. *Technical:* ability to use knowledge, methods, and equipment necessary for the performance of specific tasks in such activities as screening, diagnostics, remediation, consultation, reporting, budgeting, recruitment, supervision, or evaluation.
B. *Human:* ability to use proper judgment and interpersonal communication methods required to direct, motivate, and lead people effectively, including children and adults.
C. *Conceptual:* ability to understand the needs and complexities of a total organization, in addition to the unit for which the manager is responsible; and to create goals, objectives, and procedures that will meet the needs of the unit in such a manner that they complement those of the overall organization.

Program managers in industry and in the schools increasingly are relying on organized management systems to serve as the "work maps" that delineate the procedures to be followed in meeting goals and objectives. These management systems serve various purposes and complement the processes of planning and evaluation. In fact, "management-by-objectives" (MBO) systems are the subordinate mechanisms of overall program planning, budgeting, and evaluation concepts.

Management-By-Objectives

Management-by-objectives (MBO) involves the SLP's or manager's use of instructional or program objectives and criteria-referenced measures in or beyond the classroom in a complete and sophisticated way. For example, pupils operating under the intelligent application of an MBO system should know exactly what is expected of them and should have their learning enhanced. Many SLPs and teachers actually have their pupils participate in setting the instructional (learning) objectives. In one sense, MBO provides the bridge that joins the better concepts of skinnerian psychology (behaviorism) and piagetian psychology (heuristicism), or *programmed* learning and *open* learning. At other levels of management, the logical, clear, and orderly purposes of MBO certainly can help subordinates understand what is expected of them in fulfilling their responsibilities and in being accountable. Figure 6–9 depicts the cycle of management-by-objectives.

It is beyond the scope of this chapter to do little more than acquaint the reader with some of the emerging management theories, techniques, and procedures. The bibliography, however, offers the reader a list of suggested titles that cover each aspect of management (also see Chapter 5 on Supervision). In the space available, four examples of management systems are described briefly, including the Delphi Technique (used in planning and establishing goals and objectives), PPBS (a program planning budgeting system), PERT (a program evaluation and review technique), and MIS (a system for obtaining information needed in making management decisions).

Delphi Technique

The Delphi Technique is one method for determining individual and collective opinions about goals, objectives, and priorities. It has become a desirable method for managers to use in pursuing consensus, especially for long-range goals and objectives. Use of the Delphi Technique generally is not helpful in making quick or relatively short-term decisions.

When a school program in communication disorders wants to forecast the future, reorganize, design new curricula, recommend new building or room design changes, create new service or schedule models, or establish new procedures, the Delphi Technique is a rather objective method for determining "what is" and "what should be." It provides a means for (a) internal and external participants (staff and community constituents) to recommend

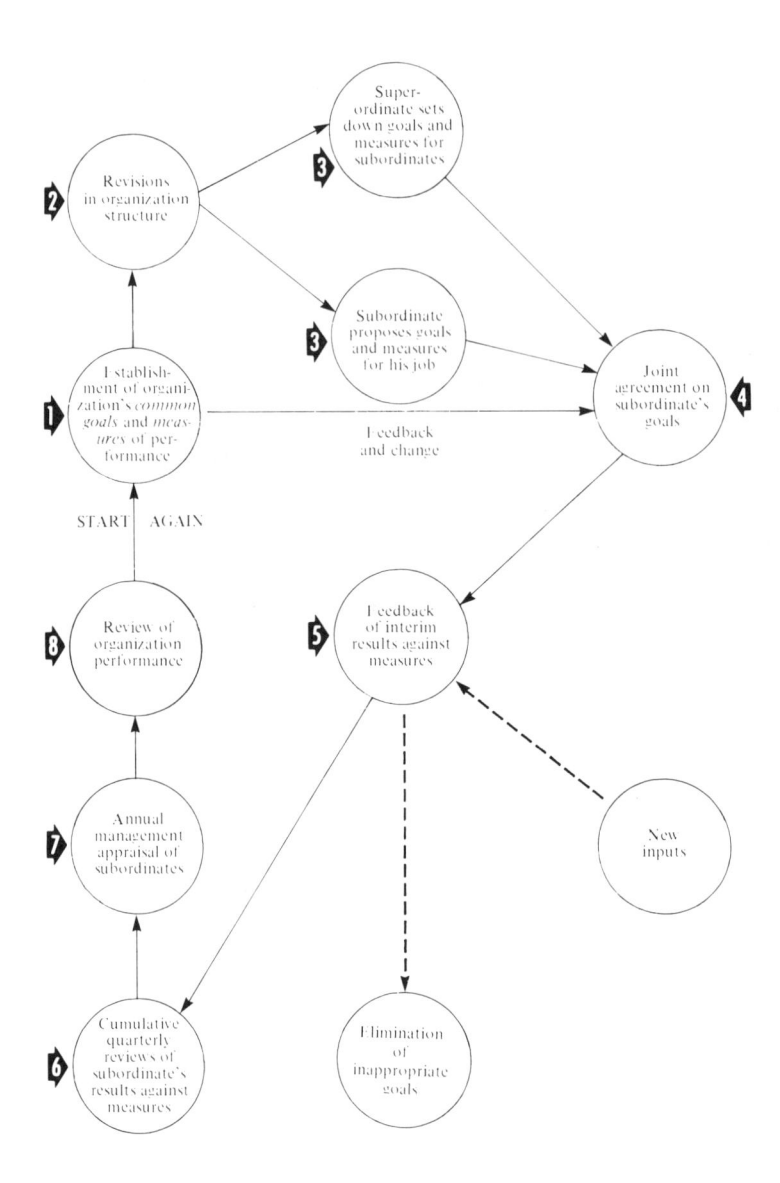

Figure 6-9. Management-by-objectives cycle.

and react to new goals and objectives; (b) each person's opinion and rationale to be heard and studied; (c) determining the will and magnitude of minority positions; and (d) ranking the importance and potential impact of proposed decisions. Participatory management, such as this, responds to people's desire to have their opinions solicited and taps the various levels of expertise that exist among interested parties.

The Delphi Technique (named after Apollo's oracle at Delphi in Greece) is designed to reduce the undesirable interactions that frequently can occur in a less-structured approach to planning and employs the following procedures:

- A. A questionnaire with briefly written statements of recommended activities or predictions of the future is given to all participants.
- B. Participants are asked to list their opinions about the activity or prediction in such terms as degree of desirability, feasibility or chance of success, timing or period of possible occurrence, if ever, and rationale.
- C. Participant responses are tabulated by a coordinator, and statements that were unclear or subject to several interpretations are clarified.
- D. The coordinator submits a refined list and summary of responses to the participants for a second probe. Persons in the minority are asked if they want to revise their opinion and, if not, are encouraged to state or elaborate on their reasons for maintaining a minority position.
- E. These responses are returned to the coordinator for further summarization and refinement.
- F. Each participant receives an updated list of summarized views for a final opportunity to revise opinion.
- G. Finally, the coordinator receives the last round of questionnaires and summarizes the responses in a final report that is distributed to all personnel involved in the process of planning and decision making. Some users prefer to assemble the participants at this point to discuss the results and review the rationale statements made by the majority and minority respondents as another step before making final decisions.

Experience with the Delphi Technique shows that two rounds are essential, but four rounds are seldom required to derive a rather clear understanding of majority and minority points of view. Figure 6–10 represents one format that can be used in managing the Delphi probe.

The Delphi Technique, which requires time, creative thinking, and the use of futuristic experts, has many practical uses in planning comprehensive instructional/clinical services for the handicapped. Unfortunately, educational program managers tend to have had little preparation or experience in using this technique as a means of participatory planning.

	In each box below, write down the projected date (1982 – 2000) for the occurrence of each event, given a 60% probability of occurrence	In each box below, assign a value to each event by circling a numerical value. +5 = highly desirable for handicapped -5 = totally undesirable JUSTIFY EACH ANSWER
1. "Super agencies" that assume all educational, medical, and social responsibilities for the handicapped individual exist in 80% of the cities of over 100,000 population.		+5 +4 +3 +2 +1 0 -1 -2 -3 -4 -5
2. Pre-service training of special educators includes one academic and one clinical course on the basic concepts of medicine.	⇧	+5 +4 +3 +2 +1 0 -1 -2 -3 -4 -5
3. Non-habit forming drugs which accelerate learning are administered daily by school personnel to 40% of the public school student population.	⇧	+5 +4 +3 +2 +1 0 -1 -2 -3 -4 -5
4. A national stockpile of instructional materials and equipment useful in the education and training of handicapped individuals is available through a remote access computerized ordering service to all professional personnel.	⇧	+5 +4 +3 +2 +1 0 -1 -2 -3 -4 -5
5. All preservice teachers will be taught how to work with children who have each type of handicapping condition.	⇧	+5 +4 +3 +2 +1 0 -1 -2 -3 -4 -5
6. 70% of all educational preparatory programs require six credit hours of course work with the exceptional child.		+5 +4 +3 +2 +1 0 -1 -2 -3 -4 -5

Figure 6-10. A possible format for a Delphi Probe.

Planning-Programming-Budgeting System (PPBS)

While the Delphi Technique is a procedure for setting goals and objectives, the PPBS (Planning-Programming-Budgeting-System) is a method for projecting the costs of meeting goals and objectives. The method gained national recognition in the mid-1960s when President Lyndon B. Johnson insisted that governmental agency administrators and program managers adopt the system as a means of effecting some uniformity in planning, managing, and budgeting federal projects. Figure 6–11 shows the PPBS, model which differs slightly from the general planning/management/evaluation model presented in Figure 6–1 at the beginning of this chapter. Notice that the insert at Step 7 illustrates The Concept of Program Budgeting by showing both the interdependencies among programs and the total budget needed to operate all programs for each of five years (Hostrop, 1973).

PPBS, like management by objectives, begins with the identification of goals and objectives. Activities are grouped into programs that encompass each of the objectives and emphasize the output or product(s) that will be accomplished. PPBS focuses on *what* and *how* something will be produced. This procedure is different from traditional line-item type budgets that primarily list anticipated expenditures without necessarily describing the expected outcome(s) and proposed effectiveness. For example, the department director in communication disorders could develop a new program to meet the language modification needs of kindergarten children identified as having language disorders. The director would explain how the new program contributes to the department's five-year plan (intermediate goals), identify the anticipated outcomes, summarize the budget request, and assign a priority ranking to the program proposal. One format for such a program request is outlined in Figure 6–12.

Implementing the PPBS system allows the department director to describe each program and its costs within an overall organizational structure and plan. In contrast, the line-item budget simply uses such categories as administration, instruction, supplies, maintenance, and department requirement for all programs combined. This procedure makes it difficult to identify what programs exist or which organizational unit is responsible for the costs and outcomes.

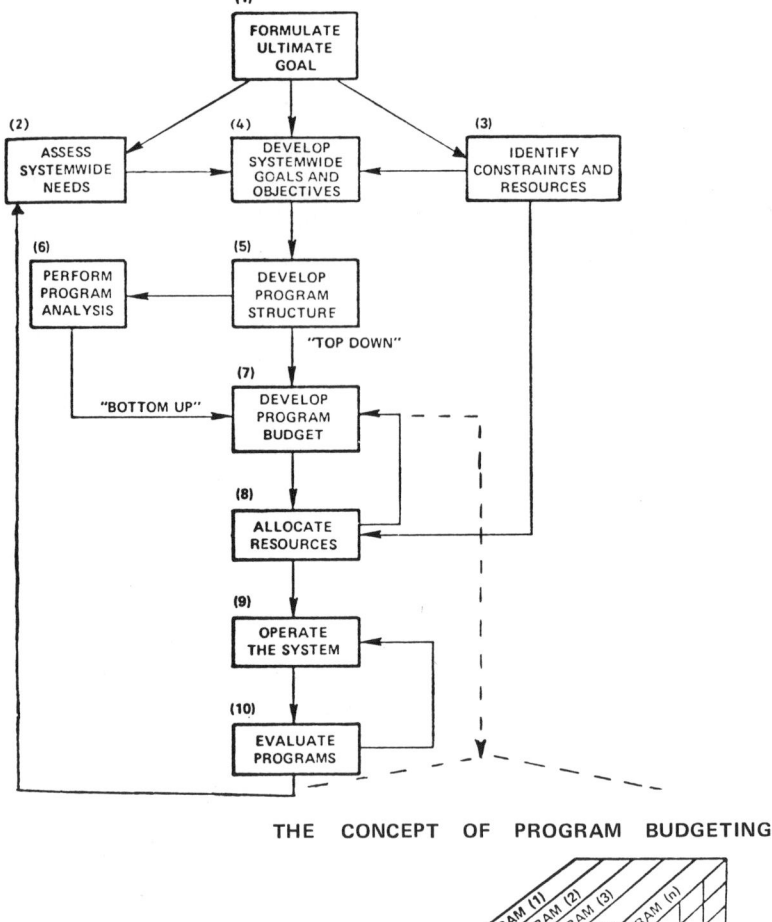

282 Speech-Language Programming in the Schools

Figure 6-11. Implementation steps for PPBS.

PPBS provides school personnel and the public with information about the resources that are allocated toward the goals and objectives

Name of Submitter	Title	Department	Date

Program description:
(new or existing one)

Describe how this program will, if approved, contribute to implementing the system's Five-Year Plan:

List additional budget needs if request is approved:

                                    <u>Personnel Services</u>   <u>Equipment</u>   <u>Space Needs</u>

Numbers:

Kinds:

Support Services:
(eg, travel, supplies, etc.)

Total dollars needed:

PROGRAM
GRAND TOTAL: $

Rank the program proposal as to necessity in order to implement the system's Five Year Plan: (Circle one)

    1. Essential   2. Highly desirable   3. Desirable

Justify your ranking:

Figure 6-12. Program request.

of a program. It shows the relationship between programmatic and budget decisions; it can facilitate eventual evaluations of expenditures associated with outcomes.

Identifying the procedures that will be followed and estimating the amount of time required to meet program objectives in a PPBS also can be formalized by using a Program Evaluation and Review Technique (PERT).

Program Evaluation and Review Technique

PERT is an acronym for a program evaluation and review technique that permits managers and staff to identify each task that must be completed to meet an objective and the estimated time(s) for completing the task(s). Sophisticated users of the PERT are interested especially in identifying the "critical path," which is the direction or route to be followed from initiation to completion of a task and requires the shortest possible time with the least amount of cost. Program efficiency is related directly to the critical path concept. For example, speech-language pathologists in schools frequently voice consternation over the time involved in effecting medical or psychological assessment referrals and receiving the results of these supportive examinations. Too often, the referral system follows a circuitous route rather than a critical path. In large school districts, state education departments, and other bureaucratic organizations, the simple task of ordering, purchasing, and receiving materials and supplies needed to complete a project can emerge as a cumbersome, frustrating process that impedes the efficiency and effectiveness desired in meeting a program objective.

PERT also recognizes that the work of one individual or group often impinges on the ability of others to initiate and terminate tasks on time. For instance, the program manager cannot assemble and complete child count reports for the state and federal education agencies until each SLP has reported her case load. Fortunately, these reporting dates can be established, and each participant can schedule respective dates for appropriate completion of the task. In planning new projects, the process of projecting task initiation and completion times can involve numerous variables that make events and times uncertain and make absolutes or time specifics impossible. For example, to begin new classes for severely language impaired children may involve such events as approval of the plan; recruitment, employment, and arrival of the SLPs; completion of a curriculum by a writing task force; and appropriately equipping two classrooms. The various tasks of the program manager, SLPs, writing team, and physical resource personnel constitute a rather elaborate network of integrated and interdependent relationships. These interrelationships will govern the time, cost, and quality associated with meeting each objective under the goal for a new program to serve kindergarten children with language disorders. Conceptualizing and orchestrating this network of events and activities is the foundation of the PERT system.

Imagine the complex interactions of events and activities involved with putting a person on the moon and charting this network to make certain that the work of all persons associated with the project is coordinated and complementary. The charting of *events* might be represented by a circle while the *activities* are depicted by using arrows. Time estimates, initially, should be estimated as a given number of work days or weeks. Accordingly, a time estimate of 0.1 week would be the equivalent of one-half day; an estimate of 0.2 equals one day. Some PERT systems provide each staff member or project participant with work activity forms that are used for listing each task in sequence and assigning estimated start and stop times. The forms generally have columns for entering "expected start" and "actual start" with similar columns for designating expected and actual completion dates. Elaborate systems might use three time estimates: Optimistic Time; Most Likely Time; and Pessimistic Time. Optimistic Time obviously constitutes the earliest possible estimate for task initiation or completion under optimum conditions. Most Likely Time represents the amount of time the activity will consume under normal circumstances. Pessimistic Time assumes adverse conditions or failures that could require new starts.

Once the tasks are listed and times are estimated for each person and group, their events and activities can be collated, coordinated, and plotted on an implementation calendar as shown in Figure 6–13. The events are numbered, and the arrows indicate the activity sequence.

The format for plotting personnel activities is shown in Figure 6–14. The codes *P, M, O* represent the pessimistic (P), most likely (M), and optimistic (O) estimates of time, cost, and number of personnel required to manage each task. As all staff become familiar with the PERT process, they generally discover that time is saved, resources are optimized, and movement through a project is orderly, productive, and reinforcing. Additional examples and details on use of these systems can be found in *Managing Education for Results* (Hostrop, 1973).

All of the systems discussed (Delphi, MBO, PPBS, PERT) are dependent on the availability of a comprehensive data or man-

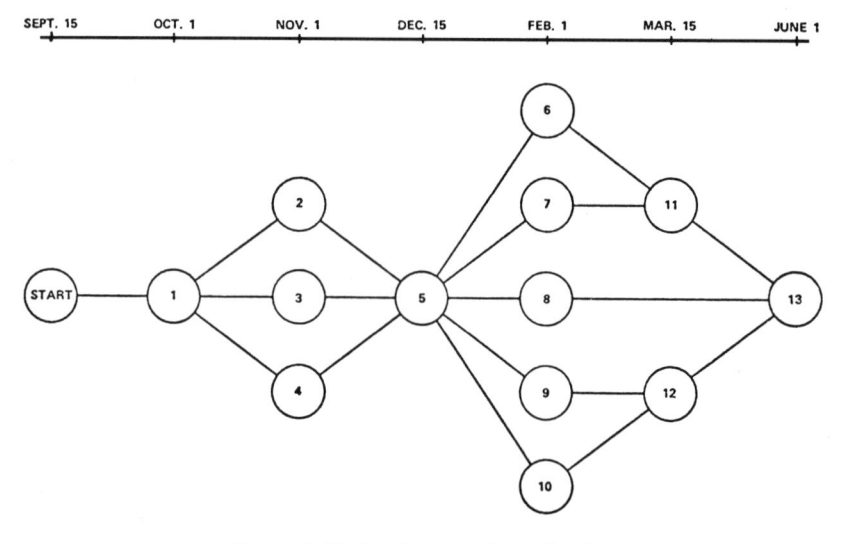

286   Speech-Language Programming in the Schools

SEPT. 15   OCT. 1   NOV. 1   DEC. 15   FEB. 1   MAR. 15   JUNE 1

Figure 6-13. Implementation calendar.

Objective: Language Curriculum   Task Leader: Ima Good   Date: May 15, 19__

No.	Task Elements	Time (weeks) P	M	O	Money P	M	O	Personnel P	M	O	Comments
1	Review	2.0	1.0	0.2	50	25	0	10	4	2	Library may have some information but doubtful there is enough.
2	Visit other institutions who have such programs	3.0	1.0	0.4	1,000	200	40	10	2	1	The best program I have heard of is out-of-state, but 2 fairly good ones are nearby. Nearby ones will be visited first.
3	Etc.										
4	Etc.										
5	Etc.										
End	Total	20.0	12.0	10.0	2,000	650	350	12	4	2	

Figure 6-14. Plotting personnel activities.

agement information system (MIS) that provides program directors and staff with the information needed to make decisions.

Management Information System (MIS)

The development of a comprehensive management information system (MIS) for use in conducting and *evaluating* speech-language-hearing programs represents a new and somewhat controversial concept. The major controversy arises over the value of quantifying the plans, procedures, and results in programs providing services for the communication handicapped. More specifically, the question is posed in this manner: can quantification of relevant data enhance service delivery and professional growth? This issue has emerged over the past decade as efforts toward achieving accountability have grown in the fields of Speech-Language Pathology, Audiology and other educational and health-related professions. For instance, the state education departments of Pennsylvania, Maryland, and West Virginia have had differing and difficult experiences in implementing uniform management information systems in school district programs serving handicapped children. Although their efforts have met with varying levels of success and failure, it is true that most school programs have some type of record-keeping and data-oriented information system. Just as school districts vary in size, staffing patterns, sociologic status, and economic ability, so does their use of management information or data systems.

In the National Evaluation of Education District Services Project (ASHA, 1974), the following results of a study on *data available* and *data needed* for proper program management were reported:

A. Record-keeping systems varied greatly among the four school districts and from clinician to clinician within two of the districts surveyed. Systems of program planning, and evaluation of services, using case management and cost data to determine program effectiveness across districts were non-existent and were minimal within a single school district.

B. The difficulty in locating case records in two of the four school districts due to the lack of a central filing system and incomplete case management data in all of the districts suggested a need to develop more specific guidelines and procedures for managing data related to pupil services. However, the differences between information required in

the individual school district records and information recorded by staff indicated that, in many instances, SLPs were not using the established procedures and guidelines.
C. Some demographic and other types of data that would be of value when making individual child service decisions as well as programmatic decisions were not included in the existing record-keeping systems. For example, diagnostic test results were not present in 47.8 percent of the records surveyed.
D. Retrieval of data regarding school district sources of funds and expenditures was difficult due to imprecise methods of collecting and reporting this information.
E. A more uniform method of collecting information regarding cost-effectiveness of various services was needed. Percentages of staff time spent in various activities varied greatly among the school districts depending on the delivery service model used, ratio of SLPs to school population served, geographical size of the district, and so forth.
F. There was a need to correlate various facets of programs to better analyze treatment effectiveness. Two items (pretreatment severity of the primary disorder and duration of treatment for the primary disorder) were computer cross-tabulated from data of the smallest and largest districts to assess whether or not such tabulations would yield information on treatment progress. It was found that treatment effectiveness for these two variables could be assessed readily. It also was determined that, with the development of a more precise record-keeping system and data retrieval procedure, many such cross-tabulations could be made that would result in better analysis of treatment effectiveness and provide the data needed to make programmatic decisions.
G. An evaluation-oriented program and case management data system are required before the effectiveness of services provided to handicapped children can be determined at the local, state, or national levels.
H. No state department of education or federal agency had developed a case management data system that would permit the systematic collection of data to evaluate the progress made by handicapped pupils receiving special services.
I. Terminology and definitions of handicapping conditions were

found to be incomplete, inadequate, and inconsistent as used in data systems at the national, state, and local levels.
J. Case management data too often were nonexistent, even in the local school district program.
K. Few school districts routinely used any formal system to summarize and evaluate program and case management data.

The use of a uniform data system for compiling information on screening, assessment, and intervention creates the capacity for continuous and more objective program and staff evaluations. In an output-oriented system, these data also assist staff in evaluating both the effect of *case management procedures* and *student progress.* However, for output data to become available, a uniform data system and uniform program procedures must be maintained over an extended period of time.

The recognized need for a uniform case management data system in speech-language-hearing programs in schools has been accentuated by the passage of Public Law 94-142. This legislation presents a mandate to providers of special services in the schools to develop accurate and reliable methods of reporting data on handicapped children.

A prototype MIS system has been developed by the American Speech-Language-Hearing Association and is entitled "Comprehensive Assessment and Service Evaluation (CASE) Information System." It is designed to assist speech-language-hearing programs in maintaining adequate and accurate evaluation-oriented record-keeping procedures. The information to be managed through the system can be categorized under the following processes: referral; screening; diagnostic assessment; placement decisions; intervention programs; coordination of service delivery; and program management. Inherent in the CASE Information System is the premise that data or information needs are greatest at the direct service level. These data are reduced increasingly and summarized in appropriate ways as they pass from the direct service provider through the supervisory and administrative levels in the local, state, and federal agencies (see Figure 6–15). For example, *case level* information may contain data elements on *individual* students and document screening, assessment, placement or intervention services. *Program level processes and data forms* deal with various aspects of the *total* language, speech, and hearing program such as summary student information and cost analyses and per-

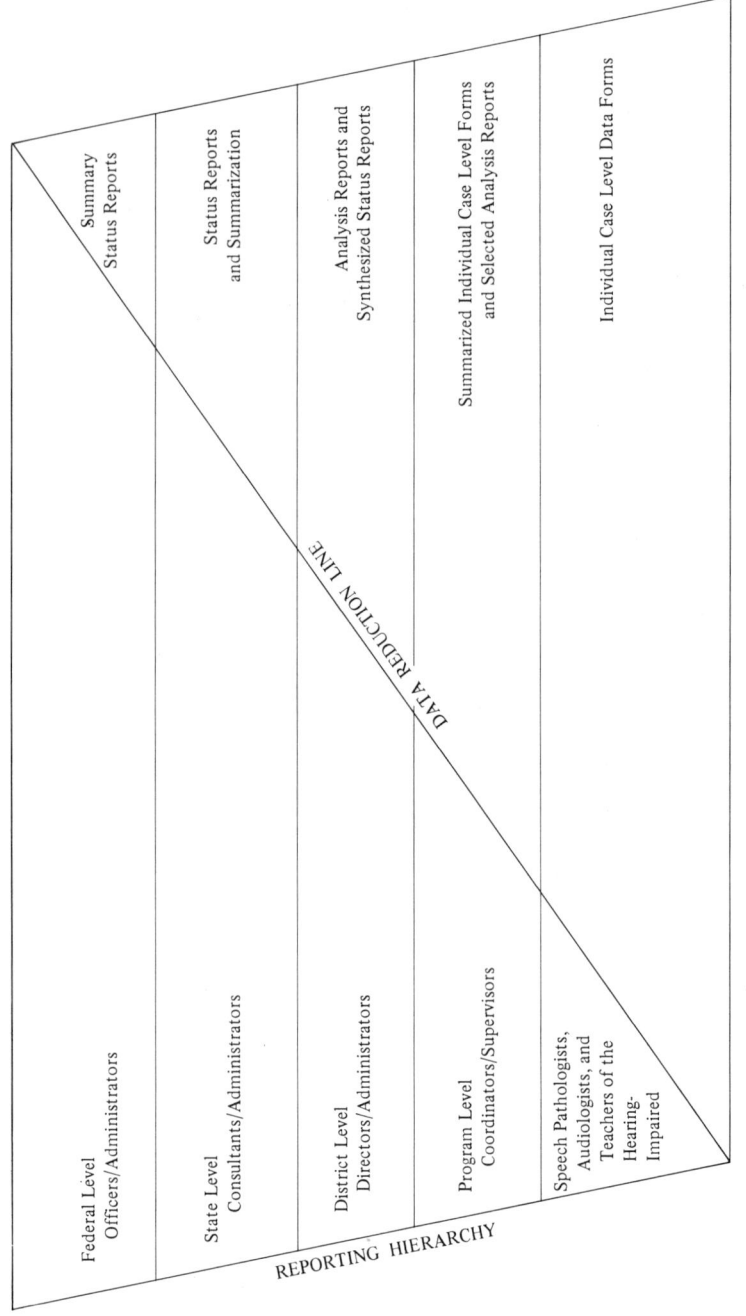

Figure 6-15. Information needs.

mit compilation of special reports that are of evaluative interest to local, state, or federal personnel.

In creating or evaluating an existing MIS, program staff need to understand the following basic principles that should govern the design of the system:
- A. The data collection procedures should be tied to those processes through which a student passes as he/she is identified, assessed, and placed in a speech-language-hearing program.
- B. Data collection should reflect the decisions made at critical points within the processes at both the case management and program management levels.
- C. The overall system design should permit the collection of data necessary for managing an accountable speech-language-hearing program.
- D. The system should be designed to meet the record-keeping needs of specialists at the direct service level.
- E. The data system should recognize the variation in information needs among programs and accommodate for those variations through a component or additive design.
- F. The system should provide for the data needs of supervisory and administrative personnel.
- G. The system should be practical to use, but comprehensive.
- H. The system should be designed to permit appropriate reduction of the data as the information is reported from the direct service level to local, state, and federal administrative levels.
- I. The system should be designed to ensure the protection of confidentiality.
- J. The system should reflect the concept that written documentation is necessary for all critical decisions.
- K. The system should incorporate those data elements necessary for use in hearings and legal actions and for determining fiscal accountability.
- L. The system should be oriented to the individual student and designed to meet the unique staff needs in keeping data on each student with a communication handicap or special need.
- M. The system should be behaviorally oriented. While not prescribing a particular methodology, this approach should focus on the communication performances of a student and emphasize the development of management programs that

are based on observation and assessment of a student's performance.

N. The system should be evaluation or output oriented. This approach is an outgrowth of the need for data that facilitate continuous evaluation of decisions made and procedures used in the identification and management of communicatively handicapped students. An output orientation addresses the need for more objective and accurate evaluations of speech-language-hearing services provided in schools. As designed, the system provides a means for recording and organizing pertinent data so that information needed for evaluating the *quality* of services provided can be retrieved and used in all decision-making processes, e.g. program planning and determination of appropriate placement.

These principles should guide developers in the design of a management information system that complements and becomes an integral component of the more comprehensive planning, management, and evaluation system. The MIS can be inserted into each of the models previously described (PDME, MBO, PPBS, PERT) and is presented as a system coordination device in Figure 6-16.

Program Management Processes

Discussion of the MIS nearly completes the listing of management procedures that can be used in school programs for the communicatively handicapped. A remaining system, that of EVALUATION, is discussed under a separate heading in the final section of this chapter.

In summarizing management processes, it appears necessary to show the relationship of management to the more umbrellalike concept of program planning, management, and evaluation. Such a relationship can be described more clearly, perhaps, by showing the management cycle (Fig. 6-17), concluding with the *Purpose, Who, What,* and *When* components of the program management process:

PURPOSE   To plan, monitor, and evaluate speech-language-hearing programs and services.

Systems for Program Planning, Management, and Evaluation 293

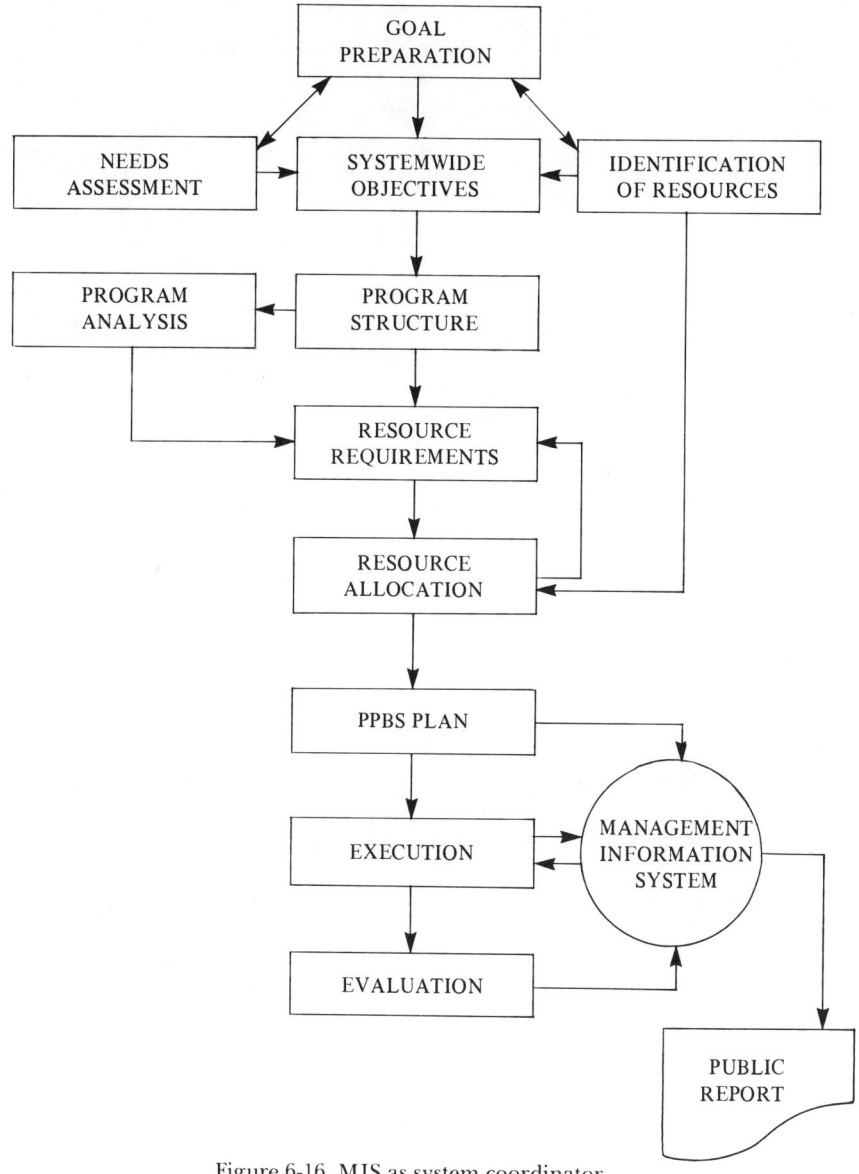

```
                    ┌──────────────┐
                    │     GOAL     │
                    │ PREPARATION  │
                    └──────────────┘
┌──────────────┐    ┌──────────────┐    ┌──────────────────┐
│    NEEDS     │───▶│  SYSTEMWIDE  │◀───│  IDENTIFICATION  │
│ ASSESSMENT   │    │  OBJECTIVES  │    │   OF RESOURCES   │
└──────────────┘    └──────────────┘    └──────────────────┘

┌──────────────┐    ┌──────────────┐
│   PROGRAM    │◀───│   PROGRAM    │
│   ANALYSIS   │    │  STRUCTURE   │
└──────────────┘    └──────────────┘
        │                   │
        │           ┌──────────────┐
        └──────────▶│   RESOURCE   │◀───┐
                    │ REQUIREMENTS │    │
                    └──────────────┘    │
                            │           │
                    ┌──────────────┐    │
                    │   RESOURCE   │◀───┘
                    │  ALLOCATION  │
                    └──────────────┘
                            │
                    ┌──────────────┐
                    │  PPBS PLAN   │──────┐
                    └──────────────┘      │
                            │             ▼
                    ┌──────────────┐   ╱MANAGEMENT╲
                    │  EXECUTION   │◀──│INFORMATION│
                    └──────────────┘   ╲  SYSTEM  ╱
                            │             │
                    ┌──────────────┐      │
                    │  EVALUATION  │─────▶│
                    └──────────────┘      │
                                          ▼
                                   ┌──────────────┐
                                   │   PUBLIC     │
                                   │   REPORT     │
                                   └──────────────┘
```

Figure 6-16. MIS as system coordinator.

WHO   Participants in the program management process include
- direct service speech-language-hearing

specialists
- supervisor(s) and/or program coordinator(s) of local speech-language-hearing program(s)
- Director(s) of speech-language-hearing program or Special Education Director(s)
- State Administrative Personnel

WHAT IS DONE   Formal program planning and evaluation systems provide the means for
- assessing the special needs of students and parents
- assessing the comprehensiveness of service delivery

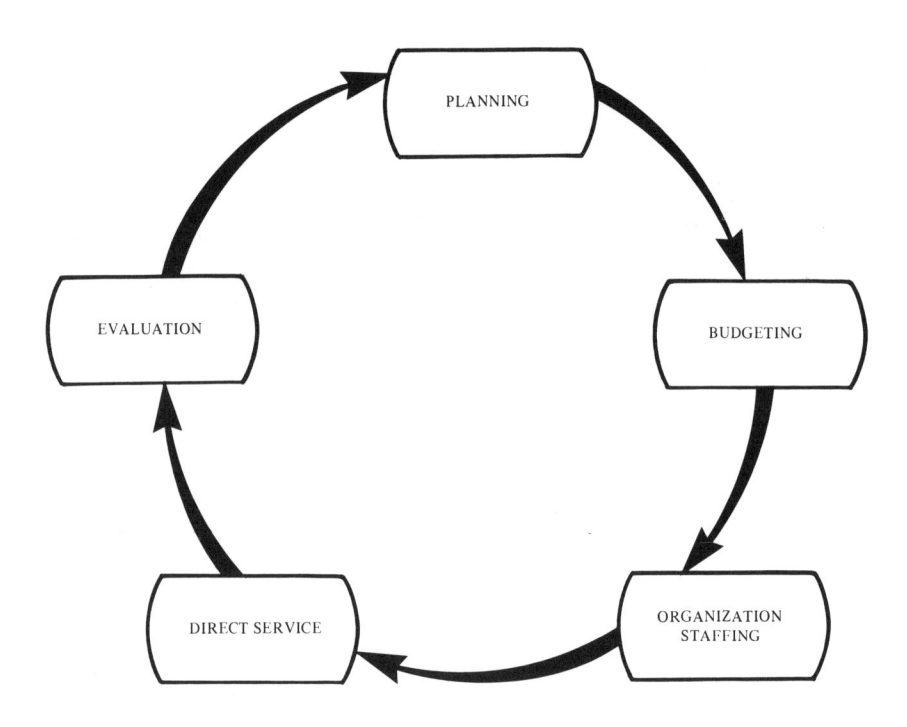

Figure 6-17. Management cycle.

- insuring efficient and effective program management
- evaluating student progress
- demonstrating accountability to Boards of Education, parents, state and federal agencies, and the public

In any management information system, data for program planning and evaluation can be generated in the following three categories:
- Student Information Analysis (SI)
- Cost Analysis (CA)
- Special Reports (SR)

Student Information Analysis provides for the collection of data including
- total enrollment by school and total number of students with communication disorders and differences
- total number of students screened and screening results
- total number of students assessed and assessment results by communication disorder/difference
- total number of students needing placement versus placed in the speech-language-hearing program by disorder/difference
- student progress information by disorder/difference

Much of the information used in completing the Student Reports comes from a central card file. Cost Analyses provide for the collection of data including
- program funding sources
- staff time distribution by Direct and - Indirect service activities, e.g. Direct—screening, assessment, consultation; Indirect—in-service provided, travel, in-service received
- staff time distribution by program area,

e.g. hearing, language, speech
- total costs and expenditures by program or department
- summary cost information for budget planning

Special Reports provide for the collection of data on
- cost information for equipment and materials by program and by service activity
- facilities to determine their appropriateness to program needs and objectives

These reports represent one way of collecting case and program information to help administrators plan and evaluate program goals and objectives and their compliance with federal and state legislative mandates. A broad data base has the potential for providing a wide variety of additional comparisons, correlations, studies, and reports. These data can be generated from the information contained in the program level reports and from the information collected at the direct service level. Examples include
- assessment results by estimated severity level
- total number of assessments performed
- student progress and dismissal rate by placement/service model and by staff member
- student progress and length of intervention by disorder and severity
- student progress and duration of intervention by group size
- educational/clinical placement by disorder/difference severity
- ratio of clinical staff to student(s) in speech-language-hearing program

- principal intervention methods and instructional materials
- staff characteristics

WHEN Program management activities occur at various times with differing frequencies. Most phases of management activity are annual, monthly, or tied to a local, state, or federal reporting period.

Most speech-language-hearing programs in the schools have had to rely on manual procedures when using any of the aforementioned management systems. However, each of these systems can be operated more efficiently and economically in many school districts when they are computerized. It is interesting to note that districts, increasingly, are using computers to manage the payroll, schedule students into classes, and operate bus routes, but few make their computer facilities and personnel available to providers of instructional/clinical services. Hopefully, this practice will change as program managers implement new management procedures that deal with the complexities inherent in formal planning, management, and evaluation systems. This hope (and recommendation) is based on two supporting premises: (1) existing computer technology offers superior processing capabilities at an economically justifiable price; and (2) only a computer can offer the manipulative and analytic mechanisms necessary to gain a comprehensive understanding of the underlying, complex processes that characterize the provision of services for the handicapped. Automated management systems offer the following advantages:

a. Allow superior data storage capabilities, greater processing speed, and quicker information access
b. Provide greater operational cost-effectiveness for large transaction volumes
c. Offer a powerful tool for responding to complex and dynamic information needs
d. Facilitate the generation of different data stratifications, reports, summarizations, and relationships
e. Furnish a sophisticated data base for conducting research,

outcome measures, program evaluation, and quality assurance studies
f. Facilitate improved record-keeping practices
g. Free speech-language-hearing personnel for more productive service activities

Finally, automated processing of information not only generates more time for evaluation activities but also facilitates the process of program and case management evaluation. The steps required in assessing needs, determining problems, designing programs, implementing service procedures, and effecting proper evaluations cannot be achieved without special information and data systems required to support each of the aforementioned steps. Each step requires decision making based on the most comprehensive information available. Making policy or procedural decisions on the basis of inadequate information is irresponsible behavior.

EVALUATION

Achieving congruence between a program's goals and its results can be the crux of accountability. The process required for determining the degree to which congruence exists is *evaluation*. Evaluation is a review of performance that should take place at various intervals along the route to meeting a goal. Interim or continuous evaluation permits program personnel to take corrective action at any time effectiveness and efficiency fail to meet the criteria established for student or program management.

Management systems simply are incomplete if they fail to establish procedures for evaluating programmatic effects on students receiving services, parents, and personnel. The lack of appropriate evaluation procedures has represented the single greatest failure of education, including programs providing special instruction and related services for children and youth with handicaps.

The goal of evaluation is to assure quality management and, consequently, high quality end products. Educational systems are just beginning to implement systems of "quality assurance." For example, quality assurance strategies enable the staff of a speech-language-hearing program to assess and improve the effectiveness of the services they provide to communication handicapped pupils. The goal is to have staff demonstrate that services meet identified standards of quality and improve the communication abilities of pupils receiving those services. One set of procedures for setting standards and evaluating quality is described in the Child Services Review System (ASHA, 1978).

Child Services Review System (CSRS)

Use of the Child Services Review System by a speech-language-hearing program can facilitate professional accountability and growth in any area of program management or direct service delivery. As a quality assurance mechanism, CSRS assesses the quality of present performance and commitment to corrective action when a need is indicated by the assessment. The assessment component of CSRS is the measurement aspect, conducted through a record review (audit) according to predetermined standards, problem identification, and problem analysis. The assurance component of CSRS involves developing a solution to the problem, implementing corrective action, and reassessing the same information to document improvement.

Although the primary application of the system is at the case management level, CSRS may be incorporated into the comprehensive design of a speech-language-hearing program at the administrative or program level. For those programs using other planning and evaluation procedures developed by the American Speech-Language-Hearing Association (ASHA), the audit process on which CSRS is based may serve as an effective evaluative instrument. After acquiring skill in using CSRS at the case management level, staff may use the CSRS process in assessing the effectiveness of administrative procedures. Standards and Guidelines for Comprehensive Language, Speech and Hearing Programs in the Schools (Healey, 1973) was published by ASHA as a resource on professionally accepted standards for program quality and serves as a guide for assessing the quality of each component in a communication disorders program.

For those school districts already using the ASHA planning system, Essentials of Program Planning, Development, Management and Evaluation (PDME) which was described earlier in this chapter, CSRS can be used as a needs identification procedure or as an evaluation technique. It also may be used to identify problem areas in service delivery and to assess the degree of compliance with criteria stated in specific goals and objectives. Additionally, the concepts included in the PDME Manual can be used in developing the Remedial Action Plan, which is one quality assurance component of CSRS.

Finally, CSRS requires the availability of a Management Information System (MIS), such as Comprehensive Assessment and Service Evaluation (CASE) Information System previously presented in this chapter. The CASE Information System, or a similar formal system for collecting, storing and retrieving pupil and program information, will provide an adequate data base for a CSRS Audit.

The CSRS Audit incorporates a series of sequential activities that involve the following:

a. identifying a program area for review
b. establishing standards of quality within the program area
c. retrospectively reviewing (auditing) selected records of services delivered to a specific population for a given period of time
d. identifying trends in service delivery to reveal deficient and superior procedures and outcomes
e. improving the quality of services provided to communication handicapped pupils

CSRS Audit procedures are designed to identify and correct discrepancies between expected performance levels and actual performance levels through an application of the audit cycle depicted in Figure 6-18.

The Child Services Review System begins with the selection of an Audit Committee. This committee is comprised of four or five communication disorder specialists in a speech-language-hearing program. As other staff members learn the CSRS process, membership on the Audit Committee may change so that all staff members eventually can have the opportunity to serve on the

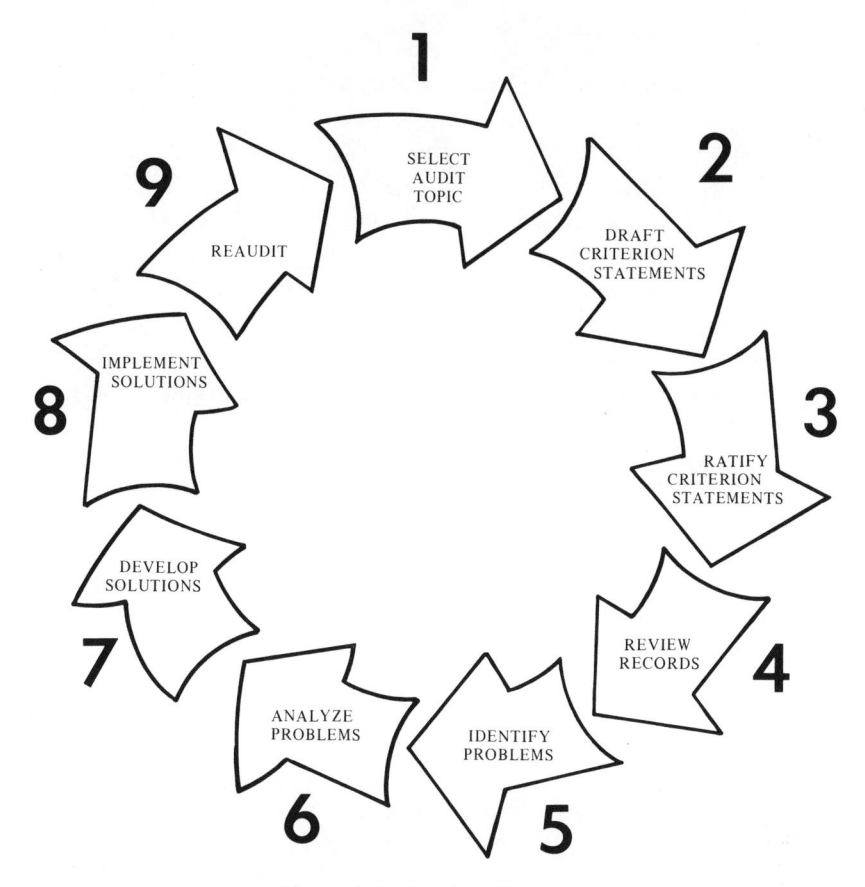

Systems for Program Planning, Management, and Evaluation 301

Figure 6-18. CSRS audit cycle.

committee. Once the Audit Committee is selected, the following nine-step audit cycle occurs:

STEP 1. Select a Topic

The Audit Committee selects an area of service delivery for review. The *topic* may be any area in which services are delivered regularly, any area in which changes would upgrade the quality of pupil services, or any area identified by staff as needing improvement.

Following the selection of the audit topic, the Audit Committee specifies an audit *focus* that states the group's purpose for doing the audit. Wording of the focus usually begins: "To improve;" "To assess;" or "To evaluate" some aspect of the selected topic. The focus limits the scope of the audit topic so that specific statements can be developed that identify the critical components of quality services to communication handicapped pupils.

Next, the Audit Committee identifies the pupil *population* from which a sample of records will be drawn. The population is defined by pupil age; primary communication disorder; type of intervention setting; length, intensity, or frequency of intervention; or any combination of these variables. Finally, the time period during which records were generated will limit variations due to staff or administrative changes within the program.

This process represents step one in the cycle. Examples for each step described are used with permission of ASHA and are taken from the CSRS Manual:

STEP 1 EXAMPLE

Audit Committee *selects a topic* **and** *identifies a focus*, *a population*, **and a** *time period* **for the audit.**

TOPIC: Language Impairment

FOCUS: To improve the criteria for termination of services to pupils in a language-impaired class setting.

POPULATION: All pupils ages four through six who were dismissed from language classes and placed in regular classroom settings.

TIME PERIOD: Dismissal occurred within the past six months.

Step 2. Draft Criterion Statements

The Audit Committee usually drafts fewer than ten *Criterion Statements* that represent their concepts of quality service delivery for the audit Topic, Focus, and Population. These Criterion Statements are determined from professional expertise, review of the literature, or consultation with experts in the area under review. The Criterion Statements identify staff procedures that should be followed or expected pupil behaviors following intervention including a 100 percent *Expected Level of Performance*. The Criterion Statements serve as standards of quality against which the actual performance of pupils or staff is measured.

Next, the Audit Committee sets a *Threshold for Action,* which identifies the percentage of records that must meet the Expected

Level of Performance. If the actual level of performance falls below the Threshold for Action, the group should take corrective action to improve intervention procedures or outcomes. Setting a Threshold for Action ensures that all staff members know the degree to which each Criterion Statement must be met.

These processes constitute Step 2 in the audit cycle and are summarized in the example below:

STEP 2 EXAMPLE

Audit Committee drafts criterion statements and specifies a threshold for action for each statement.

Criterion Statement	Expected Level of Performance	Threshold for Action
1. Each pupil exhibits language comprehension abilities six months or less below age level.	100%	95%
2. Each pupil exhibits expressive vocabulary usage six months or less below age level.	100%	95%
3. Each pupil exhibits syntactical skills 12 months or less below age level.	100%	90%
4. Each pupil exhibits morphological skills six months or less below age level.	100%	90%
5. Each pupil exhibits spontaneous utterances of four words or more.	100%	95%

Step 3. Ratify Criterion Statements

Staff whose records will be reviewed must accept/ratify each Criterion Statement and Threshold for Action drafted by the Audit Committee. If a staff member does not agree, she may propose changes in either the Criterion Statement or the Threshold for Action percentage. Ratification means that no staff member's records will be reviewed against standards that she has not accepted. See the example of Step 3 and compare the "performance" and "action" percentages with those in the Step 2 Example.

STEP 3 EXAMPLE

All speech-language pathologists and audiologists whose records will be reviewed MODIFY and ACCEPT/RATIFY CRITERION STATEMENTS.

Criterion Statement	Expected Level of Performance	Threshold for Action
1. Each pupil exhibits language comprehension abilities six months or less below age level.	100%	95%
2. Each pupil exhibits expressive vocabulary usage six months or less below age level.	100%	90%
3. Each pupil exhibits syntactical skills *six months or less* below age level.	100%	90%
4. Each pupil exhibits morphological skills *12 months or less* below age level.	100%	90%
5. Each pupil exhibits spontaneous utterances of four words or more	100%	90%

Step 4. Review Records

Staff members review pupil records from the target population to determine whether or not the Criterion Statements have been met. Using an initial screening level of 100 percent or 0 percent, all records that do not comply with Criterion Statements are referred to the Audit Committee for verification of failure. The Audit Committee computes an *Actual Level of Performance* that is expressed as a ratio of the number of records that meet the Expected Level of Performance in each Criterion Statement compared to the total number of records reviewed:

STEP 4 EXAMPLE

The Audit Committee *reviews records* of target population to determine whether or not the Criterion Statements have been met.

Criterion Statement	Expected Level of Performance	Threshold for Action	Actual Level of Performance
1. Each pupil exhibits language comprehension abilities six months or less below age level.	100%	95%	75%
2. Each pupil exhibits expressive vocabulary usage six months or less below age level.	100%	90%	92%
3. Each pupil exhibits syntactical skills 12 months or less below age level.	100%	90%	90%

4. Each pupil exhibits morphological skills 12 months or less below age level.	100%	90%	36%
5. Each pupil exhibits spontaneous utterances of four words or more.	100%	90%	54%

Step 5. Identify Problems

The Audit Committee compares the *Actual Level of Performance* to the *Threshold for Action* for each *Criterion Statement* to identify possible problems. The example of Step 5 that follows shows that problems can be identified when the Actual Level of Performance is lower than the Threshold for Action for any Criterion Statement. This constitutes a performance deficiency that must be verified by the Audit Committee.

STEP 5 EXAMPLE

The Audit Committee compares Actual Levels of Performance to Thresholds for Action to *identify problems.*

Criterion Statement	Expected Level of Performance	Threshold for Action	Actual Level of Performance
1. Language comprehension	100%	95%	75%
2. Expressive vocabulary usage	100%	90%	92%
3. Syntactical skills	100%	90%	90%
4. Morphological skills	100%	90%	36%
5. Spontaneous speech	100%	90%	54%

Problems are identified in the areas of language comprehension, morphological skills, and spontaneous speech. The Audit Committee selects Criterion 4, "Each pupil exhibits morpholgoical skills 12 months or less below age level," as the first audit problem for analysis. This problem is selected as most critical because of the large discrepancy between the Threshold For Action and Actual Performance Level. In an actual audit in a school district, all three problems would be analyzed, but for workshop purposes, only one problem is used.

Step 6. Analyze Problems

In the example given for this step, note that the Audit Committee identifies problems, develops a list of possible causes for each deficiency, and ranks the probable causes by priority.

STEP 6 EXAMPLE

The Audit Committee *analyzes the problem*

Reasons for the discrepancy between the Threshold for Action and the Actual Level of Performance in the assessment and documentation of pupil's morphological skills:

1. Some staff members do not include morphological assessment as part of a diagnostic evaluation because they do not consider morphology to be an important indicator of linguistic competence.
2. Some staff members measure morphological skills but do not document results.
3. Some staff members are not familiar with methods for assessment of morphological skills.
4. Some staff members do not have the time available that is required for morphological assessment.

Step 7. Develop Solutions

The Audit Committee develops a *Remedial Action Plan* that specifies the corrective actions to be taken, the responsible individuals, the completion time for each action, and a specific date for Reaudit of the same problem. The Remedial Action Plan must be ratified by all staff members prior to implementation.

STEP 7 EXAMPLE

The Audit Committee *develops a solution*

Remedial Action Plan

What	Who	When
1. Staff development committee will present *in-service* training about development and assessment of morphological skills	Staff Development Chairperson	Next Staff Meeting
2. Staff will review currently available tests of morphology and *order new tests*, on approval.	Materials Chairperson	By Next Month
3. Staff will *conduct an audit* to improve the total diagnostic evaluation of pupils with language impairment	Audit Chairperson	In Two Weeks
4. Staff will *Reaudit* the same problem	Audit Chairperson	In Six Months

Step 8. Implement Solutions

The staff *takes the corrective actions* agreed upon in the Remedial

Action Plan. As the staff generates new records, the Audit Committee monitors the records and procedures to see that positive modifications are occuring in service delivery.

STEP 8 EXAMPLE

The speech-language pathology and audiology staff *implements the solution.*

The individuals designated in the Remedial Action Plan complete the specified tasks by the date indicated in the plan.

At this point in an actual audit, the Audit Committee returns to the additional problems identified in the record review and completes steps 6–9 for those discrepancies.

Step 9. Reaudit

The staff performs a *Reaudit* of the same Topic, Focus, and Population at the time specified in the Remedial Action Plan. The original Criterion Statements are applied to records developed after implementation of the Remedial Action Plan. Using the reaudit process, the Committee can determine the degree to which services have improved. New levels of performance are recorded as shown below.

STEP 9 EXAMPLE

The speech-language pathology and audiology staff *reaudits* the same problem.

The staff applies the same Criterion Statements developed in the original audit to a new set of records generated after the implementation of the Remedial Action Plan. The new Actual Level of Performance for each Criterion Statement demonstrates the effectiveness of the remedial action and the improvement of criteria used to terminate language class placement for language-impaired pupils.

Criterion Statement	Expected Level of Performance	Threshold for Action	Original Actual Level of Performance	New Actual Level of Performance
1. Language comprehension	100%	95%	75%	95%
2. Expressive vocabulary	100%	90%	92%	93%
3. Syntactical skills	100%	90%	90%	93%

4. Morphological skills	100%	90%	36%	94%
5. Spontaneous speech	100%	90%	54%	93%

The preceding audit example assesses the end result of an intervention process. To identify specific reasons for the deficits, the actual intervention procedures must be reviewed. This can be accomplished by conducting a CSRS audit using Process Criterion Statements which enable a speech-language-hearing staff to assess the methods and procedures being used in intervention. Examples for this type of audit appear in the CSRS Manual that may be obtained from the American Speech-Language-Hearing Association.

In addition to the case management evaluation system, like CSRS, some evaluation procedures are designed to assist school personnel in assessing total program effectiveness. The Bi-Cycle Evaluation System is one example.

Bi-Cycle Evaluation System

The Bi-Cycle Evaluation System[2] uses a scientific problem-solving process to evaluate each component of a delivery system and makes visible one of the conceptual models of evaluation that may be used in programs serving the handicapped.

Thirteen steps are taken to formulate a practical evaluation system, explain the interrelational processes that should be followed, and present the information in a manner that permits wide application of the system. For example, state or local groups and individuals should be able to use the system for evaluative research in demonstration programs or inservice programs.

Figure 6-19 represents the concept and procedures used in an evaluation system that parallels the planning system depicted earlier in Figure 6-1.

The Bi-Cycle Evaluation system uses "competent performance" concepts, procedures, and criteria. Each step is summarized and

---

[2]Originally called the Bi-Cycle Concept and developed by Clement Brown, M.D., Chestnut Hill Hospital, Philadelphia (see Brown, C. R., Jr. and Fleisher, D. S., The Bi-Cycle Concept—Relating Continuing Education Directly to Patient Care. *New England Journal of Medicine*, May, 88–97, 1971).

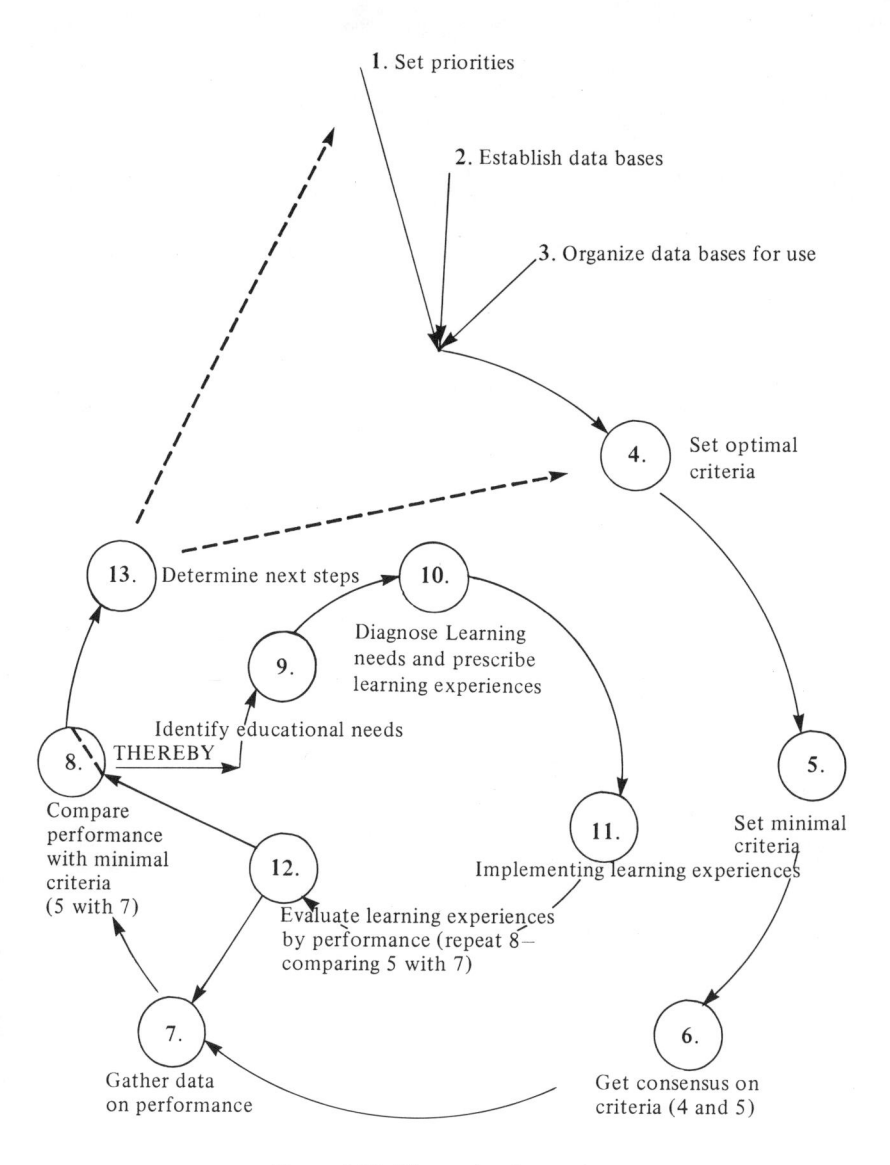

Systems for Program Planning, Management, and Evaluation 309

1. Set priorities
2. Establish data bases
3. Organize data bases for use
4. Set optimal criteria
5. Set minimal criteria
6. Get consensus on criteria (4 and 5)
7. Gather data on performance
8. Compare performance with minimal criteria (5 with 7)
9. Identify educational needs THEREBY
10. Diagnose Learning needs and prescribe learning experiences
11. Implementing learning experiences
12. Evaluate learning experiences by performance (repeat 8 — comparing 5 with 7)
13. Determine next steps

Figure 6-19. The evaluation cycle.

permits the staff to use skills developed during the application of the planning and management systems outlined previously in this chapter.

Step 1: Setting Priorities (based on identified needs)
Step 2: Identifying and/or Establishing Data Systems (MIS)
Step 3: Organizing Data Sources (computerization and alternatives)
Step 4: Setting Optimal Criteria
Step 5: Setting Minimal Criteria
Step 6: Gaining Staff (Consumer) Consensus and Approval
Step 7: Gathering Data on Performance in Current Service Activities
Step 8: Comparing Performance Date with Minimal Criteria
Step 9: Identifying Educational Needs (strengths and deficits; sequence and continuity)
Step 10: Assessing Individual and Group Learning Needs and Prescribing Future Instruction
Step 11: Implementing Appropriate Activities
Step 12: Monitoring and Evaluating Performance (repeat 8 and compare 5 with 7)
Step 13: Obtaining External Validation of Criteria Through Cross-Auditing Procedures to Determine Next Steps (as in CSRS)
Step 14: Returning to Step 1 or Step 4

Any evaluation system must be reviewed and updated as (a) results indicate directions for change, (b) technology improves, and (c) standards for service are upgraded. The staff or a panel can formulate recommended procedures for updating the system or, at least, various components of the system. These recommended procedures for revision, upgrading, and revalidation should be incorporated into a manual describing the evaluation system concept and procedures that are to be used by all speech-language-hearing staff.

Ideally, systems of evaluation should use *explicit criteria* in determining whether or not performance standards have been met. There should be scientific procedures to determine whether or not the observation of program activities based on individual judgments (implicit criteria) correlates highly with the explicit criteria that have been established and are more objective.

To date, criteria used in judging the performance of professional personnel or the quality of services provided generally have been based on professional judgment (*consensus criteria*) rather than on data concerning actual empirically based criteria in providing services. Regardless of the way the panel or staff establish criteria for evaluating in-services and projects, the criteria must be (1) understandable; (2) free from interpretation; (3) based on data acquired through records or other evaluative sources or objective data; (4) specific to the service or project components being evaluated; and (5) reasonable to use in terms of time and cost. In the systematic evaluation of *services* provided, criteria can be applied to the evaluation of structure, process, or outcome. *Structure* includes the tools necessary to provide instructional facilities, services, and staff or peer consultants. Structural appraisal is a major part of any evaluation system. The intended outcome is one of certification that the program has met the necessary level of quality within the standards established. *Process* includes the activities of professionals or aides in the management of their respective roles. These studies often focus on process data and determine such things as "were pre- and posttests of performance provided?" *Outcome* studies include intermediate and long-term results of service provision in terms of both learning and a determination of the satisfaction for the end results of services provided. Outcomes are the most direct measures of quality but are complicated because other factors besides the type of services provided can affect them. Outcome evaluation should be a part of any comprehensive service educational program for pupils with communication and other handicapping conditions.

It is necessary to put the use of norms, criteria, and standards in the context of a comprehensive evaluation system designed to review the appropriateness and effect of service provided in local and state agencies. The following definitions of norms, criteria, and standards may be used in establishing evaluative procedures:

1. *Norms*—Numerical or statistical measures of usual observed performance.
2. *Criteria*—Predetermined standards of performance against which aspects of the quality of service may be compared. Criteria will be developed by the panel or staff relying on professional expertise and on the data provided or acquired

during each step in the evaluative process.
3. *Standards*—Professionally developed expressions of the range of acceptable variation from a norm or criterion.

Unfortunately, school personnel frequently feel they have neither the time nor the system required for completing comprehensive analyses of existing data or implementing procedures that have been requested by parents, technical assistance consultants, teachers, and administrators for evaluating those variables which determine service accessibility, appropriateness, or effectiveness.

Answers to critical questions about the quality and quantity of services contribute to both immediate and long-term improvement of the education system. Obtaining comprehensive evaluations to identify such information as personnel characteristics, geographic distribution, service frequency, and other basic demographics are important but primarily are issues of design and management. Creating a system to evaluate appropriateness and effectiveness is complex and confronts staff with both philosophic and practical issues involving the acquisition of objective and judgmental information.

Administrators may need to elicit the assistance of expert consultants to complement staff expertise and balance any staff bias when designing their evaluation system. A panel might be composed of representatives from the following groups:

1. state university professors
2. school district teachers and administrators
3. state education coordinators
4. consultants from national projects such as the National Inservice Network and the Evaluation Training Consortium[3]
5. handicapped advocates or education consumers

Panel members and staff review all components of the current program and conceptualize a system designed to increase competent performance of educators serving handicapped children. Next, the panel should summarize their concepts of system evaluation, identify program components that require the establishment of standards, evaluative measures, or analytic procedures, and elicit

---

[3] Sponsored by the Office of Special Education and Rehabilitation (formerly the Bureau of Education for the Handicapped), 400 Maryland Avenue, S.W., Washington, D.C. 20202

staff recommendations for effecting a comprehensive evaluation system.

The panel must deal with many of the constraints discussed previously. For example, any system that evaluates professional and paraprofessional personnel must establish standards for performance, criteria to judge the quality with which those standards are met, and norms indicating those measures which will be used to determine the range of performance judged as being acceptable within the criteria established for the standards of operation.

In summary, evaluation should (1) provide feedback information for the decision making required to upgrade services, (2) provide baseline data for future planning, and (3) describe the strengths and weaknesses of a program in a manner that quality can be advanced.

THE FUTURE OF FORMAL PLANNING, MANAGEMENT, AND EVALUATION SYSTEMS

Education of the handicapped, because of the range and depth of its services, has become increasingly expensive to the American society. This occurs at the same time when society is discovering additional needs for energy control, urban readjustment, and comprehensive health insurance, all of which carry unprecedented high price tags. More frequently, program administrators and individual service providers are being told that their needs exceed the resources available and that priorities must be reordered. A somewhat fickle taxpaying public tends to demand more service than it is willing or able to pay for. The recent challenge to be accountable, in many ways, has represented a smokescreen for what actually constitutes a demand to reduce, or at least hold level, expenditures for educational services. Parents and others often want quick, inexpensive and simple solutions to the very time-consuming, complex issues. Resolving issues and solving problems in programs for the future requires formal and not voluntary coordination in planning and evaluating the quality of managerial services. The process of decision making adopted by program coordinators is of central importance to the ultimate quality of special educational and related services that will be available to children with communication and related disorders.

Effective coordination among individuals within the district and from the authoritative top to the level of practitioner is critical if decisions are to be based on adequate information. Even though such coordination frequently can make the decision-making process within a program or school district complicated, such procedures are necessary and represent an effort to respect the information available through those who really know what needs and problems exist at all levels. The complexity of the educational enterprise and the subtleties in the knowledge base require, as a matter of wisdom if not right, this respect for informed opinion.

The call for formal program planning, management, and evaluation systems should not be perceived as a threat by school personnel but as an appeal—an appeal to recognize the weight of responsibility carried by SLPs, teachers, and program administrators.

STUDY ACTIVITIES

1. You have conducted a needs assessment and determined that only 10 percent of the staff participates in any type of continuing or in-service education annually. Write a goal statement that would result in at least 50 percent of the staff completing group or individual educational experiences each year. Include the *When*, *What*, and *Criterion* components in your goal statement.
2. In the following program objective, identify the *When, Who, What, To Whom, Criterion,* and *Evaluation* components:
    By June 1, 19••, the speech and language pathologist will have revised the formal referral form to be used by regular classroom teachers. A copy of the form will be submitted to the Director of Special Education for fund approval.
  Now write your own program or instructional objective and make certain you have incorporated each component.
3. Using the prevalence data (Figure 6-4), estimate the high-

est and lowest numbers of hearing handicapped pupils in school districts that have 10,000, 30,000, and 60,000 pupils. Now, compute similar numbers for "speech handicapped" pupils.
4. If about 30 percent of all pupils in special education have communication disorders, how can you use the prevalence data to estimate the number of handicapped pupils who might need the special services of a speech-language pathologist in a school district with 10,000 people?
5. In a school district of 20,000 pupils, use the prevalence data to estimate the number of pupils with hearing loss. Assign 50 percent of these pupils to classes having a staff:pupil ratio of 8. Assign the remaining 50 percent to audiologists. How many teachers and audiologists would you need to employ?
6. If you will receive local, state, and federal funding totaling $2,500 per each speech and language handicapped pupil in a district of 30,000 pupils, determine the estimated prevalence and compute your total potential income. Now, if each specialist is to be paid an average salary of $15,000, how many specialists can be employed when 85 percent of the income is allotted to salaries?
7. You have 400 language handicapped pupils. About 10 percent will spend one to three hours per day in a resource room, and the remainder will be served by itinerant personnel. Assign what you consider to be appropriate staff:pupil ratios for each type of placement and determine the number of staff required for each.
8. Review the program processes listed in the *CASE Information System* and determine how a problem occurring in each process could be evaluated and solved by using the Child Service Review System or the Bi-Cycle Evaluation System.

REFERENCES

Abeson, Alan et al. *A Primer on Due Process.* Reston, Virginia: The Council for Exceptional Children, 1975.

Adair, Melanie et al. *The Peer Review Manual of the Iowa Speech and Hearing Association.* Cedar Rapids, Iowa: St. Lukes Methodist Hospital, Department of Speech Pathology and Audiology, 1975.

Anderson, J. (Ed.). *Conference on Supervision of Speech and Hearing Programs in the Schools.* Bloomington, Indiana: Indiana University, 1970.

Anderson, J. Status of college and university programs of practicum in the schools, *Asha, 15*, 60–68, 1973.

Anderson, J. Supervision: The Neglected Component of our Profession. In L. J. Turton, (Ed.), *Proceedings of a Workshop on Supervision in Speech Pathology.* Ann Arbor: University of Michigan, 1974.

Andrews, J. R. Applying Principles of Instructional Technology in Evaluating Speech and Language Services. *Language, Speech and Hearing Services in Schools, 6,* 66–71, 1973.

Annual Survey of Hearing Impaired Children and Youth. Washington, D.C.: Gallaudet College, October, 1975.

Ansoff, H. Igor and Brandenburg, R. G. The General Manager of the Future, *California Management Review,* Spring, 1969.

Audette, Robert H. *CORE Evaluation Manual.* Bedford, Massachusetts: The Institute for Educational Services, 1974.

Bernstein, C. D. et al. *Financing Educational Services for the Handicapped: An Analysis of Current Research and Practices.* Palo Alto, California: Management Analysis Center, Inc., 1974.

Blaschke, Charles. Performance Contracting Costs, Management Reform, and John Q. Citizen, *Phi Delta Kappan,* December, 1971.

Bloom, B. S., Hastings, J. T., and Madaus, G. F., *Handbook on Formative and Summative Evaluation of Student Learning.* New York: McGraw-Hill, 1971.

Bloomer, H. H. Professional Training in Speech Correction and Clinical Audiology. *Journal of Speech and Hearing Disorders, 21,* 5–11, 1956.

Boone, D., and Prescott, T. Content and sequence analysis of speech and hearing therapy. *Asha, 14,* 58–62, 1972.

Borton, Terry. Reform without Politics in Louisville. *Saturday Review,* February 5, 1972.

Brooks, R., and Hannah, E. A tool for clinical supervision. *Journal of Speech and Hearing Disorders, 31,* 383–387, 1966.

Bullock, L. M. and Whelan, R. J. Competencies Needed by Teachers of the Emotionally Disturbed and Socially Maladjusted. *Exceptional Children, 30.* 67–73, 1971.

Caccamo, J. M. Accountability—A Matter of Ethics? *Asha, 15,* 411–412, 1973.

Calvert, D. O. and Bruder, E. J. *Determining Cost of Speech and Hearing Services.* Washington,. D.C.: American Speech, Language and Hearing Association, 1971.

Chronology of Development of New Definitions of Hearing Impairment, Deaf, and Hard of Hearing. Proceedings from the Conference of Executives of American Schools for the Deaf. Greensboro, North Carolina, June, 1975.

Conway, M. E., Sherertz, D. D., Lazarus, C. B. et al. *Massachusetts General Hospital*

Utility Multi-Programming System (MUMPS). Rockville, Maryland: Health, Education and Welfare, Public Health Service, National Resources Administration, 1975.

Coombs, Philip H. *The World Educational Crisis: A Systems Analysis.* New York: Oxford University Press, 1968.

Cooper, E. B. Client-clinician relationships and concomitant factors in stuttering therapy. *Journal of Speech and Hearing Research, 9,* 194–207, 1966.

Crystal, D. *Linguistics.* Baltimore, Maryland: Penguin Books, Inc., 1971.

Cullata, R., Colucci, S., and Wiggins, E. Communication between clinician and supervisor. Unpublished paper, University of Pittsburgh, 1974.

Curlee, R. A. A Computer-Assisted PSRO. *Asha, 15,* 415–421, 1973.

Dale, P. S. *Language Development: Structure and Function.* Hinsdale, Ill.: The Dryden Press, Inc., 1972.

Davis, G. An examination of dialogue and certain other factors and their influence on interaction between the client and the therapist in the therapeutic process in speech and hearing. Unpublished Ph.D. dissertation, Ohio State University, 1968.

Dempsey, D. The Right to Read. *Saturday Review,* April 17, 1971.

Diebold, J. *Business Decisions and Technological Change.* New York: Praeger Publishers, 1970.

Diedrich, W. Assessment of the Clinical Process. *Journal of the Kansas Speech and Hearing Association,* 1969.

Diedrich, W. *Counting and charting target phonemes from conversation.* University of Kansas; Audio-visual Center, 1972. (16mm film)

DiGiammarino, F. P. *CORE Evaluation Manual: Project LEADS.* Lexington, Massachusetts: Massachusetts Department of Education, Division of Special Education and Lexington Public School System, 1976.

Dorwood, B. A comparison of the Competencies for Regular Classroom Teachers and Teachers of Emotionally Disturbed Children. *Exceptional Children, 30,* 67–73, 1963.

Drucker, Peter F. *The Effective Executive.* New York: Harper and Row, 1966.

Drucker, P. F. *The Practice of Management.* New York: Harper and Row, 1954.

Drucker, P. F. *Technology, Management and Society.* New York: Harper and Row, 1970.

Dublinske, S. *Program Goals and Objectives: State of Vermont's Supervisory Unions and Districts.* Montpelier, Vermont: Vermont State Department of Education, 1975.

Dublinske, S. and Grimes, J. *Program Planning Evaluation.* Montpelier, Vermont: Vermont State Department of Education, 1971.

Dublinske, S. and Grimes, J. *PPE: Program Planning and Evaluation.* Des Moines, Iowa: Iowa State Department of Public Instruction, 1970.

Dyer, M., Competency-Based Teacher Education. *American Education,* November, 38–39, 1974.

Education for All Handicapped Children's Act. P.L. 94–142. 94th Session, U.S. Congress, Washington, D.C., 1975.

Education of the Handicapped Act. P.L. 93-380. 93rd Session, U.S. Congress, Washington,

D.C., 1974.

Elliot, Lois et al. Description of a Computer-Oriented Record-Keeping system. *Asha, 13,* 435–443, (1971).

Elliot, L. and Vegley, A. Notes on clinical record-keeping systems. *Asha, 13,* 444–446, 1971.

Emerick, L. L. and Hatten, J. T. *Diagnosis and Evaluation in Speech Pathology.* Englewood Cliffs: Prentice-Hall, 1974.

Fink, A. J. Teacher-Pupil Interaction in Classes for the Emotionally Handicapped. *Exceptional Children, 30,* 67–73, 1963.

Flanders, N. A. *Teacher Influence, Pupil Attitudes and Achievement.* Washington, D.C.: USGPO, (1965).

Fleisher, D. S. Priorities and Data Bases: Their Relationship to Continuing Education. *Fostering the Growing Need to Learn,* 1974.

Forbes, R. F. Cost Effectiveness Analysis Primer and Guidelines. *Educational Technology, 14,* 21–27, 1974.

Fourth Regional Workshop on Rehabilitation Codes and Communication Disorders. Carmel Valley, California, 1966.

Freire, Paulo. *Pedagogy of the Oppressed.* New York: Herder and Herder, 1970.

Gallager, J., Surles, R., and Hayes, A. *Program Planning and Evaluation.* Chapel Hill, North Carolina: First Chance for Children, 1973.

Geers, A. V. and Coaker, F. W. *The Computer-Oriented Record-Keeping System (CORKS).* St. Louis, Missouri: Privately printed, 1974.

Grady, M. J., Jr. *Cooperative Accountability Project: Using Educational Indicators for Program Accountability,* Madison, Wisconsin: Wisconsin Department of Public Instruction, 1974.

Granger, C. *A System for Management of Selected Data in Medical Rehabilitation.* Boston, Massachusetts: Privately printed, 1973.

Griffin, K. M., Rogin, C. M., and Stormer, J. *Child Services Review System.* Rockville, Md.: American Speech, Language and Hearing Association, 1976.

Halfond, M. Clinical Supervision—Stepchild in Training. *Asha, 6,* 441–447, 1964.

Hartman, E. The Cost of Computer Assisted Instruction. *Educational Technology Magazine,* December, 1971.

Havelock, R., Benne, K. An Exploratory Study of Knowledge Utilization. In G. Watson (Ed.), *Concepts for Social Change.* Washington, D.C.: National Training Laboratory, N.E.A., 1967.

Hawthorne, P. *Characteristics of and Proposed Models for State Accountability Legislation.* State Education Accountability Repository (SEAR) Cooperative Accountability Project, Denver, Colorado, 1973.

Hawthorne, P. *Cooperative Accountability Project: Legislation by the States: Accountability and Assessment in Education.* Madison, Wisconsin: Wisconsin Department of Public Instruction, 1974.

Healey, W. C. and Karp-Nortman, D. S. *The Hearing Impaired Mentally Retarded.* Washington, D.C.: American Speech and Hearing Association, 1975.

Healey, W. C. *Standards and Guidelines for Comprehensive Language, Speech and Hearing Programs in the Schools.* Washington, D.C.: American Speech, Lan-

guage and Hearing Association, 1974.
Healey, W. C. and Jones, S. *Guidelines for Evaluating State Education Laws and Regulations.* Washington, D.C.: American Speech, Language and Hearing Association, 1975.
Healey, W. C. and Jones, S. *Program Development and Management Evaluation.* Washington, D.C.: American Speech, Language and Hearing Association, 1973.
Healey, W. C., Ludlow, C., and Glassman, L. *National Evaluation of Educational District Needs Final Report.* Washington, D.C.: American Speech, Language and Hearing Association, 1975.
Healey, W. C., Pikus, A., Roth, F., and O'Reilly, A. *Comprehensive Assessment and Service Evaluation Information System.* Washington, D.C.: American Speech and Hearing Association, 1973.
Holderman, J. B. Executive director's Report No. 86, State of Illinois, Board of Higher Education, May 5, 1970.
Hostrop, R. W. *Managing Education for Results.* Homewood, Illinois: ETC Publications, 1973.
Hostrop, R. W. *Teaching and the Community College Library.* Hamden, Connecticut: The Shoe String Press, Inc., 1968.
Hubbard, C., Jahoda, G., and Torter, R. A systems approach to library problem-solving. *Educational Technology Magazine,* February, 1972.
Irwin, R. B. Microsupervision: A study of the behaviors of supervisors of speech clinicians. Presented at the American Speech, Language and Hearing National Convention, Chicago, 1971.
Jeffers, J. *Audiology Services Needed by Public Schools, Competencies Needed by Audiologists to Perform Services.* California State University, 1973.
Johnson, T. S. The Development of a Multidimensional Scoring System for Observing in the Clinical Process in Pathology. In T. S. Johnson (Ed.), *Clinical Interaction and Its Measurement.* Department of Communicative Disorders, Utah State University, 1971.
Jones, R. Accountability in Special Education: Some Problems. *Exceptional Children, 39,* 631–642, 1973.
Journot, V. *The Tabulated Accountability Plan for Speech Therapy Services.* Hurst, Texas: Privately printed, 1973.
Kakalik, J. et al. *Services for Handicapped Youth: A Program Overview.* Santa Monica, California: Rand Corporation, 1973.
Kent, L. R. *Language Acquisition Program.* Michigan: Privately printed, 1972.
Kerr, C. Four Decades of Educational Commissions. *Change, 9,* 4–5, 64, November, 1973.
Klevens, D. R. and Volz, H. B. The Development of a Clinical Evaluation Procedure. Presented at the American Speech, Language and Hearing Association National Convention, Detroit, 1973.
Konon, M. J. A Program Management Oriented Documentation System for CCS Program Automated Support. *MCH Exchange, 2,* 1–7, 1972.
Landry, L. *The Scope, Purpose and Procedures of Accreditation by Contract.* Denver,

Colorado: Colorado Department of Education, 1971.
Lawrence, P. R. and Lorsch, J. W. *Organization and Environment.* Homewood, Illinois: Richard D. Irwin, 1969.
Livingston, S. A. Will a Simulation Game Improve Student Learning of Related Factual Material? *Educational Technology Magazine,* December, 1971.
Lorentz, J. A Computer System for Behaviorally Oriented Curriculum Objectives. *Educational Technology, 15,* 26–31, 1975.
Lyons, J. (Ed.), *New Horizons in Linguistics.* Baltimore, Maryland: Penguin Books, 1970.
Mackenzie, R. A. The Management Process in 3-D. *Harvard Business Review,* November–December, 1969.
Mackie, R. P., Kvaraceus, W., and Williams, H. *Teachers of Children Who Are Socially and Emotionally Handicapped.* Washington, D.C.: U.S. Govt. Print. Office, 1957.
Marland, S. P., Jr. Accountability in Education. *Teachers College Record,* February, 1972.
McGregor, D. M. *The Human Side of the Enterprise.* New York: McGraw-Hill, 1960.
Meyen, E. L., Connolly, A. J., Chandler, M. R., and Altman, R. Prototype Training Program for the Preparation of Curriculum Consultants for Exceptional Children. Department of Health, Education, and Welfare, United States Office of Education, Bureau of Education for the Handicapped, Division of Training, November, 1971.
Mowrer, D. Accountability and Speech Therapy in the Public Schools. *Asha, 14,* 111–115, 1972.
Nelson, G. Supervised Training in Clinical Supervision. Presented at the American Speech, Language and Hearing Association National Convention, San Francisco, 1972.
Nelson, G. University Supervision of Clinical Practicum in Speech and Language Pathology: Let's Set Some Standards! Presented at the American Speech, Language and Hearing Association National Convention, Detroit, 1973.
Odiorne, G. S. *Management by Objectives.* New York: Pitman, 1965.
O'Toole, T. Accountability and the Clinician in the Schools. *Language, Speech and Hearing Services in Schools, 2,* 14–32, 1970.
Perkins, W., Shelton, R., Studebaker, G., and Goldstein, R. The National Examination in Speech Pathology and Audiology: Philosophy and Operation. *Asha, 12,* 175–181, 1970.
Peter, L. J and Hull, R. *The Peter Principle.* New York: William Morrow, 1969.
Prather, E. An Approach to Clinical Supervision. *Asha, 9,* 471–481, 1967.
Privacy Act. P.L. 93-579 (U.S. Code Section 552-a), 93rd Session, U.S. Congress, Washington, D.C., 1974.
PSRO Management Information System. Rockville, Maryland: Bureau of Quality Assurance, Health Service Administration, Department of Health, Education and Welfare, September, 1975.
PSRO Data Routing and Processing Policies: Memorandum to PSRO Planning, Conditional and Support Center Organizations. Director of Quality Assurance, Depart-

ment of Health, Education and Welfare, Health Services Administration, Bureau of Quality Assurance, Washington, D.C.: unpublished, 1975.

Putnam, J. F. *Student/Pupil Accounting: Standard Terminology and Guide for Managing Student Data in Elementary and Secondary Schools, Community Junior Colleges and Adult Education.* Washington, D.C.: U.S. Govt. Print. Office, 1974.

Quay, H. C. Special education: Assumptions, Techniques, and Evaluative Criteria. *Exceptional Children, 40,* 165–170, 1973.

Reynolds, M. C. and Balow, B. Categories and Variables in Special Education. *Exceptional Children, 38,* 357–366, 1972.

Roberts, C. T. and Lichtenberger, A. R. *Financial Accounting: Classifications and Standard Technology for Local and State School Systems.* Washington, D.C.: U.S. Govt. Print. Office, 1973.

Rosenshine, B. and Furst, N. Research on Teacher Performance Criteria. In B. O. Smith (Ed.), *Research in Teacher Education—A Symposium.* Englewood Cliffs: Prentice-Hall, 1971.

Rossmiller, R. A., Hale, J. A., and Frohreich, L. F. Educational Programs for Exceptional Children: Resource Configurations and Costs (National Educational Finance Project Special Study No. 2). Madison: University of Wisconsin, 1970.

Roth, B. Research Needs in Supervision. In L. J. Turton (Ed.), *Proceedings of a Workshop on Supervision in Speech Pathology.* Ann Arbor: University of Michigan, 1974.

Ruebhausen, O. N. Preface, In *Guidelines for the collection maintenance and dissemination of pupil records.* Hartford, Connecticut: Russell Sage Foundation, 1970, pp. 5–7.

Schalk, M. C. Consistency and reliability of supervisory evaluations at university training centers. Presented at the American Speech and Hearing Association National Convention, San Francisco, 1972.

Schubert, G. W. *The Analysis of Behavior of Clinicians (ABC) System.* Grand Forks, North Dakota: University of North Dakota, 1974.

Shores, R., Cegelka, P., and Nelson, C. M. Competency-Based Special Education Teacher Training. *Exceptional Children, 40,* 192–198, 1973.

Shriberg, L. D. Study of Supervisory Effectiveness and Efficiency. Unpublished paper, Madison: University of Wisconsin, 1972.

Steck, E. L. Base Rate of Reinforcer Use in Clinical Practice: Inventory, Modulation, and Frequency of Use of Reinforcers in Speech Pathology. Presented at the American Speech and Hearing Association National Convention, Chicago, 1971.

Stinson, J. E. and Robertson, J. H. Follower-Maturity and Preference of Leader Behavior Style. *Psychological Reports, 32,* 247–250, 1973.

Task Force Report on Data Collection and Information Systems, American Speech and Hearing Association. *Language, Speech and Hearing Services in Schools, 4,* 57–77, 1976.

Task Force on Learning Disabilities. Position Statement of the American Speech and Hearing Association. *Asha, 18,* 282–290, 1976.

Thompson, R. B. *A Systems Approach to Instruction.* Hamden, Conn.: The Shoe

String Press, 1971.
Toffler, Alvin. *Future Shock.* New York: Random House, 1970.
Townsend, R. *Up the Organization.* New York: Alfred A. Knopf, 1970.
Trudeau, E. et al. *Digest of State Laws and Regulations for School Language, Speech and Hearing Programs.* Washington, D.C.: State-Federal Information Clearing House for Children of the Council of Exceptional Children and the American Speech and Hearing Association, 1973.
Van Dusseldorp, R. Some principles for the development of management information systems. *Management Information Systems in Higher Education: The State of the Art.* Durham, North Carolina: Duke University Press, 1969.
Van Riper, C. *WMU Journal of Speech Therapy, 8, (3),* 1–9, 1971.
Ward, L. and Webster, E. The training of clinical personnel: I. Issues in conceptualization. *Asha, 7,* 38–40, 1965a.
Ward, L. and Webster, E. The Training of Clinical Personnel: II. A Concept of Clinical Preparation. *Asha, 7,* 103–106, (1965b).
White, O. R. *A Glossary of Behavioral Terminology.* Champaign, Illinois: Research Press, 1971.
White, R. et al. *Anne Arundel County Special Service Information System.* Baltimore, Maryland: Maryland State Department of Education, 1975.
White, R. et al. *Special Service Information System.* Baltimore, Maryland State Department of Education, 1974.
Wing, D. M., A data recording form for case management and accountability. *Language, Speech and Hearing Services in Schools, 6,* 38–40, 1975.
Woodbury County. *Program Goals and Objectives.* Des Moines, Iowa: Iowa State Department of Public Instruction, 1973.
Work, R. S., Hutchinson, E. C., Healey, W. C., Sommers, R. K., and Stevens, E. I. Accountability in a School Speech and Language Program: Part I: Cost Accounting. *Language, Speech and Hearing Services in Schools, 7(1),* January, 1975.
Work, R. S., Hutchinson, E. C., Healey, W. C., Sommers, R. K., and Stevens, E. I. Accountability in a School Speech and Language Program: Part II: Instructional Materials Analysis. *Language, Speech, and Hearing Services in Schools, 7(4),* October, 1976.
Zani, W. M. Blueprint for MIS. *Harvard Business Review,* November–December, 1970.

Chapter 7

COMMUNICATING: IN THE SCHOOLS, TO THE COMMUNITY

Thelma P. Albritton

COMMUNICATING THROUGH RECORDS AND REPORTS

Records and reports are essential documents in communicating in schools by speech-language pathologists. They are the official documents that contain all information about individuals enrolled for speech-language treatment by the SLP. Records are maintained in a systematic file that describes evaluation results and treatment plans.

In recent years, records and reports have become the accountability instrument for the SLP. The written accounts of the needs of speech-language handicapped children and the services provided for them have been a measurable device whereby justifiably interested school administrators can see what has been done for children in their school systems. Experience has taught speech-language pathologists that their work can no longer be viewed and implemented only as the individual SLP views it, but that they must have records and reports to verify the services provided. Never in the history of the profession have records and reports been more essential to the work of the SLP in schools than they are in this decade.

Historically, record keeping and reporting by the SLP have ranged from a simple listing of names of school children on the case load to a complete individual file for each client of all services provided including detailed reporting of evaluation, treatment, correspondence and progress notes. Where minimum recording keeping has occurred in the past, it has been a poor index to growth in clients served and has provided little in the way of accountability for speech-language pathologists. Complete records, on the other hand, have been an excellent yardstick of progress made by clients and a means of measuring how, why, and when improvement was made.

Some speech-language pathologists argue that the practice of speech-language therapy in the schools does not require the record keeping that "clinics" in other environments require because of the nature of the speech-language disorders or because of the size of the case load being served. Neither argument can be substantiated any longer. Services to clients must be equal in quality, including records and reports, regardless of work environment.

The advent of state mandates for special services for children in schools and the federal mandate under P.L. 94-142 have established requirements for speech-language pathologists in certain managerial aspects of their work and particularly in the record-keeping area. Certain written documents now required by law no longer allow the SLP to decide independently how much or how little will be done in the record-keeping and reporting areas. While the "paperwork" aspect of the state and federal mandates appears to some to be awesome, to others it is a reasonable requirement and one that will be a critical indicator of how, why, and when services are provided.

In summary, the importance of the development and maintenance of complete records for each client served in the schools and the regular reporting of client progress and of other pertinent information to the schools are critical indicators of accountability of the SLP and of services provided to children. To better define and describe the record-keeping tasks and the reporting tasks of the speech-language pathologists, each topic will be treated as a separate function rather than as one single function. The first part of this chapter is devoted to the record-keeping procedures, and the second part will describe the essential reporting aspects in the management of speech-language-hearing programs in schools.

Records as Documentation

Records that detail all services provided to the school client from admission to discharge become the official document for each client receiving services from the SLP. These individual documents are a means of preserving the written accounts of what has been done for a client. The records must be sufficiently complete to enable any authorized person to understand the diagnosis of the client, treatment plans developed for the client, progress made by the client, and, when appropriate, reasons for dismissal. The records must be easily readable with terminology familiar to speech-language pathologists and other specialists who may review the records. This is especially true when multiple services are provided to the same client.

Records may be viewed as verification of what has been done, by whom, for what purpose, how often, and the known outcomes. The charting is quite similar to the familiar charts of patients in a hospital. The major differences are those of style, information desired, and general appearance.

The individual speech-language-hearing record becomes a document usable by school administrators, school health specialists, teachers, special educators, and as a resource for referral purposes. The document should be developed in an orderly manner so that the most recent information appears first in the file. All information should be concise and to the point. All material must be *dated* to have any significant meaning to the reader. The accounts should be entered into the record on a systematic and regular basis so that it becomes a cumulative record of services.

As the individual student record develops and enlarges as services are continued over a long period of time, the record becomes an increasingly useful tool for some of the following purposes: (1) data for administrators for projection of estimated length of services needed by certain clients, (2) data for research projects, (3) projecting staff needs, (4) cost accounting, (5) speech-language pathologist accountability, (6) verification of services rendered, (7) data for determining educational planning and placement, and (8) essential data in case of litigation. The possibility of litigation is far more prevalent today then ever before, which requires the SLP to produce documents for evidence of diagnosis of and services for clients. In this day of "rights" for every person, every group, and every cause, records are essential for the protection of the persons responsible for delivering speech-language-hearing services. Never has any aspect of the work of the SLP been more important, more useful, and more protective for both client and specialist as is the document that openly and honestly verifies everything that has been done for a client. Again, it should be emphasized that it is for the SLP's protection as well as that of the client that a complete individual record be developed and maintained on any client for which any service is provided.

CONTENTS OF RECORDS

Whether the records are referred to as files, charts, folders, cumulative records, cards, or case records, the contents should be basically the same. All records for clients enrolled or admitted to programs for speech-language-hearing services should contain the following:
1. Personal identification data
2. A clear, concise statement regarding diagnosis
3. Referral source
4. Case history
5. Individual Education Plan that includes: evaluation reports, treatment plans and/or educational plans, and appropriate signatures
6. Correspondence and reports to and from medical, psychological, and educational specialists
7. Chronological logs of all services (these should include attendance records and progress notes)
8. Audiological reports
9. Progress reports
10. Discharge reports, letters, or notices
11. Optional: Recorded speech-language samples and analysis
12. Signed release forms

The above record contents will ensure and facilitate easy retrieval of information about each student as well as provide an excellent monitoring device for managing the case. One may argue the merits of including all of the above information for the mild articulation client while seeing the merits of including all of the above for the severe language disordered client. If a client's speech is sufficiently deficient to merit the time and services of the SLP, then the development of the individual record is equally meritorious. If one can see the individual client record as a useful tool rather than a useless motion in paperwork, then the development of the record will be done with greater acceptance and ease.

Description of Content

Each of the following twelve areas of information contained in the speech-language-hearing record is representative of a complete record for clients in speech-language-hearing programs. The accuracy and completeness of each record are dependent on the entries made by the SLP.

1. The *Personal Identification Data* include the name of the student, current address, name of parents and/or guardian, phone numbers, emergency phone numbers, school name, teacher's name and grade, brothers and sisters (if desired), and any other desired information felt to be pertinent to the identification of the client. This information is usually entered on a prepared form that carries the name of the school system. Some personal preferences may be considered in the design of the format so that it may be used more efficiently. (See Chapter 3, Appendix E for an example of an I.E.P. form.)

2. The *Diagnosis*, although included in the I.E.P., should be conspicuously placed in the record.

3. The *Referral Source* may appear on some of the Personal Identification Data forms, although these are most often separate forms. Figure 7-1 is a referral form for teachers. The referral source or form should contain sufficient information to assist the speech-language pathologist in selecting appropriate evaluation instruments to conduct the evaluation. The Referral Source should include the reason for referral, i.e. a brief description of the speech-language of concern to the referring person. It should contain the name of the referral source and the name and location of the client. Appendix A includes this.

4. The *Case History* used for school records may be an abbreviated version of what is often used in nonschool clinics. Essentially the information needed is a profile of the child's family, his developmental history, his medical history, his social history, and his educational history. The format should be simple in requesting the above information in that the Case History may be obtained

REFERRAL

Name of Child _____ Grade _____
                last   first

Date of Referral _____ School _____ Room No. ____

Reason(s) for Referral _____

_____

_____

_____

_____

Referred by _____
           signature   title

- -

EVALUATION

Name of Child _____ Grade _____
                last   first

Date of Evaluation _____ School _____ Room No. ____

Referred by _____ Date of Referral _____

Reason(s) for Referral _____

_____

Findings _____

_____

_____

Disposition _____

Evaluated by _____
           signature   title

_____

Figure 7-1. Speech-Language-Hearing Referral Form.

by sending a form such as that in Appendix A to the parents or guardian and having it completed at home and returned to the SLP. The value of obtaining the history is based on the belief that it is helpful to have knowledge of a child's family along with information about the child's development. The SLP has no other way of obtaining this information if the case history is not used. In practice, most school speech-language pathologists do not include a case history. The reasons given for not including this practice are generally based on time and value of the case history. The

SPECIAL EDUCATION UNIT
Printed Here

Date _____

Dear Parent (s) or Guardian:

Your child, _____ , has received a speech-language evaluation at school. At this time your child's speech-language is considered to be:

☐ adequate.
☐ in need of reevaluation at a later date.
☐ in need of speech service.

Your child is enrolled for speech-language class at _____

_____ on _____
and _____ from _____
to _____ . This service is a part of your school's educational program provided at no extra cost to you.

I would appreciate your completing the enclosed form and returning it to me.

I may contact you at a later date for a conference appointment. At that time we will discuss your child's speech-language and how your child may be helped at home.

Feel welcome to attend speech-language class on any day when your child is scheduled to receive therapy. Please contact me if you have any questions regarding your child's speech. I shall appreciate your cooperation.

Sincerely,

Figure 7-2. A form for notifying parents.

suggestion here is to make it a simple format and simple procedure by sending a form home to obtain the information desired. The information obtained should be placed in the file and used appropriately in the management of the client. Figure 7-2 is an example of a form letter that can accompany the history form and also informs the parents that their child is scheduled for assistance.

5. The *Individual Education Plan (I.E.P.)* requires very specific information. The format used is at the discretion of the school system with adherence to the federal mandate. Basically, the information that is included on the IEP is a statement of the problem or present level of performance; goals and objectives, both short-term and long-term; specific placement in a special education program; evaluation procedures to be used and when completed the evaluation tools used and a report of the outcomes. It is essential that the I.E.P. be signed by the speech-language pathologist, the parent or guardian, the supervisor, and a classroom teacher where applicable. The I.E.P. is invalid without the proper signatures. It is not legal to "sign off" for any of the above persons in the I.E.P. procedure. School specialists have developed a variety of useful tools that amplify the I.E.P., particularly in the charting of performance of clients to indicate progress. These tools, such as charts for success and failure performances, are critical indicators of both the value of the treatment provided and the response of the client to the treatment procedures. Use of performance charts permits modification of methods and techniques of treatment when failure rates outnumber success rates. Another important component of the file is to develop a narrative report of the diagnosis and evaluation procedures, findings, outcomes and recommendations. This indepth diagnostic report may be brief, yet it is indispensable in understanding the problem of the student and documenting how the diagnosis was reached. The clear, concise, and succinct description of the evaluation and of the treatment plans will enable parents and other professionals to understand the goals set for the client. The least the record or IEP should show is a compendious effort to identify client needs and plans established to meet the client's needs.

6. *Correspondence and Professional Reports* to and from specialists such as medicine, psychology, and education must be placed in the

client's record. These documents often pertain to critical decisions made by related professions, which enable the SLP to reach appropriate decisions about clients. Such correspondence is considered essential in preparing a complete speech-language record.

7. The *Chronological Logs* are regular written accounts of that which takes place between the client and the SLP. These logs include attendance records, progress notes, communications between concerned parties such as phone calls and visits. The chronology provides the reader of the speech-language record an ongoing account of how the case is being managed. The format for logs varies from a plain sheet of paper with entries logged by dates to the inclusion of information entered in the log on special forms and special books such as a teacher plan book. The format for the log is not as important as maintaining the log on a regular basis.

8. *Audiological Reports*, when available, must be placed in the file. It is inconsequential that the report is negative, it is significant that an audiological assessment was made and is recorded in the file.

9. *Progress Reports* are prepared at periodic intervals to inform parents, guardians, teachers, and related disciplines of the progress toward the goals set forth in the I.E.P. Figure 7–3 is an example. The progress report should reflect growth and improvement in the client from one period to the next. These reports must not contain statements which may be misleading about the prognosis of the client. The report must simply contain current status of the success and failure of the client from period to period. When progress reports are issued regularly and contain factual information which includes failure along with success, concerned parents will have been informed. Then, in the event parents are dissatisfied and raise questions about the progress, the SLP will have sufficient documentation to defend the program. A related report is that prepared at the end of each year. Appendices G and H are examples of forms that can be used for such reports.

10. The *Dismissal Report* may be a simple letter or a prepared form notice. The information should be straightforward in saying exactly why the client was dismissed from the program. There are categories of conditions for dismissal, which include statements or conditions such as *reached maximum potential, speech-language prob-*

PROGRESS REPORT

Name of Child _____ Grade _____

School _____ Report To _____

Type of Service _____

Date of Report _____ Period Covered _____

OBJECTIVES:

OBSERVED CHANGES:

CURRENT DIAGNOSIS:

RECOMMENDATIONS:

CONTINUE SERVICE: ____ Yes ____ No ____ Recheck ____ Other

_____
Specialist

Figure 7-3. Progress Report.

lem corrected, treatment discontinued for reasons of..., moved from school, referred to another agency, and post-school age. Whatever the condition for discharge it should be accurate and defensible through the speech-language-hearing record.

11. Another component of the speech-language-hearing record is optional but highly recommended for severe speech-language-hearing problems. That is the option of making *audio and/or video recordings* of speech-language from admission to the program through discharge from the program. Recorded samples and analysis of speech-language behavior are far more concrete registers of the speech-language behavior than all of the written *perceptions* of

the speech-language problem by specialists. This practice is recommended for students presenting multiple handicaps who will require long-term care and a variety of special services. It is also recommended for short-term success rates. Audio and video recordings are indisputable documents that, if ever needed, provide the critical chronical data of the problem and the treatment. They are invaluable tools for the SLP working in schools today.

12. Finally, the *Signed Release Form* is a step that is necessary to obtain records from or send records to medical or nonschool specialities. Parents and/or guardians must sign for you to request records from other nonschool specialists, and they must sign for you to release materials to other nonschool specialists. Even if the school has blanket permission from parents and guardians to carry out this exchange of information, it is suggested that you further protect yourself by requesting the signed release forms as they are needed.

Packaging the Speech-Language-Hearing Record

The speech-language record is a compilation of many pieces of information. Appendix B is an example of a cumulative speech-language-hearing record. The assembly of the contents should be indexed in such a way that information is easily retrievable. Usually, the standard manilla folder is used to store or package the contents, as these can be stored in standard filing cabinets. To assure that contents are indexed in an orderly way, a system should be agreed upon by all speech-language pathologists working in the same school system to establish uniformity in records. Contents are grouped according to the list of contents previously provided and within each group the documents are entered in the record with the most recent entry in front. When this practice is used, uniformity is achieved, and a chronology of services is preserved.

In summary, the contents of the individual speech-language-hearing records must be developed for every admission to the speech-language program or case load as required by P.L. 94-142. Each student must have an Individual Education Plan developed specifically for him based on the evaluation data. No longer can some school specialists group types of disorders on a single sheet of paper with a minimum amount of information—limited generally to name, age, grade, teacher, disorder, admission and dismissal dates. It is no longer legal to operate with group reports. Group files are not allowed. Any state receiving federal financial assistance for schools must comply with P.L. 94-142. Put another way, any state's schools that receive federal assistance must comply with Public Law 94-142 and the record keeping requirement through the use of the Individual Education Plan (I.E.P.). In retrospect, it is unfortunate that our federal government had to mandate a procedure that should have been implemented in school programs, as in other clinic programs, many years ago. The predicted positive outcome of the record-keeping requirement (over the years) will provide valuable information that will be more readily available and more readily retrievable than ever before. One can assume that the practice of speech-language pathology in schools will be viewed more positively in years to come because of the documentation of the work. Accountability will be provided by the Speech-Language-Hearing Record.

Interrelationship of the Speech-Language-Hearing Record and the School Cumulative Record

The speech-language-hearing record as described in the previous pages is a complete written account of all services provided to the student and maintained by the SLP. The school cumulative record is a record of all data related to the child's years spent in school. The cumulative record contains such items as names of teachers grade by grade, promotions from grade to grade, health record, educational record overall, and any special services rendered during the school years. The cumulative record has limited space for entries related to special services such as speech-language-hearing services. An entry is made in the cumulative record that the service was provided, by whom, and for how long. It does not provide a full account of services. Cumulative records accompany a child from school to school, while the speech-language-hearing record usually remains in the school system, and only a summary of services is abstracted from the record and forwarded with the cumulative record. It is a most important and essential function of the SLP to forward a summary of information from the speech-language-hearing record along with the child's cumulative record when the child moves to another school. Communication between school officials, principals and teachers, and speech-language pathologists must be open and current so that the SLP is made aware that a report of the speech-language services will be needed for a child leaving a school.

The interrelationship of the speech-language-hearing record and the cumulative school record must be that of coordination, data entries, and follow-up for clients moving from one school to another. Communication between all professionals is essential to the efficiency with which these tasks are accomplished.

Security, Confidentiality, and Access to Records

Files and records of all kinds must be secured to the extent that confidentiality of the student is assured. The most secure system is one that can be locked. A filing cabinet that locks is ideal; however, all schools cannot provide locked cabinets, drawers, or desks for their clinicians, so they must often settle for having files in a locked room.

Access to the confidential files maintained by the speech-language specialist is limited to the SLP and other designated professionals. Under current laws, some files are open for inspection by parents, guardians, and even clients; however, this practice is interpreted differently by different professionals and in different environments. The safest policy regarding access to confidential records is to comply with district policy.

Security, confidentiality, and access to student records are interrelated in that to protect the confidentiality of the information written about the client the files must be guarded to the degree that confidentiality is assured. Access to the files by anyone other than authorized professionals is currently interpreted in a variety of ways. To be certain that unauthorized persons do not have access to the files, local school policy regarding the speech-language record should be followed.

Storage of Records and Length of Maintenance After Discharge

Records should be stored in a place that gives the SLP the easiest access to the files. The best place for each child's file is in the building where he receives speech-language therapy. The reason for this is that files must be readily available for clinicians to enter session or therapy notes following the session. If records are stored in a central office and access is limited to weekly entries, the efficiency of the record-keeping process is diminished and the task made more difficult for the SLP. The complete speech-language-hearing record for each individual must be easily accessible to the clinician *at the time* services are rendered. This practice does not preclude having an abbreviated summary of services for children admitted to the program in a central location. It is quite common to find statistical and abbreviated records in a central office in school systems.

The length of time that records are maintained after clients are discharged is determined by state regulations, SLP discretion, and school system policy. All schools maintain records on an active and inactive basis. The length of time that inactive files are maintained may be determined by reason for discharge in the first place, such as lack of progress; or other services necessary before proceeding with speech therapy; or discharged with maximum expected improvement achieved; or moved from school district; or graduated from school district; or moved to another program. Storage of bulky manilla folders that contain most of the speech-language-hearing records can be a space-consuming problem. For whatever reason a student is dismissed from the program, inactive records are usually maintained for a three-year period. If the student does not return to the school system within three years, the individual record should be reduced to a summary of the contents and forwarded to a central depository.

Caution should be exercised in the disposal of any records. There have been instances of clients who have made claims that a speech, language, or hearing disorder was due to an accident or the fault of an employer or work environment in the postschool years when the disorder was a matter of record during the elementary and secondary school years. Preserved records can provide valuable assistance to persons faced with such circumstances. A system for storing at least a summary of the diagnosis and treatment provided for school age children, which can be retrieved indefinitely, should be developed. In so doing the integrity of the SLP's work will have been preserved.

USE OF REPORTS IN COMMUNICATING TO THE SCHOOL AND COMMUNITY

Communicating to the school and community through written and verbal reports is the topic of this part of this chapter. There are a variety of ways to make known to others the work of the speech-language pathologist in the schools. The variety of ways in which reporting is done, as discussed here, are in no way the only methods by which reporting is accomplished. These are suggested modes with strong emphasis on some of them.

Purpose of Reporting

Reporting to teachers, principals, school administrators, school boards, parents, and to the public in general is a means of enunciating and documenting your work to others. The mystery of the itinerant SLP who, according to some school personnel, appears and disappears from one hour to the next, would be solved if regular communication through written and verbal reporting were as routine as providing speech-language therapy for students. Speech-language pathologists who are assigned to only one building do not always receive the same criticism as the itinerant SLP because their presence in a building is more evident. Being stationed in one school does not, however, relieve the SLP of reporting responsibility.

The purpose of reporting is to display professional accountability to professional colleagues, to the employer, and to the community at large. It may seem unfortunate to many speech-language pathologists to feel that they must *justify* their work to any extent. This author views reporting in our profession as one of the weakest areas of function. It is weak because the reporting aspects have been almost totally ignored in the schools except for documents that are required by a school system, state, or federal policy. It is regrettable that the excellent work of the school SLP has been so poorly reported over the years that the recognition of the superb accomplishments of so many have been virtually lost because of a lack of written and verbal reporting.

Routine reporting gives the SLP the much needed *recognition* for the work that has been accomplished. The excellent work of the SLP goes unrecognized because the work is known only to the SLP and to a lesser degree to parents and teachers.

Routine reporting also gives the SLP *visibility* through written reports and verbal presentations. Too many speech-language pathologists maintain a low profile and "don't make waves" attitude. Visibility is a powerful and influential component of the SLP that is often too obscure and too lacking to create any influence at all. One must plan and design methods to become visible in her or his work environment. Visibility in one's own profession is not only desirable but is a marketable component as well. In the profession of speech-language pathology and audiology there are no representatives to present or communicate the profession to the public except the individual herself. The only public representation that speech-language pathologists and audiologists have is through the American Speech-Language-Hearing Association (ASHA). ASHA has been expected to function in ways that are far beyond an organization's scope and purpose. The individual professional must contribute routinely to her own recognition and visibility if each professional is to have the respect and authority that are deserved.

The purpose of communicating our work to others seems quite clear. If we are to survive the professional competitiveness and criticism from colleagues, employers, and the community we serve, then it is incumbent upon all of us to improve and expand our communications through the use of widely distributed written accounts of our work and through a variety of personal appearances to represent our work.

Modes of Communication in Schools

There are a variety of modes of communication available to professionals working in schools. These include the use of *written reports* that are issued on a regular basis; direct interaction with parents, teachers, and administrators through face to face conferences and telephone conferences; *verbal presentations,* such as talks and workshops, for teachers, principals, parents, administrators, boards of education; and *direct communication* through the use of the public media: radio, television, and newspapers. Each of these modes will be discussed to encourage SLPs to improve their current practices in communicating regarding this profession and the services provided by a given SLP to others.

Written Reports

In a world where most information is obtained and reported on a "form" of some kind, from obtaining a driver's license to an individual's income tax report, the focus on written reports issued by SLPs will not emphasize forms. Forms are convenient packages of information that are efficient for storing information but are less efficient for conveying messages. You will find in this chapter a lack of emphasis on forms; the reason for that is the emphasis is placed on communication. The messages conveyed to persons to whom reports are sent must be written in such a way that they draw attention to the message and influence the reader with the message.

Let us consider the variety of statistical reports that are forwarded to administrators in school programs. Unfortunately these data, as important as they are, go forward with numbers only. The statistical reports must carry an interpretation of the data. The interpretation of the statistics being reported must reflect actualities of a given situation. If the statistics show a need for additional staff, then this should be stated in a paragraph or two, circled in red to draw attention to the significance of the data, and then forwarded. School administrators must plan and govern their budgets based on documented needs. Speech-language pathologists have neglected to provide the necessary documentation to help alleviate their needs and further develop their programs. Statistical reports are critical documents in justifying increases in personnel; in gaining support for space, materials, and supplies; and in supplying factual data for determining all components of programs. The only person responsible for providing this data is the SLP. The independence of the SLP permits her to provide only that which is required, while the emphasis should be on using every opportunity available to place the program in the eyes of those who control the existence of the program.

Other types of reports that are issued at least twice a year are progress reports to parents and teachers, with copies to principals and/or the immediate supervisor; disposition reports; and therapy schedules. This latter report is generated usually on request by other disciplines such as educational specialists and medical specialists. All of these reports should be presented in narrative form to gain the attention of the receiver of the report. When checklists are used to describe behaviors, accomplishments, and special needs, they are insufficient. The clear, readable, understandable narrative that describes exactly the message the SLP wishes to convey is by far the superior form of reporting. Good examples of this are the customary letters received from the medical profession, which simply describe the findings and recommendations. Figure 7-4 is an example of a yearly statistical summary and Figure 7-5 an end-of-year disposition report. These should not replace the suggested narrative reports but can serve as summaries.

The use of the everyday memorandum has never become standard practice with school SLPs. Using the memorandum to apprise, advise, influence, or gain support is a most efficient means of communicating speech-language program progress and needs to others. The memorandum need not be lengthy. Copies of all memos must be retained by the SLP as her personal documentation that a communiqué was made on a certain date about a certain matter. Using memos is highly recommended as standard practice in the schools.

Verbal Presentations and Workshops

Informing the school and community through the use of personal appearances at meetings and through workshops creates a high level of visibility for the speech-language pathologist. The personal appearance, when done well, can gain significant respect and understanding for the work of the SLP. It is acknowledged that not all people are skilled in public speaking, and many are so fearful of making public addresses that this opportunity for visibility and recognition is often lost. For those who are willing to put

Area Served _____

Period from _____ to _____ 19____

Total School Enrollment in Areas Served _____

	SPEECH	HEARING
Total Number of Students Evaluated	_____	_____
Number Evaluated as a Result of Previously Known Problems	_____	_____
Number Evaluated as a Result of Referral	_____	_____
Number Evaluated as a Result of Screening	_____	_____
Identify Grades Screened	_____	_____
Total Number of Students Receiving Service	_____	_____
Regularly Scheduled Service	_____	_____
Intermittently Scheduled Service	_____	_____
Indirect Service	_____	_____
Other	_____	_____
Total Number of Students on Waiting List	_____	_____
Total Number of Conferences	_____	_____
Total Number of Observations	_____	_____
Disposition of Students Receiving Service		
Continue	_____	_____
Dismissed as Satisfactory	_____	_____
Dismissed for Other Reasons _____	_____	_____
Other _____	_____	_____

Distribution of Students

Receiving Speech Services	Grades 1-6	Grades 7-12	Ungraded
Language	_____	_____	_____
Articulation	_____	_____	_____
Cleft Palate	_____	_____	_____
Cerebral Palsy	_____	_____	_____
Hearing	_____	_____	_____
Stuttering	_____	_____	_____
Voice	_____	_____	_____
Other	_____	_____	_____

Summary Submitted by _____ Date _____

Figure 7-4. Statistical Summary.

END OF YEAR DISPOSITION
FOR CHILDREN RECEIVING SPEECH-LANGUAGE-HEARING SERVICE

School _____ Date _____ Specialist _____

Name of Child	Grade	HEARING			SPEECH					
		Continue	Other	Remark	Continue	Dismissed Satisfactory	Dismissed Other	Recheck	Disorder (See Code)	Remark
last first										
Totals										

Disorder Code   Hearing Handicapped (HH);   Articulation (A);   Cleft Palate (CL P);
                 Cerebral Palsy (CP);   Stuttering (S);   Voice (V);   Other (O)

Figure 7-5. End of Year Disposition for Children Receiving Speech-Language-Hearing Services and Annual Report.

themselves in the speaker's spotlight with a well-articulated message and an interesting and meaningful message, the benefits gained are incredibly positive. Appearing before teachers at their regular meetings is an easy approach to this mode of communicating program goals and operations. Extensive planning should go into any presentation to ensure that the messages are clear and concise and that the amount of time needed to convey the messages is held to a minimum. When presentations are ill prepared and more time is taken than is needed to say what needed to be said, then this means of communicating the program has been defeated and criticism will follow. One basic principle must be respected when taking up valuable time of teachers and administrators: the SLP must present verbal material that could not be very well presented in a written form, or the verbal presentation must enhance something that was presented in the written form. It would be a great mistake to distribute a written report and then proceed to read it to the audience.

The SLP must not wait for an invitation to make a personal appearance before meetings of teachers, parents, administrators, and the community at large. She must seek out the opportunities to appear and be scheduled properly to appear before a particular group. For addressing teachers, such arrangements are made through the building principal. Inform the principal of your desire to have some time at teacher meetings to report to them on a regular basis. Appeal to officers of Parent Organizations to permit you to be the speaker at one of their meetings. When it is felt appropriate, seek the approval of your supervisor to make presentations to administrative personnel and boards of education. An amazing change can take place when well constructed presentations are made to the latter group. It is emphasized here that the presentations must be made by the SLP rather than assuming that the SLP has been properly represented by a supervisor who is not a member of the profession.

Workshops designed to provide in-depth information about speech-language-hearing disorders are an excellent means of gaining recognition and visibility. Workshops for teachers have never been so needed as they are now in implementing P.L. 94-142. Confusion may be reduced if workshops are instituted to help teachers to become educated about special children and their needs. In almost all school calendars there are designated days for teachers for workshops and institutes in which the activities are considered continuing education. The author has participated in many of these over the country and can say with great confidence that much of this activity could and perhaps should have been handled by the clinicians employed in the schools. The SLP must plan her calendar along with that of the teachers and offer to provide a workshop for teachers when the opportunity arises.

Workshops for parents should be a part of the program and responsibilities of the SLP as well as for teachers. The experience of the author in this activity has been to establish parent education workshops and classes through the school system's Adult or Community Education Programs. Almost all school systems have these programs now, and it is quite easy to establish a class or workshop under the auspices of the Adult Education Program. In the first place, most of the classes are offered in the evening when parents are free to attend. Second, the SLP may be paid additionally to teach these classes or workshops, and third, parents must register and pay a fee to take the classes or workshops, which tends to make parents committed to attending. The author found this opportunity for parent education to be one of the most challenging and the most rewarding of all of her work in school programs.

The opportunities for personal appearances to communicate with the school and with the community are virtually untapped. The challenge is there and must be sought by the SLP. The rewards gained from personal appearances far exceed rewards gained from other, less personal means of communicating. The SLP should be encouraged and go forward with a new and dynamic approach to communicating.

Communicating Through the Media

The greatest influence on people today seems to come through public media: radio, television, and newspapers. If the media are such powerful tools for conveying messages to the public, then they should be considered powerful tools for describing speech-language disorders, programs, and services to the public. Again, the SLP must take the responsibility and aggressively seek ways to use the media.

Radio interviews with local radio personalities about the SLP's work or about special problems creates interest and provides information to local listeners. Prepared radio spots may be distributed to highlight an upcoming program or to announce availability of services offered in schools. The author participated in a radio talk show in which speech disorders were discussed and listeners could call in questions and receive immediate answers. This experience proved that there is public interest in a field that is little known outside of the profession itself and that SLPs should pursue this medium more vigorously.

Television is an even more powerful means of communicating. If speech-language-hearing professionals can arrange appearances on local or national television to present information about speech-language disorders, ways of referring students, and about services in general, a larger audience will be reached and the messages made more visible and dramatic.

The use of the newspaper in communicating to the school and community is more readily available than either radio or television. Newspapers, bulletins, flyers, or any of a variety of written accounts that are distributed on a regular basis to the school and community are to be sought for getting an item released about the work of the SLP. Often local school systems have their own newspapers, which will offer space to the SLP for including information pertinent to her program. Finding a newspaper that will have interest in the material you wish to have published is the first step in the process. Preparing the material to be released is the second step. Planning feature articles for newspapers that have large circulations will attract the attention of thousands of readers in some instances. However, even small circulation local newspapers provide a good method for distributing information. Photographers and writers from the paper that is publishing the article should be invited to do the photography work and, through interview with the SLP, prepare the article. When a reporter prepares an article about the SLP and her program, the material should be received prior to publication to correct any errors in the information contained in the article. Newspaper releases containing inaccurate information or erroneous impressions about a program can do more harm than good.

ASHA can provide the speech-language pathologist with help in the media area, and persons interested in obtaining professional assistance should write the Director of Public Information, American Speech-Language-Hearing Association, 10801 Rockville Pike, Rockville, Maryland 20852.

SUMMARY

Communicating is an essential role of the speech-language pathologist. The written accounts of services to students are preserved through the speech-language record and become a critical instrument of accountability for the SLP.

The speech-language-hearing record is a complete document about an individual admitted to the speech-language program and the treatment that is provided until discharge. Each item in the speech-language-hearing record is placed in an orderly manner for easy retrieval of information. Files and records are confidential and are to be secured, with information provided to only authorized persons. Records are stored and maintained after discharge of clients for a period specified by the local school, state, or federal policy.

Reporting to the school and community on a regular basis through a variety of communication modes is recommended. The written report issued through attention-gaining narratives is emphasized. Use of the memorandum is highly recommended as a means of keeping school personnel informed on a regular basis and gaining support for the SLP's needs. Personal appearances to communicate with the school and with the community are included. Verbal presentations through meetings and workshops for school personnel and parents are suggested. The use of the media is viewed as a powerful and influential tool for communicating the work of the school professional in speech-language pathology.

The reporting role of the SLP is regarded as a significant means of accomplishing recognition and visibility for work in the schools. Reporting in a variety of ways is urged in aggressively seeking a mode of reporting that will gain the greatest advantage in conveying important messages to the school and to the community.

Each school speech-language pathologist is her or his own public relations person. In successfully accomplishing the missions outlined in this chapter the SLP needs to move from the current static position of only meeting the minimum required record-keeping and reporting functions to a dynamic and aggressive role expansion in these areas.

STUDY ACTIVITIES

1. Develop a format that will include the twelve items included in the Speech-language Record. Using a manilla folder, establish a mini-file for a given student.
2. Prepare a letter of referral to a medical specialist to refer a client with a voice disorder. Include in the letter your reason for referral and a description of the problem.
3. Using a local school form for Individual Education Plans, develop an I.E.P. for a student.
4. Prepare a narrative report to a parent for dismissing a child from therapy. Include in the report a summary of the diagnosis and treatment provided, the goals that were accomplished, and the reason for being discharged.
5. Make an audio recording of a client's speech. Analyze the speech and describe the problem.
6. Prepare a memorandum to the Supervisor of Speech Pathology and Audiology to defend a position that staff increases are needed. In your defense include data that will support your position. Make the memorandum convince and influence the reader to take positive action. Include exhibits.
7. Prepare an outline for a workshop for parents. Include in the outline the mode of presentation, the content, the requirements in terms of time and money commitments, and the expected outcomes.
8. Prepare a newspaper release for a program of your own or for one that you have visited. Describe the program in detail.

SOURCES OF INFORMATION

Information on the topics presented in this chapter is available from the American Speech-Language-Hearing Association, 10801 Rockville Pike, Rockville, Maryland 20852 and from Interstate Printers and Publishers, Inc., Danville, Illinois 61832.

REFERENCES

Collins, P. C. and Cunningham, G. *Writing Individualized Programs.* Tigard, Oregon: C.C. Publications, 1979.

Nation, James E. and Aram, D. M. *Diagnosis of Speech and Language Disorders.* St. Louis: Mosby, 1977.

Van Hattum, R. J. (Ed.). *Communication Disorders.* New York: Macmillan, 1980.

APPENDICES
FORMS

The following appendices are samples of forms used in a typical school program. These forms may be varied to serve individual needs.

APPENDIX A
INITIAL PARENT QUESTIONNAIRE

Date _____

Child's Name _____ Birthdate _____

Address _____ City _____ Zip _____

Person responsible for child _____ Mother _____ Father _____ Guardian _____ other

Name _____ Phone _____

Address (if different) _____ City _____ Zip _____

Person to be contacted in emergency

(other than listed above) _____ Relationship _____ Phone _____

Child's doctor _____ Phone _____

Address _____ City _____ Zip _____

School District in which you live _____ Nearest School _____

Who referred you to the Clinic? _____

List any previous speech, language, hearing or psychological evaluations or training received by the child _____

_____

_____

Please list other children in the family

Name	Age	Sex	School	Grade

_____

Please list others living in the home

Name		Relationship

_____

Are you a Medicaid recipient? _____ Yes _____ No Number _____

Are you a Medicare recipient? _____ Yes _____ No Number _____

Does your insurance cover _____ Speech Evaluation _____ Speech therapy

Company _____

Number _____

Initial Parent Questionnaire

BIRTH HISTORY

Health of mother during pregnancy _____

Any unusual illnesses
(measles, RH factor, etc.) _____

Any history of miscarriage _____ Pregnancy _____ months

Labor _____ hours Birthweight _____ lbs., _____ ozs. Birthlength _____ inches

Circle any of the following which applied:

    breech birth   instruments used
    dry birth   caesarean section
    trouble breathing at birth   unusual scars or bruises
    unusual color at birth   incubator used

DEVELOPMENTAL HISTORY

Sat alone _____ months   walked alone _____ months/years

Toilet trained day _____ months/years   toilet trained night _____ months/years

Physical development has been _____ rapid _____ normal _____ slow

Coordination is _____ good _____ clumsy

Feeding difficulty _____ yes _____ no If "yes," explain _____

_____

Swallowing or choking difficulty _____ Yes _____ No If "yes," explain _____

_____

Serious illnesses _____ Yes _____ No If "yes," explain _____

_____

History of _____ high fevers _____ seizures/convulsions _____ earaches _____ sore throats

Explain those checked _____

Serious accidents _____ Surgical operations _____ Tonsils or adenoids removed _____

Explain those checked _____

Allergic reactions _____ Eye problems _____ Loss of consciousness _____

Explain those checked _____

Is the child receiving medication? _____ Yes _____ No _____ Type _____ Dosage

Please describe briefly any medical or behavior problems not listed above _____

_____

Initial Parent Questionnaire

SPEECH and LANGUAGE HISTORY

Generally describe the child's behavior as an infant _____ good baby _____ demanding baby

Was the child responsive as an infant (cry or smile appropriately)? _____ Yes _____ No

If "no," explain _____

First words _____ months First sentence _____ months

Age at which you were first concerned about the child's speech _____ months

Briefly describe the child's present speech and what caused your concern _____

_____

_____

_____

_____

_____

_____

Can the child be understood by
    Mother _____   Strangers _____
    Father _____   Other children _____
    Relatives _____

Is the child aware of his speech problem _____ Yes _____ No

Does any other member of the family have a speech or hearing problem _____ Yes _____ No

If "yes," explain _____

PRESENT BEHAVIOR

Please write two or three sentences which characterize the child's behavior _____

_____

_____

_____

_____

Would the child separate easily for therapy _____ Yes _____ No

APPENDIX B

Speech-Language Programming in the Schools

CUMULATIVE SPEECH AND HEARING RECORD

Name _____ (Ink)   Sex _____ School _____ Address _____ Phone _____ Pupil No. _____
                                                                          (Pencil)   (Pencil)

Birthdate _____ month _____ day _____ year   Form Initiated by _____ Name _____ Title _____ Date Original Diagnosis _____ Completion Date Initial History _____

INSTRUCTIONS FOR ENTRY: Enter information in boxed sections for every child regularly scheduled. Collect and record additional information in each area as needed.

INITIAL   SPEECH AND HEARING   ENVIRONMENTAL   HISTORY

Problem _____

           Father or Guardian _____ Age _____ Occupation _____ Education _____
           Mother _____ Age _____ Occupation _____ Education _____

Date of Original Examination _____ Examiner _____ Title _____

           Brother(s) _____ Age(s) _____ Sister(s) _____ Age(s) _____

Previous Speech or Hearing Evaluations _____

           Influence of Other Individuals Living in the Home _____
           Influence of Paternal and Maternal Relatives _____
           Marital Status of Parents _____ Separated, divorced, dissension _____

Problem first noticed _____ Action Taken _____

           Family problem _____ Speech problems, deafness, alcoholism, mental health, etc.

           Siblings _____ Interaction, parental preference, total family relationships

Language Readiness _____ Auditory and pre-speech Behavior _____

           Methods of Discipline Used _____ Parental agreement on method _____

Meaningful Language Usage _____ Age—first word _____ two & three word combinations _____ sentences _____

           Socio-Economic Status _____ Size of house, ownership, play space, neighborhood, church membership, leisure time activities, etc.

Amount of Verbalization _____

PHYSIOLOGICAL — DEVELOPMENT

           Physical Anomalies _____ Mouth, ears, nose, eyes, teeth, etc.

Examination Results

           Chronic or Acute Conditions _____ Discharging ears, head noises, earache, mouth breathing

AUDIOLOGIC: _____

           Neuromuscular Condition _____ Coordination _____
           Age (months) at: first tooth _____ sitting _____ standing _____ walking _____
           feeding self _____ dressing self _____ bowel control _____ bladder control _____

ARTICULATION: _____

           Pregnancy _____ Duration and mother's health
           Birth _____ Normal, instrumental, premature, etc.

CONVERSATIONAL SPEECH: _____

           Feeding _____ Breast, bottle, problems, etc.

FLUENCY: _____

           Diseases: Age _____ Injuries: Age _____ Operations: Age _____

VERBAL OUTPUT: _____

           Sequale: _____

ABILITY TO COMMUNICATE: _____

           Health Habits _____ Diet, exercise, sleep, etc.

VOICE: _____ Pitch, quality, rate, loudness

Peripheral Speech Mechanism Deviations _____

           Physical and Dental Examinations _____
           Date _____ Doctor's Name _____ Address _____ Findings _____ Recommendations _____

Communicating: In the Schools, To the Community

BEHAVIORAL

Pupil Attitude Toward Problem
Parent Attitude Toward Problem
Social Behavior
  Peers (classroom, playground), siblings, adults

Teacher Description of Behavior

Observations of Behavior   Observations made by
Fears
Withdrawal
Habits
  Thumbsucking, etc.
Tantrums
Attention Span
Distractibility
Perseveration
Awareness of Environment
Consistency of Behavior Pattern
Psychologist Interpretation

Personality and Projective Tests	Date and Examiner	Results

EDUCATIONAL

Language Arts   Strengths and weaknesses
Attendance Record   Reason(s) for Frequent Absences

Test Results

Date Administered	Grade Level	Tests of Mental Ability	C.A.	Verbal M.A.	Non-Verbal M.A.	M.A.	IQ	Grade Place

Date Administered	Grade Level	Tests of Achievement Aptitude, Interest, etc.	Form	Findings

Age at entering School   Level at which entered (preschool, kindergarten, etc.)
Grades Repeated   Reason(s)
Likes   Dislikes
Most Difficult Subject(s)
Least Difficult Subject(s)
Teacher(s) Evaluation of Progress

Extra-curricular Activities

Work Experience   Outside School
Post-High School Plans   Complete for students in grade 9 or above

353

Chapter 8

ESTABLISHING THE THERAPY PROGRAM: CASE FINDING, CASE SELECTION, AND CASE LOAD

RONALD K. SOMMERS

MARGARET E. HATTON

Prior to the initiation of the therapy program, the speech-language pathologist is called upon to make a number of important professional decisions regarding program organization. What methods should be used to locate those children in need of help? Which of those identified should be selected for inclusion in the therapy program? How many children should be scheduled? These decisions will influence the type of therapy program significantly and, in the opinion of the experts, will influence the degree to which the program is successful in meeting the needs of children.

In professional terminology the method employed to locate children in need of services is called *case finding*, the system used to determine which children are scheduled is called *case selection*, and the number of children scheduled is called *case load*.

CASE FINDING

Locating those children who require clinical speech-language services is a type of problem solving. Of the many proposed methods for solving this problem, those used must meet the criteria of effectiveness and efficiency. The term *effectiveness* denotes the successful arrival at intended goals, while the term *efficiency* refers to techniques or procedures that are used competently and are not wasteful of time, effort, or information. Of the many case finding techniques that have been suggested or used by speech-language pathologists in the schools, most fail to meet one or both of these criteria. One technique, the survey method, appears most capable of being modified for specific circumstances, thus making it more effective and efficient than other approaches to the case finding problem.

THE SCREENING PROGRAM

The Education Amendments of 1974 (P.L. 93-380), requiring states to identify and evaluate all handicapped children, and the subsequent Education for all Handicapped Children Act of 1975 (P.L. 94-142), guaranteeing the right of all handicapped children to free and appropriate public education, require that the communication status of all school children should be assessed. "As a consequence the ASHA School Services Program recommends that all pupils suspected of being handicapped be screened by a speech-language pathologist and audiologist to determine the presence or absence of communicative disorders" (Dublinske and Healey, 1978).

Because considerable numbers of children, of preschool and school age, are involved, the clinician must determine the most effective and efficient procedures for locating speech-language defective children within the schools, i.e. case finding.

The ASHA Task Force on Screening Procedures in the Schools (1973) suggests three major steps in analyzing communication behavior problems of school children: rapid screening of the entire school population or of selected segments, extensive screening procedures for those whose initial tests indicate possible problems, followed by complete diagnostic evaluation of those apparent candidates for clinical intervention. Screening should be thought of as a quick general testing procedure, the purpose being that of eliminating children determined to have "normal" speech and language, leaving to be dealt with only those children needing further diagnostic evaluation.

Careful organization of the screening program is essential. Basic decisions to be made are what groups are to be screened, with rationale for choosing these groups over others; who will do the screening; what procedures will be used; how much time will be alloted; what materials will be used; where the screening will be done; what forms are to be used for recording and reporting.

Groups to Be Screened

Whether or not one would screen the entire population of the schools served would depend upon a number of factors, including available time and personnel. If there has been an ongoing and effective program of speech-language remediation, the yearly screening of all children in all grades would not seem necessary. Typically, selected grades are screened each year with suspected speech-language handicapped students from the remaining grades being referred by their classroom teachers. All children previously enrolled in therapy are evaluated.

There is a lack of agreement as to which grades should be selected for screening. Some SLPs would screen all kindergarten and first grade children with the rationale that the sooner the deviations are identified and remediated the better. Many clinicians would prefer to take advantage of the maturation that occurs during these early years and would choose to start screening at the third grade level, relying on classroom teachers of lower grades to refer those children with handicapping problems. Screening eighth or ninth graders might well be based on the rationale of finding and correcting problems before the child enters high school. Similarly eleventh or twelfth graders would be screened with the idea that students should have the advantage of optimal speech as they graduate from school to take jobs or go on to college.

Who Will Screen

Speech-language pathologists are responsible for the evaluation of verbal communication skills of children who may have such problems. This responsibility may be fulfilled in a variety of ways. The clinician may elect to set up and carry through the screening program in the assigned schools alone. SLPs in a given school system may combine their efforts and work as a team going from school to school in a concentrated effort to complete the screening in as short a time and as effectively as possible.

A third alternative is to train nonprofessional aides to assist with the screening. Alpiner, Ogden and Wiggins (1970) recommend, as a result of their study, that although supportive personnel can make effective contributions to the speech-language program in the schools, they should not be used in the screening program. However, the 1973 Task Force on School Speech, Hearing and Language Screening Procedures (1973) encourages the use of trained supportive personnel working under the supervision of speech-language professionals. Pickering and Dopheide (1976) discuss the training strategies and evaluation procedures they used in a two-day, competency-based workshop for training aides, mostly classroom teachers, to conduct large scale screening of speech-language problems in elementary aged children. Although the study showed a strong tendency on the part of the trained aide group to overrefer, it was felt that the training of existing school personnel could reduce significantly the large block of time routinely required by the clinician to do the screening. It appears that the best use of the trained nonprofessional would be as part of a professional team whose members could be consulted when the aide needed advice or confirmation of a judgment.

Whether or not the classroom teacher is trained as an aide, the teacher should be considered an important member of the team. The alert clinician will cut down on the margin of error in the screening program by looking to the classroom teacher to call attention to children with problems that may have been missed in the necessarily brief screening sample. Sommers (1970) reported studies performed in Montgomery County, Pennsylvania, that supported earlier studies done by Diehl and Stinnet (1956) questioning the ability of classroom teachers to effectively identify speech problems. Both studies showed that teachers overlooked 20 percent to 40 percent of the children with significant deviations. Wertz and Mead (1975) confirmed the earlier findings of James and Cooper (1966) that teachers did best in identifying stuttering problems and poorest in recognizing voice disorders. However, the cooperation of a knowledgeable classroom teacher is vital, particularly in the referral of children from classes not screened. When the speech-language pathologist asks classroom teachers to make referrals of articulation, language, voice, and fluency problems, the clinician must make certain that the teacher knows what constitutes such problems. Although many universities require their teacher training graduates to take a survey course in speech-language-hearing problems, many classroom teachers are hesitant to make referrals, perhaps fearing the embarrassment of making the "wrong" referrals. Van Hattum (1977) suggests the use of descriptive phrases, such as "produces sounds incorrectly," on the referral form provided teachers rather than "articulation disorder." The SLP should know each classroom teacher and provide the level of help that each needs to elicit the greatest cooperation in identifying and serving the child with a problem. The clinician who wishes to encourage this cooperation must show respect and appreciation for each referral made by the teacher and take advantage of these contacts as means of helping the teacher to better understand the issues. If the referred child is not to be enrolled for therapy, the SLP must carefully explain to the referring teacher why not and what disposition has been made of the case.

Freeman has written a helpful book that the clinician may wish to supply to the classroom teacher: *Speech and Language Services and the Classroom Teacher* (1977), available from the Council for Exceptional Children.

Procedures Used in Screening

Careful planning is essential to locate, with maximum efficiency and economy, those children whose speech-language differences may be educationally handicapping. Once it has been decided who will comprise the screening team, the principal of each school involved should be informed. The SLP should first make certain that the principal understands the importance and organization of the screening, then consult with the principal to plan convenient time and space. The principal then apprises the classroom teachers of the plans. Either the classroom teachers or the school secretary will supply lists of names and birthdates of children in each room to be screened. Use of such lists saves the examiner's time in trying to identify the child whose intelligibility may be limited and serves as a means of insuring that all children in each class have been seen. The list should provide space after each child's name for notations regarding test results. The clinician should provide the forms for these rosters. Figure 8-1 is an example of such a roster.

Establishing the Therapy Program 359

SPECIAL EDUCATION UNIT
School _____   Printed Here   Teacher _____
Specialist _____   Grade _____ Room No. _____

SPEECH-LANGUAGE OR HEARING EVALUATION ROSTER

_____ Speech _____ Hearing   Screening Date _____ Diagnostic Test Date _____

Name of Child		Screening Results		Diagnostic Test Results				Remark
last	first	Adequate	Retest	Adequate	Referred	Service	Other	

Totals

Figure 8-1. Speech-Language-Hearing Evaluation Roster.

The screening procedure may be carried out in a quiet corner of the classroom if the room is fairly large and the class is involved in a quiet activity. In many schools the halls are quiet enough for screening, with several chairs set up just outside the classroom. A quiet room (or space) as close as possible to the class being checked cuts down on time lost. If the testing is done outside the classroom, it is wise to take three or four children at a time. The child who is finished goes back to the classroom and sends the next child, thus maintaining a steady flow of children. As the child learns from watching those ahead, little time is needed for explanation. The young child who may be apprehensive about the situation may gain confidence from the presence of his peers. If young children must be tested in a room far removed from the classroom, an older student may be delegated as "runner" to see them back and forth.

Time Allotted for Screening

Irwin (1953) suggested that an average of two minutes per child be allowed for speech screening. The ASHA Task Force on screening procedures in the schools (1973) found that the procedure averages about five minutes per child. Multiplying the number of children to be screened by five should provide a good estimate as to how much time should be alloted.

Materials Used for Screening

The experienced clinician may not feel the need for formal testing materials, recognizing almost as soon as the child begins to talk whether or not there is a problem needing further investigation. The less experienced SLP needs the help of a structured evaluation procedure to insure that all sources of potential error are covered. In most cases screening routines similar to that suggested by the ASHA Task Force (1973) are used: The child is asked to —
1. Tell full name, address, and age;
2. Describe an action picture to test for sentence use and fluency;
3. Follow a one-step and then a two-step command to test memory span and knowledge of prepositions and verbs;
4. Point to parts of body, describe clothing;
5. Name objects as shown in a test such as the Templin-Darley Screening Test.

A screening test of articulation does not include all phonemes. The /p/, /b/, /m/, for example, need not be included in the sample: if the child's articulation is so deviant that these sounds are defective, no test is necessary to show the need for intervention. Roe and Milisen (1942) suggest that the phonemes to be included in a screening are /s/, /z/, /ʃ/, /tʃ/, /l/, /f/, /v/, /r/.

Validity of articulation evaluation based on the child's recitation of the pledge of allegiance or other memorized material is highly suspect. Such samples may represent memorized production rather than the child's functional speech.

For prereaders and beginning readers, picture cards are used to elicit the phoneme and/or language patterns to be checked. Lee (1974) found that representative samples of the child's language could be obtained by having the child repeat phrases or sentences presented by the examiner. If articulation is checked in like manner, use of the target sound in phrases or sentences gives a more valid sample than asking the child to repeat a single word. The upper elementary or junior high school student may be asked to read words or sentences containing the phoneme to be checked. Similar materials or a selected paragraph such as "My Grandfather" (Van Riper, 1963) may be used with high school students.

SCREENING IN THE SECONDARY SCHOOLS

One Day per Week

There is reason to believe that the teacher referral method of case finding at the junior and senior high school level is rather ineffective. Assuming that these findings are valid, the clinician responsible for children at these grade levels should develop specific screening procedures. It is particularly important that these children be examined if they were not screened as elementary students. High schools frequently include children from private and parochial elementary schools where speech help was not available. As before, a number of various plans can be developed. One of these will meet the clinician's and the school's requirements best. Two principle plans will be suggested. One is predicated on the SLP working by himself; the other is based upon a team approach in which a number of speech-language clinicians from one administrative organization, or several neighboring ones, work together to accomplish this task.

As an example, an individual clinician wished to screen a combined junior-senior high school by working one period daily. The choice was to try to use the homeroom or activity period. Unfortunately, many other activities occurred during this time, e.g. the teacher did guidance work, the chorus practiced, special clubs met, and there were multiple interruptions of various types. In general, it was difficult to coordinate the testing; interruptions were frequent and the atmosphere was too informal for controlled screening. The clinician then reviewed the program of instructions for all the students and consulted the master schedule. It was subsequently determined that each student was scheduled for English every day (a common requirement for many states). The high school principal and SLP conferred and ultimately planned a schedule that allowed a screening of the entire school body of 1,000 students in five working days. This plan had the following features: (1) there were eight fifty-five minute periods of instruction each day with a minimum of four and a maximum of six English classes taught each period; (2) testing would be done in the English classes for an entire day, one day each week over a five-week period; (3) the English teachers would be alerted according to a schedule concerning when a particular class would be screened and prepare seatwork accordingly; (4) the clinician would sit in the back of each classroom and indicate to each of the students when he or she was to walk over and read the screening material—which would take approximately one and one-half minutes to read; (5) a brief phonetic analysis was completed for students revealing errors; all others were not listed (but the attendance in each class was carefully noted); and (6) between class periods the clinician moved to the next scheduled English class until the day's screening was completed.

During the conference with the principal, it was decided that all testing would be scheduled on Mondays, since this was more stable in the sense of fewer interruptions in school routine. It will be noted in the hypothetical example contained in Figure 8-2 that almost all testing could be accomplished over a five-week period except for three classes (periods one, two and three). These were planned another time.

A One-Day Program

It can be seen quite readily that the plan for screening in English classes can be adapted so that an entire school can be completed in one day if a sufficiently large group of testers is available. Six speech-language clinicians working on a Monday, for example, could test the entire school of 1,000 pupils. Although arrangements for such mass testing might appear to be formida-

Period	English Classes Scheduled on Mondays
1	Rooms: 210, 212, 214, 216, 217, 210
2	Rooms: 211, 212, 214, 109, 306, 307
3	Rooms: 209, 210, 212, 111, 214, 306
*4	Rooms: 212, 210, 208, 209
*5	Rooms: 207, 208, 210, 209
6	Rooms: 209, 211, 212, 306, 208
7	Rooms: 211, 210, 111, 306, 212
8	Rooms: 206, 209, 306, 111, 211

*Lunch periods of ninety minutes each, forty-five for lunch and forty-five for a class.

Figure 8-2. Hypothetical schedule of high school English classes.

ble, experience shows that this is not so. The advantages of completing a school in one day are obvious. Testing plans are particularly simplified if all the participating speech-language clinicians are employed by one administrative unit, i.e. a county or city school program. In such instances, permission to leave assigned schools for a day is easier to obtain, since the screening service is part of a total program. Clinicians working by nature of being employed by an independent school district might find that neighboring SLPs similarly employed would be willing to participate in screening their secondary schools if reciprocity were agreed upon.

A number of ways of screening secondary students for speech-language problems also may prove efficient. For example, a junior high school with an enrollment of 925 students was screened by a staff of seven speech-language clinicians in less than three hours. This was accomplished as a result of careful planning, a most cooperative principal, and the use of one of the facilities in the school, the Audion. This amphitheater-type room with multiple entrances and exits and seating accommodations for 200 students was particularly suitable for organized, quiet reading. Clinicians were spaced four to six rows apart, and as many as fifteen students were seated adjacent to them. After each student was screened, he left the Audion by an exit and returned to his class. The principal and her assistant kept whole classes of students flowing into the Audion and to the testers without interruption and with excellent control over noise and extraneous movement. The soundproofing of the Audion was also of significant value. In this case, the disruption to junior high classes was minimized due to rapid flow of students examined and their quick return to their assigned classes. The principal was willing to allow a major change in a morning's activities to complete this screening. The auditoriums of most junior and senior high schools are almost as efficient for this type of testing as the Audion proved to be in this case. In summary, a number of efficient ways can be developed for screening secondary schools. Each of these should probably be tailored to a particular school's program and can be developed jointly by key school personnel and the SLP.

Decision Making

The listening sophistication of the examiner must be considered in determining the type of test to be used. The beginning clinician may need the help of carefully explicit test items if errors are to be recognized. King and Berger (1971) warn against the clinician doing too much talking during the testing. With experience, the clinician learns to guard against using questions that are answered with yes or no and questions that the SLP answers but credits to the child. Opportunity for checking the child's spontaneous language must always be provided.

Although the ASHA School Services Program stresses the primacy of the speech-language pathologist in the diagnostic and intervention program, P.L. 94-142 requires the involvement of a team including the child's classroom teacher. Input of the classroom teacher and other non–speech-language personnel should be welcomed as a balancing factor in the determination of what children are "handicapped." Clase, in a cogent discussion of the "Ethical Implications of Screening" (1976) questions at what point deviant speech becomes a speech problem. She suggest that in the zeal to recruit clients, the clinician labels as defective speech that is deviant but that does not interfere or handicap enough to concern the speaker. Do we create, by labeling, the problems we help to "cure"? Clase related therapeutic failure to this lack of concern on the part of the client and questions whether there is a problem present when there is no felt need. She notes that it becomes exceedingly important for the SLP to distinguish between the person's own needs and values and those the professional thinks he ought to have. Two entire issues of *Seminars in Speech, Language and Hearing* (Van Hattum, 1981) are devoted to screening in the schools. They are recommended reading.

CASE SELECTION

As school speech-language-hearing case loads have declined nationally, the importance of proper case selection has increased. It can be stated that the most effective SLP in the schools cannot be considered effective if case selection procedures are poor. All the best therapy techniques and skills in the world are of no consequence if wasted on those not needing them and denied those who do. The case selection problem is a familiar one to speech-language pathologists in other working settings, but it is a fundamental problem for the clinician who must sort through hundreds of children to identify the best choices for inclusion in the therapy program.

Diagnostic Procedures

Federal regulations do not require the parent's written permission prior to the general screening of whole classes of children. Because written permission must be obtained prior to the conducting of individual diagnostic assessment, the speech-language pathologist should be as precise and complete as possible in the screening process so that valuable time is not lost in seeking permission for diagnostic testing, which may prove not to be necessary. P.L. 94-142 indicates that a qualified speech-language pathologist must evaluate each speech impaired child using procedures that are appropriate for the diagnosis and appraisal of speech disorders.

Language

Berry (1969) emphasizes that the evaluation of language disorders must be an ongoing process and that children picked up in the screening survey should be admitted to a program of diagnostic teaching. Such an educational plan would be based on group instruction conducted by a team made up of language teachers, classroom teachers, medical, psychological, and social workers in a program that encompasses both the child and family. Whether or not the clinician chooses to develop such a desirable and exciting program, there is an immediacy to the necessity of providing objective evidence justifying the child's enrollment.

Sommers et al. (1978) question the validity of many of the language tests being used, finding that, in fact, they frequently do not give valid information in the areas that they purport to assess. As a result of their investigations, the authors recommend the use of a battery of tests in evaluating the linguistic performance of young children: the Menyuk Sentence Repetition Task (1969) as a cross-modality measure, Carrow's Test for Auditory Comprehension of Language (1973) as a measure of the more general auditory receptive abilities, and McCarthy's Mean Length of Utterance (1930) or Lee's Developmental Sentence Analysis (1974) to measure expressive levels.

Other tests widely used are Lee's Northwestern Syntax Test (1969), The Illinois Test of Psycholinguistic Abilities (1968), and The Peabody Picture Vocabulary Test (1965). Hearing must also be evaluated. Results of these various tests provide pieces in the jigsaw puzzle, which ultimately gives the picture of the speech-language handicapped child. Very important pieces of the puzzle result from parent interviews and the clinician's observation of the child's behavior. As the picture never quite reaches completion, diagnosis must be an ongoing part of therapy.

Articulation

Although there are those who would not discriminate disorders of articulation from the general disorders of language, a national survey of speech-language clinicians in the schools across the United States (Sommers and Hatton, 1979) reveals that an average of 48.9 percent of speech therapy case loads were children whose problems were diagnosed primarily as defective articulation. Neal's survey of school speech clinicians (1976) showed a 65.6 percent prevalence of articulation disorders. In her six-year overview of speech therapy services in the Montgomery County (Maryland) Public Schools, DesRoches (1976) found gradually increasing percentages of case loads designated as language with a concomitant decrease in those coded as articulation. However, articulation problems continue to account for nearly half of many school case loads. Children having exhibited deviant articulation in the preliminary screening must then be diagnosed to determine the specific type and severity and, if possible, the cause of the problem. There are several ways of obtaining the speech sample. Perhaps the most commonly used way of eliciting "spontaneous" samples, particularly with young children, is not truly spontaneous but rather the response to a series of pictures such as the Templin-Darley (1960), Goldman-Fristoe (1969), and the Photo Articulation Test (1965). Mullen and Whitehead (1977) report that another test, the Arizona Proficiency Scale (Fudala, 1970) is a more efficient instrument than the Goldman-Fristoe, requiring less time to administer. There is no shortage of articulation tests from which the clinician may choose. Many clinicians prefer to develop their own. These picture tests usually elicit one word responses and are selected so that each of the phonemes of English appears in initial, medial, and final positions within the word. Because such tests sample isolated words, they do not represent true samples of spontaneous speech. The examiner must be alert to the possibility that the child may produce all the phonemes acceptably in such one-word responses even though his conversational patterns may be virtually nonintelligible. Additionally, there is good reason to believe that the consistency of phoneme defectiveness in spontaneous speech cannot be predicted from such tests (Faircloth and Faircloth, 1970; Sommers and Sitler, 1979). For the pupil who reads, testing speech by presenting selected passages also yields a systematic sample.

Regardless of which of the above methods of obtaining samples are used, the examiner must also provide for truly spontaneous sampling of the individual's conversational speech. Some tests, such as the Goldman-Fristoe (1969), include pictures from which the pupil is encouraged to tell a story. The examiner may use carefully framed questions to start the child talking. These spontaneous samples are of greatest importance in determining the adequacy of the child's articulation or the extent to which it handicaps communication.

One approach used with good success by the authors is to ask children what they like to watch on TV. This generally provides a very adequate sample of connected speech from which some judgments of articulatory and other linguistic skills can be determined. Of course, speech sounds that occur infrequently in children's speech may require additional, more structured, probing or perhaps direct testing using imitated syllables or words, picture stimuli, or similar strategies.

Prognostic Testing

Efforts to locate highly efficient, reliable, and valid predictors of children's speech and language skills have been centered heavily on articulation. Few if any prognostic tools have been identified in other related disorders including language, voice, and stuttering. Over a period of years, investigators appear to have identified three prognosticators of articulation changes in children from five to eight years of age.

The first of these and the one having the greatest number of independent investigations to support its predictive validity is the simple test of *stimulability*. This is defined as the extent to which the child can alter his defective speech sound measured spontaneously using a picture stimulus to a correct form when the same defective sound is assessed using imitated nonsense syllables. In one of the more extensive tests of the value of stimulability measures to predict children's articulation improvements and study therapy effectiveness, Sommers et al. (1967) reported that kindergarten, first, and second grade children having poor overall stimulability scores frequently required speech therapy to make significant improvements. Several other research reports support stimulability as a predictor of young children's articulation changes.

The second best tested prognostic tool appears to be measures of *consistency of misarticulation*. This common element in many children's articulation has been found to be predictive of articulation change by a number of investigators. The greatest amount of data mustered to show its effects upon young school-age children has been reported by McDonald and McDonald (1976). The extent to which consistency is predictive clearly relates to which speech sound is being studied, the age of the child, and the length of time that the phenomenon is studied to determine its prognostic strength. This statement is also applicable to the predictive strength of stimulability as well.

The final factor, *overall severity* of articulatory defectiveness, as measured by the total number of defective phonetic contexts across speech sounds, also appears to have some predictive validity. However, this severity factor, compared to measures of stimulability and consistency, is much more general and does not appear to offer specific information that is very useful for the SLP to evaluate changes in patterns of speech sound errors or to study individual speech sounds. One test that appears to measure the severity dimension of articulation and uses this information to predict articulation performances later is the Predictive Screening Test of Articulation (Van Riper and Erickson, 1969). Some children having more articulation errors on certain clusters and other commonly defective speech sounds in first grade have been reported to show residual articulation errors in third grade if no therapy has been provided for them.

Although the three prognostic indicators of children's articulation changes have been investigated in elementary-age groups (particularly in kindergarten, first and second grades), little if anything is known about prediction of change in older junior and senior high students. It seems likely that older students who show some inconsistency of error on defective sounds and a degree of stimulability for them may in fact be good responders early in therapy when production (acquisition) of sounds receives emphasis. Once acquisition has been achieved and the defective sound(s) are capable of being produced correctly in a very stable manner and under a variety of conditions, factors such as consistency and stimulability may cease to have predictive value.

Voice

Many speech-language pathologists seem to push to the bottom of the list names of those children found to have voice problems, hoping that they will disappear before they must be scheduled. However, these disorders also must be dealt with in spite of difficulties resulting from lack of objective, descriptive terms and the paucity of objective diagnostic tests.

Recent surveys (Neal, 1976; Sommers and Hatton, 1979) show that voice disorders make up 2.5 percent of case loads nationally.

The actual incidence of voice problems in the schools has been placed at 6 percent of elementary and junior high school children (Baynes, 1966; Wilson 1970).

In dealing with voice disorders one is immediately faced with difficulties in diagnosing such problems. Hyman et al. (1979) report a study supporting the earlier findings of James and Cooper (1966) showing that classroom teachers do not identify voice problems with better than 10 percent accuracy.

Deal et al. (1976) suggest a checklist that the speech-language clinician can give the classroom teacher as a guide in making voice referrals: children who (1) are hoarse for more than two weeks, (2) have laryngitis for more than two weeks, (3) have voice pitches that are too high or too low and are not appropriate for their age or sex, (4) talk through their noses, (5) have voices that are too loud or too soft, (6) have voices that are breathy, (7) have voices that sound strained, (8) have voice breaks and are younger than an age when voice changes usually occur, (9) have a monotone voice, (10) have any other voice problem that attracts attention, (11) are having tonsillectomies or adenoidectomies. This is a good checklist for the speech-language clinician as well.

Wilson (1970) presents a descriptive approach to diagnosing the voice disordered child. Adequacy of pitch, intensity, range, and nasality are charted on lines of continua from normal to unacceptable. Emerick and Hatten (1974) recommend that diagnosis include answers to who, what, when, and why. *Who* has made the referral? If the client and those around him do not consider his voice to be a problem, then there is none. *What* does the client see as the problem? *When* is it a problem? (during hay fever season?) *Why* does the client want to change the voice? It may be necessary for the speech-language pathologist to help the child and/or parents to find realistic and objective answers to the who, what, when, and why of the voice problem; but, until these questions are dealt with, the chances for successful intervention are limited.

Decisions as to whether the person's voice is normal for that individual depend upon age, sex, and physical structure. Evaluation of the speaking voice tends to be a subjective rating determined by the preference of the listener. According to Van Riper and Irwin (1958) there are three problems in evaluating voice: "(1)

We must differentiate between voice disorders or defects and the other speech disorders or defects. (2) We must differentiate between abnormal voice and normal voice. (3) We must attempt to define the various voice disorders and distinguish them one from another." In 1972 Wilson, at the Jewish Hospital in St. Louis, Missouri, developed a series of tapes demonstrating the various disorders. A comparison of the voice of the child in question with the tape should be of help in diagnosis.

We close this discussion on diagnosis of voice problems with the admonition that usually comes first in any study of this disorder: treatment should not be undertaken without medical clearance and approval. Because most schools do not have sophisticated examining equipment, the clinician should work closely with the medical specialist to gather all relevant information.

Stuttering

There is evidence that stuttering was diagnosed approximately 2,000 years before the first speech-language clinicians dropped their cassettes into place and asked Johnny to tell his name and address. Earliest evidence was recorded in Egyptian hieroglyphics. Although in the fifty to sixty years of speech research more research has been done and more articles published on stuttering than on any other type of speech defect, one wonders if significantly more is known about the disorder now than was known in the days of King Tut.

Diagnostically, "anyone" can recognize nonfluencies in speech. The problem is to distinguish normal nonfluencies from abnormal — from "stuttering." Is there a better tool for determining the difference than the ear of the trained clinician? Probably not.

With stuttering, as with language and any other speech problem, diagnosis must be ongoing. Enrolling the nonfluent child in a small group of his peers who are working on their articulation problems provides an excellent opportunity for the clinician to judge the child's fluency in conversation with peers and, incidentally, to provide experiences of success as the child models correct articulation for fellow group members. One of the most important things that can be done to help the child with fluency problems is to provide that child with experiences of success in speaking.

Dell (1980) provides some suggestions of ways to differentiate children's nonfluencies:

Speech Behavior Indicating Risk of Becoming a Stutterer
1. Facial tremors caused by excessive tension
2. Speaks cautiously
3. Speaks rapidly, almost compulsively
4. Speaks too loudly or too softly
5. Evidences of struggle and tension while speaking
6. Blocks the airflow
7. Raises the pitch or volume during dysfluencies
8. Accompanying body movements during dysfluencies
9. Signs of embarrassment while speaking
10. Uneven repetitions
11. Use of the schwa vowel on repetitions
12. Many repetitions (5 or more) during word
13. Stops in middle of word, backs up, starts over
14. Evidence of avoiding certain words
15. More than one dysfluency during a sentence

Nonspeech Behavior Indicating Risk of Becoming a Stutterer
1. Shyness, looks away especially when dysfluent
2. Low self-concept
3. Other nervous habits, e.g. nail biting, bed-wetting, hyperactivity
4. Poor socialization skills
5. Evidences of depression and sadness
6. Worry (p. 19)*

This is not to say that every shy child who speaks cautiously is a stutterer; but, as Dell points out, "when a child shows a large number of these behaviors we should be concerned." The clinician should observe the child in a variety of speaking situations and then trust his or her own judgment, perhaps in consultation with the classroom teacher, as to whether the child needs assistance. some measures of fluency assessment are described later in the chapter.

From Dell, C., *Treating the School Age Stutterer*, 1980. Courtesy of Speech Foundations of America, Memphis, Tennessee.

Tongue Thrust

Mason and Proffit (1974) define tongue thrust as one or a combination of three conditions: (1) during the initiation phase of a swallow, a forward gesture of the tongue between the anterior teeth so that the tongue tip contacts the lower lip; (2) during speech activities, fronting of the tongue between or against the anterior teeth with the mandible open (in phonetic contexts not requiring such placement); and (3) at rest, the tongue carried forward in the oral cavity with the mandible slightly open and the tongue tip against or between the anterior teeth.

Tongue thrust, sometimes called "deviant swallow" or "reverse swallow," with the accompanying myofunctional therapy, has been the cause of controversy since it began to receive increased attention in the early 1960s. In November, 1974, the Legislative Council of ASHA adopted as official policy a position statement drafted by a joint committee on Dentistry and Speech Pathology-Audiology. This statement was published in *Asha*, May, 1975, with an exhaustive bibliography on tongue thrust:

> Review of data from studies published to date has convinced the Committee that neither the validity of the diagnostic label tongue thrust nor the contention that myofunctional therapy produces significant consistent changes in oral form or function has been documented adequately. There is insufficient scientific evidence to permit differentiation between normal and abnormal or deviant patterns of deglutition, particularly as such patterns might relate to occlusion and speech. There is unsatisfactory evidence to support the belief that any patterns of movements defined as tongue thrust by any criteria suggested to date should be considered abnormal, detrimental, or representative of a syndrome. The few suitably controlled studies that have incorporated valid and reliable diagnostic criteria and appropriate quantitative assessments of therapy have demonstrated no effects on patterns of deglutition or oral structure. Thus, research is needed to establish the validity of tongue thrust as a clinical entity.
>
> In view of the above considerations and despite our recognition that some dentists call upon speech pathologists to provide myofunctional therapy, at this time, there is no acceptable evidence to support claims of significant, stable, long-term changes in the functional patterns of deglutition and significant, consistent alterations in oral form. Consequently, the Committee urges increased research efforts, but cannot recommend that speech pathologists engage in clinical management procedures with the intent of altering functional patterns of deglutition.

Mason and Proffit quote evidence that tongue thrusting is almost universal in infants. A relatively high percentage of children beginning school demonstrate these characteristics, but many of these tongue thrusters spontaneously develop normal swallow pattern by the age of twelve.

SLPs often feel pressured by the dentists to assume responsibility for retraining the swallowing pattern, dentists feeling that for them to provide the needed exercises is not the best use of their time. It is questionable whether such activity constitutes the best use of the clinician's time and talent—unless the so-called deviant swallow is accompanied by a speech problem. When tongue thrusting is accompanied by lisping, the clinician should deal with the problem as with any other lisp.

Mason and Proffit do recommend, however, that "for those older children with speech problems for whom orthodontic treatment for open bite is carried out, and in whom it is desirable to modify anterior resting posture of the tongue, the techniques of myofunctional therapy are useful. Articulation therapy techniques involving phonetic placement may also be particularly helpful in repositioning the tongue tip posteriorward."

The final decision for case selection must rest with the clinician, depending on the clinician's determination of the most effective and efficient use of time and training in meeting the speech and language needs of the children.

Case Selection: Priorities and Decision Making

The profession of speech-language pathology and audiology has experienced significant developments in the decade since the original publication of the chapter (Sommers, 1969). Language has come into its own, and the name of our professional organization has been changed to the American Speech-Language-Hearing Association. Professionals have decided that they want to be called speech-language pathologists. Perhaps the most affective event was the signing of the Education for All Handicapped Children Act, P.L. 94-142. Students preparing to work in the schools, or in any other agency, should study carefully not only the federal law but also the interpretation of that law enacted by the state in which one anticipates employment. Chapter 3 provides very helpful interpretations of the federal law as it affects the speech-language pathologist.

Some of the most far reaching changes resulting from the law concern the selection and scheduling of children. Ten years ago this chapter (Sommers, 1969) gave great emphasis to the prerogative and responsibility of the speech-language pathologist to make the decisions as to case selection. "It goes without saying that any other way of selecting children for therapy might be considered a breach of professional ethics, since only the clinician is qualified to decide on the basis of his evaluation and experience". Now, although P.L. 94-142 assigns to the speech-language pathologist the "primary responsibility to determine the assessment needs and procedures that are appropriate for the communicatively handicapped child" (121a.532), it stipulates that the assessment of the handicapped child must be completed by an interdisciplinary team comprised, in case of speech impairment, of at least the speech-language pathologist and the child's classroom teacher. Furthermore, appropriate placement of the handicapped child must be made by a team. For the speech impaired child the team could consist of the speech-language pathologist, classroom teacher, and the child's parents.

A survey in 1978 by the Public School Affairs Committee of the Ohio Speech and Hearing Association showed that of the 550 speech-language pathologists responding, 84 percent reported that selection of the case load was done by the clinician; 15 percent, by the placement team. Sixty-two percent reported that the question of educational handicap was determined by the SLP in consultation with the child's classroom teacher after the speech-language pathologist had formally assessed the speech-language-hearing problem. Other results of the adoption of due process procedures shown by this Ohio study include lowered case loads, increased diagnostic time, and the dismissal of children with minor developmental articulation errors.

It would appear that in spite of, perhaps because of, the recent federal and state legislation case selection rests largely and ultimately with the speech-language pathologist, who must be able to present convincing and documented rationale for scheduling or not scheduling each child concerned. This has resulted in a needed reevaluation of criteria for case selection. Too often the speech-language pathologist has pointed to any deviation in speech and language as a problem demanding that the child be enrolled for therapy. The results of such inclusive selection have resulted in case loads too large to be handled effectively and efficiently, not enough time to work with the severely handicapped, and lack of motivation and cooperation on the part of parents and children who are not convinced that a problem exists.

Suggesting that distinction must be made between speech impairment and a handicap, Pronovost (1971) quotes Riviere (Rehabilitation Codes 1962): "An *impairment* is any deviation from the normal that results in defective function, structure, organization, or development of the whole or any of its faculties, senses, systems, organs, members, or any part thereof. A *handicap* is the disadvantage imposed by an impairment upon a specific individual in his cultural pattern of psychological, physical, vocational, and community activities." "Most of us," Pronovost continues, "know physically impaired individuals who are in no way handicapped in their daily functioning. Other professions do not find it necessary or desirable to include every person with a detectable impairment in a therapeutic program." More careful testing leading to more discriminating case selection would result in the SLP having time to give more extensive and intensive therapy to those children who have more severe handicapping problems.

Zemmol (1977) describes a priority system of case selection based on continua of need:

First Priority

This group encompasses pupils with severely handicapping communication disorders for whom intensive programming is indicated.

    I. Language

        A. Severe delay in language acquisition

        B. Handicapping disability in reception, integration, or expression of language

    II. Organically based articulatory disorders

        A. Dysarthria, oral dyspraxia

        B. Developmental anomalies

    III. Articulatory disorders of unspecified etiology resulting in

unintelligible speech
IV. Dysfluency—severe
V. Voice disorders, particularly at the initial stages of vocal rehabilitation
VI. Speech and language problems related to moderate-to-severe loss of hearing
VII. Hypernasality
VIII. Multiple speech and language problems

Second Priority. Pupils with moderate speech and language handicaps or deviations are included. Scheduling is less frequent than for pupils falling within the first priority.
  I. Language
     A. Moderate-to-mild delay in language acquisition
     B. Moderate-to-mild deficit in reception, integration, or expression of language
     C. Residual problems of pupils previously enrolled under first priority
  II. Articulation
     A. Pupils with moderately handicapping articulatory defects—fair intelligibility
     B. Former first priority cases who can be scheduled less intensively
  III. Dysfluency—moderate
  IV. Voice deviations—moderate
  V. Speech and language problems related to mild-to-moderate loss of hearing

Third Priority. Pupils with mild speech or language handicaps or deviations are scheduled in the available time, as feasible
  I. Pupils listed previously as first or second priority who are approaching stabilization of appropriate or optimal speech patterns
  II. Pupils with poor motivation or for whom the likelihood of significant progress is highly questionable
  III. Pupils previously dismissed or at the consultative level who could benefit from supportive work
  IV. Those not previously enrolled who demonstrate developmental articulatory errors or mild speech or language deviations

Consultative Services. Scheduling allows for evaluation and consultation by appointment.
  I. Pupils not actively enrolled in the program who require periodic reevaluation
  II. Parents
     A. Counseling regarding the prevention of hearing, speech, and language handicaps
     B. Speech and language stimulation activities for preschool children
     C. Appropriate strategies for home practice
  III. In-service training for teachers
     A. Reinforcement of speech and language in the classroom
     B. Speech and language acquisition
     C. Identification of speech and language disorders for diagnostic referral
     D. Recognition of potential language-based learning disabilities
  IV. Administrators
  V. Preschool evaluations and referrals

Such a plan of case scheduling provides for adapting the program to meet the needs of each child, rather than attempting to fit the child into an existing program. It forces the speech-language pathologist to be more selective in case selection, eliminating the children with questionable "differences" to make way for those children with handicapping defects.

Other Factors

Although case selection probably should be tied closely to speech-language needs, a number of other considerations are important and, in some instances, perhaps more important. A few principles would appear to apply to guide the clinician in weighing the values involved. Since, as Johnson (1956) has said, we are dealing not with *speech defects* but with *children having speech defects,* we cannot separate the child and his problem. To paraphrase Johnson, we probably cannot also separate the child's problem from the family. If this is so, parental anxiety and reactions to a child's defective speech ought to be considered and weighed in the case selection proposition. One SLP, for example, had therapy space for an additional child in a group session. On the basis of careful assessment of all aspects of the articulatory defectiveness of two children on her waiting list, she chose the child who had more severe problems; prognostic testing had indicated a lesser likelihood for improvement without therapy. On the other hand, his teacher reported that he had many friends, talked freely in class, and did above average work in academic subject areas. The child not chosen was reported by his teacher to be withdrawn and lonely, occasionally a behavior problem in the classroom, and obviously aware of his speech problem. Furthermore, his academic work was reported to be poor. Of interest was that the mother of the unchosen child had called the clinician at least twice during the past year indicating concern about her child's speech and asking when therapy would be provided for him. Under these conditions, the concomitant factors would seem to suggest a decision to enter the second child into therapy.

A somewhat similar situation may involve two children of the type cited as "the selected one" above. Again space is currently available for only one in therapy program. One difference emerged: the parents of one child were disturbed and apparently embarrassed about his defective speech. This factor might be considered the one that tipped the scales, since a problem for a parent may in fact be a problem for the child. In summary, careful case selection demands an intensive view of the children thought to be in need of assistance. The articulatory, social, and emotional adjustment and family attitude factors should be weighed and decisions made accordingly. A few additional statements might also be presented relative to other principles of case selection.

Based on Need

Although it was found in a national study of public school speech and hearing services that three-fourths of a total of 1,462 clinicians work primarily with children in the primary grades (Darley, 1961), a few clinicians have developed a policy of working with children from third grade through twelfth and not scheduling any others. It would appear that such a practice ignores the need for service of younger children, and it is probably not the age or grade level of the child that is most important but the need for help. Conceivably, a kindergarten child may have more total need for speech-language therapy than a sixth grade child—if all aspects of the problem are viewed, i.e. the degree of communication disturbance, social and personality adjustment, educational impairment, and parental enxieties. It would appear difficult to defend such a practice also on the basis of information concerning the values of early correction, evidence to show that therapy is effective for five, six, and seven year old children (Sommers, et al., 1967), and the major emphasis on early training of exceptional children. This is not to imply that the age of a child is not a worthy consideration in case selection. Assuming that all other factors of need are determined to be equal, older children should probably be given a preference in case selection, since they have fewer opportunities as they grow older to receive this service and it is unlikely that maturation will exert any influence on their speech performance.

Etiology

A further concern centers around etiology. What preference should be given to children who are cerebral palsied, have a cleft palate, or are speech defective due to hearing loss, for example? If a basic criterion for case selection is response to careful speech-language assessment, many of these children will demonstrate a resistance to change and a consistency of error in many of the aspects of speech, e.g. articulation, voice quality, and rhythm. Second, the physical disability that accompanies many of these problems tends to increase in magnitude; therefore, an increase in problems related to social and emotional adjustments might be predicted in many instances. Finally, parental anxiety concerning total defectiveness often seems centered around the communication aspects of the total problem.

A further consideration rests upon the ability of the child to make improvements as a result of the therapy that can be provided in the school program. Assuming that further progress is indicated judging by stimulability testing, consistency measures, trial learning, past progress, and other prognostic indicators, the SLP might be well advised to continue scheduling the child. Other conditions that might tend to suggest further therapy might include the determination that past therapy was inadequate in terms of both intensity and method or that carry-over of newly learned speech-language patterns is incomplete. Obviously, the inexperienced clinician would do well on occasion to consult with more experienced clinicians who would see the child in question and make recommendations. These "consultants" might be qualified and more experienced SLPs from other schools, or from programs in hospitals, universities, or private practice.

SAMPLE GUIDELINES FROM TWO SCHOOL PROGRAMS

Staffs of school speech-language-hearing programs have developed criteria for case selection across many of the common etiologies. Almost all of these speak to an evaluation of the severity of the disorder; some include age considerations and others a wide variety of other factors. We are pleased to share criteria, guidelines, and some assessment devices used in two outstanding school programs, the speech-language and hearing program of the Montgomery County, Pennsylvania, Schools[1] and that of Broward County, Florida.[2]

We will first view some of the guidelines and principles developed and adopted by SLPs from the Montgomery County, Pennsylvania, Intermediate School Unit. We will then have an opportunity to study similar guidelines, principles, and procedures from the Broward County, Florida, Public Schools. Finally, we will present a summary and a comparison to show the reader some of the salient differences. Perhaps not surprising to many persons, it will become rather obvious that two large clinical speech-language-hearing school staffs will reflect a great deal of common thought about the evaluation and case selection process.

Montgomery County Intermediate Unit

Responding to the legislation mandating appropriate services,

---

[1] We are indebted to the members of the Montgomery County, Pennsylvania, Intermediate Schools, especially Marshall Siegel and Russell Morely, for permission to reproduce these materials.

[2] These materials were shared with us by consultant Thomas Ehren of the Broward County, Florida Schools.

accountability, and due process procedures, school districts have had to develop standards and rationale for case load selection and dismissal. One of the quality manuals is that developed by the Speech, Language, and Hearing Clinician of the Montgomery County Intermediate Unit. Following is selected information from that manual.

General Considerations in Case Selection

1. The student whose level of communicative interaction interferes with adequate functioning at home and at school should have priority.
2. The middle school or secondary school student exhibiting poor motivation and attitude should be admitted to therapy on a trial basis for six to eight months, after which time the situation is reassessed.
3. When the student's communication problem is the dialect of his environment or background, therapy is not indicated. When English is the second language, therapy is not indicated unless the deficit can be proven both in English and in the native language.
4. Selection of children under the age of eight years depends on the number and type of errors, consistency, and stimulability.

Children Who Should Not be Selected for Therapy

1. The child who has only an attending problem.
2. The child who uses slang and incorrect grammar.
3. The child weak in a discrete area of language that does not interfere with communication, i.e. child doesn't know colors or alphabet.
4. The child who malingers in articulation, language, or fluency.
5. The child whose speech is characterized by excessive rate that does not interfere with communication.
6. The child whose language is intact but who mumbles.
7. The child whose parents hold expectations beyond the child's developmental level.

Articulation

The child is considered to have an articulation *disorder* when three or more sounds are in error or, in a child seven years old or older, when a single sound is in error. The problem is considered a *developmental delay* if the development of sounds follows normal sequence but is delayed a year or more as to chronological age. If the error sound is associated with variations in dialect, bilingualism, production that is an acceptable approximation of the target sound, 70 to 90 percent accuracy or error sound, or malingering, it is classified as a *difference* and considered a pattern that does not interfere with communication.

Articulation Severity Rating Scale

Normal: Phoneme production within developmental norms.
Mild: Inconsistent misarticulation of phonemes. Sounds must be stimulable and no more than six months below the developmental range for the phoneme. Consistent misarticulation of phonemes but not interfering with intelligibility. Phonemes may be stimulable, but due to age or other factors self-correction is not expected.
Moderate: Interferes with communication. Child shows signs of frustration. Some phonemes may be stimulable.
Severe: Unintelligible all of the time or interferes with communication. Child shows signs of frustration, refuses to speak at times. Difficult to stimulate most sounds.

Articulation Assessment

Formal: McDonald Deep Test of Articulation
McDonald Screening Test
Goldman-Fristoe Test of Articulation
Fisher-Logeman Test of Articulation
Photo Articulation Test
Arizona Articulation Proficiency Test
Ling Test (for hearing impaired)
Carter-Buck Test of Sound Stimulability
Informal: Oral-facial examination

Informal stimulability assessment
Informal test of sounds in conversation

Fluency

Disorder: Disruptions in speech flow characterized by repetitions, prolongations, hesitations, interjections and/or struggle behaviors. A child with a fluency disorder is considered to have either three or more stuttered words per minute without secondary behaviors, or .5 or more stuttered words per minute with secondary behaviors such as circumlocution and/or inappropriate physical struggle.

Difference: Irregular speech flow patterns such as:
    inappropriate rate
    cluttering
    episodic stuttering (if not severe)
    developmental dysfluency
    imitative dysfluency

Fluency Severity Rating Scale

Normal: .5 or less stuttered words per minute with no secondary characteristics.

Mild: Observable nonfluent speech behavior is present (.5–1 stuttered word per minute). Child is not concerned about the nonfluent speech. Normal speech periods are observable and predominant.

Moderate: One to three stuttered words per minute. Observable nonfluent speech behaviors are present on a regular basis. Child is becoming concerned about the problem and parents, teachers, or peers are aware of it.

Severe: More than three stuttered words per minute or other stuttering behavior observable on a regular basis. Child is aware of problem in communicating. Struggle, avoidance, or other coping behaviors are observed.

Fluency Assessments

Formal: Monterey Fluency Interview
        Perception of Stuttering Inventory

              Stutterer's Self Ratings of Reactions to Speech Situations
              Iowa Scale of Attitude Toward Stuttering
              Riley Stuttering Severity Instrument
              Memphis State Assessment Battery
Informal: Parent, teacher, and student observations
              Conversational samples (5 minutes)
              Reading samples (5 minutes)
              Monologue sample (5 minutes)

Considerations for Case Selections

The SLP should select any student whose rate of stuttering exceeds normal dysfluency, including the younger stutterer.

Fluency differences must be handled on an ongoing consultative basis.

Episodic stuttering must be closely monitored and handled on an ongoing consultative or direct basis because a disorder may develop.

When the child's or parent's perception of speech is not consistent with the clinician's perception, consultative services may be employed.

Voice Disorders

Abnormality in pitch, loudness, or quality resulting from pathological conditions or inappropriate use of the vocal mechanism that interferes with communication or produces maladjustment.

Voice Difference

A distinguishable variance in pitch, loudness and quality such as
1. Various regional dialects, i.e. nasalized vowels, hoarseness
2. Episodic pitch changes
3. Acute laryngitis, i.e. screaming at a sporting event, viral infection

A voice difference should be checked periodically.

Voice Severity Rating Scale

Normal: Optimum pitch: male—⅓ from bottom of total range
female—⅓ from bottom of total range plus two to three notes
Loudness: 70dB

Mild: Inconsistent or slight deviation. Voice disorder is not noted by casual listener. Student may be aware of problem.
Moderate: Voice disorder is consistent and noted by casual listener. Student may be aware of problem.
Severe: There is a significant deviation in the voice. Voice disorder is noted by the casual listener. Parents are usually aware of problem.

Voice Assessment

Formal: Ling Test
Wilson Voice Evaluation Profile
Fisher-Logemen Voice Evaluation
Medical evaluation
Informal: Note: breathing, pitch, intensity, glottal onset, resonance, phrasing, stress patterns
Spontaneous speech sample
Oral peripheral
Review of school health records and audiometric data
Case history

Ear, Nose, and Throat Examination for Voice Disorders

1. A child must have medical clearance before enrollment in voice therapy.
2. The clinician should fill out the letter to the parents and the Clinician Referral Form.
3. The parent letter should then be given to the school nurse:
   a. It should be signed by the nurse
   b. The nurse or clinician should send it to the child's parents
4. The parents should take the child and the Clinician Referral Form and Report of Medical Evaluation Form to the physician, preferably an ear, nose, and throat specialist.

5. The forms should be returned to the clinician, and the information should be shared with the school nurse.
   6. The IEP process should be completed and therapy begun.
   7. The student should receive a medical reevaluation periodically as judged necessary by the clinician or physician.
   8. The clinician should inform the physician of therapy progress following confidentiality guidelines.

Consideration for Case Selection

   1. Children with voice disorders should be considered for direct therapy.
   2. Children with allergies should not be selected for direct therapy but may be considered for consultative services.
   3. Voice differences may be handled on a consultative basis.
   4. Children who are being treated at a hospital or clinic (repaired cleft palate or velar pharyngeal insufficiencies) should be considered for therapy after consultation with teacher, parent, physician.
   5. If home support is not present, consultation with supervisory input should precede case selection.

Language Disorders

A deviant acquisition and use of receptive, cognitive and/or expressive systems, causing a socially and/or educationally handicapping condition. Figure 8-3 presents a breakdown of language areas.

Language Delay

A pattern of language acquisition that follows a developmental sequence but is delayed by one year or more according to chronological age.

Language Differences

Atypical language patterns that may not interfere with communicative interaction, such as ethnic and regional dialect differences.

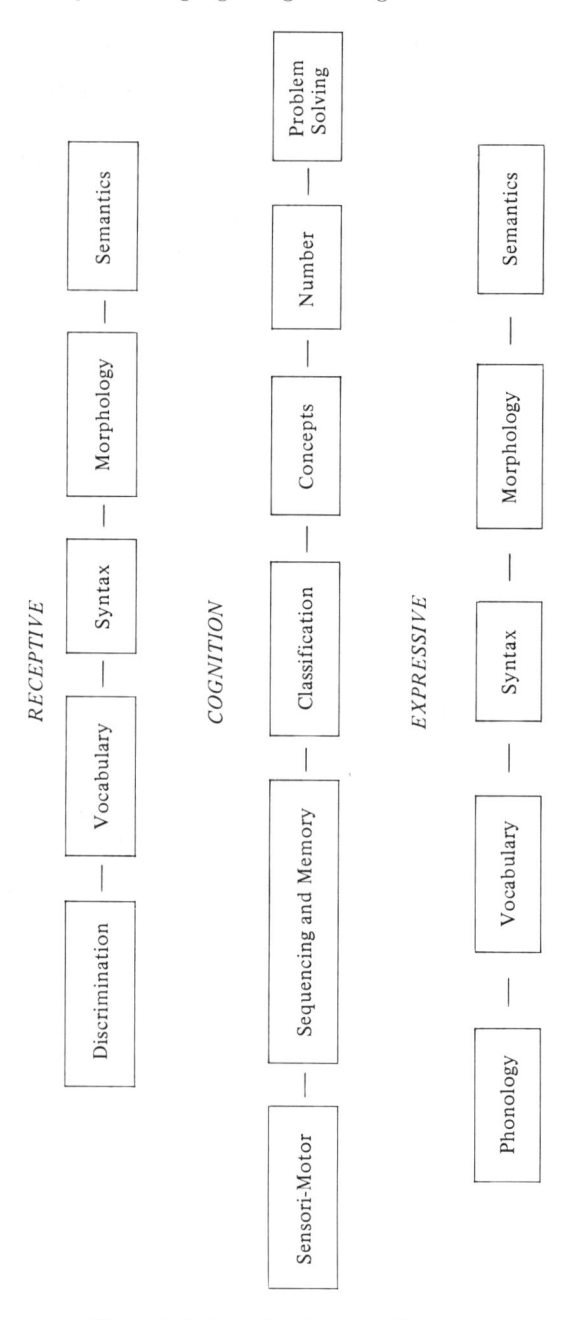

RECEPTIVE: Discrimination — Vocabulary — Syntax — Morphology — Semantics

COGNITION: Sensori-Motor — Sequencing and Memory — Classification — Concepts — Number — Problem Solving

EXPRESSIVE: Phonology — Vocabulary — Syntax — Morphology — Semantics

Figure 8-3. Functional areas of language.

Language Severity Rating Scale

Normal: Receptive and expressive language development within normal limits.

Mild: Appropriate diagnostic tests indicate a six to eighteen month delay in receptive or expressive language or both.

Moderate:[3] Expressive or receptive language disorder that limits or interferes with the student's ability to appropriately interact or respond in learning and/or social situations.

Severe:[3] Expressive or receptive language disorder that prevents the student from appropriately interacting or responding in learning and/or social situations.

Considerations for Case Selection

1. Students whose expressive language skills are not commensurate with their receptive language skills should be considered for therapy if the discrepancy is more than 12 months. The wider this discrepancy, the higher the student's priority for therapy.
2. Kindergarten, transitional first, and regular first grade students who demonstrate a 12 to 18 month language delay may be considered for the communication skills group or maintained on a developmental list.
3. Students with a language delay of more than 18 months should be selected for therapy (keeping in mind the guidelines established for various exceptionalities).
4. Language disordered students should be selected for therapy.
5. Students who are unable to express basic needs or unable to perform basic classroom tasks due to language disorder or delay should be selected for therapy intervention.
6. As indicated earlier in the general considerations section, a student who is weak in a discrete area of language that does

---

[3]Adapted from California State Department of Education Proposed Guidelines, Criteria of Eligibility for Services: Communicatively Handicapped—Appendix B (1979).

not interfere with communicative interaction should not be selected for therapy, i.e. the child doesn't know alphabet, colors.
7. Students whose emotional or behavioral characteristics interfere with the therapy process to such a degree that direct therapy is not feasible may be best handled through a consultant mode until direct intervention for language is appropriate.
8. Language deficient students may be seen on a consultative basis. When English is a second language, the clinician should check with the District to see if tutorial services are available.

Broward County Schools (Florida)

According to the curriculum supervisor for speech and language, Thomas C. Ehren, the Broward County School program has developed and revised guidelines for case selection and submitted them to the Florida State Department of Education for approval each year since 1974. The material that follows represents that in use during the 1980–81 school year.

SLPs in this program have used some severity scales developed elsewhere and, quite uniquely, have matched them for many disorders with the contact hours recommended to assist clinicians in establishing their therapy schedules. As expected, case load guidelines and concepts of severity of speech-language disorders are under continuous evaluation by staff members in light of national and local trends, new research evidence, and improved therapeutic techniques. Thus, current guidelines and concepts may be somewhat different in years to come.

Articulation

Articulation Severity Rating

	RATING	CHARACTERISTICS
	0	Normal
MILD	1	Inconsistent misarticulation of phonemes, whether substituted, omitted, or distorted. Sounds must be stimulable and within the expected range of developmental acquisition for the phoneme.

MODERATE	2	Consistent misarticulation of 1 to 4 phonemes may interfere with intelligibility, depending upon number of phonemes misarticulated. Phonemes may be stimulable, but due to age or other factors self-correction is not expected.
SEVERE	3	Interferes with communication. Shows signs of frustration. Some phonemes may be stimulable. Distractible to a listener. Intelligibility often affected.
VERY SEVERE	4	Unintelligible most of time. Interferes with communication. Pupil shows signs of frustration and refuses to speak at times. Difficult to stimulate most sounds. Distracting to a listener.

Intelligibility Severity Rating

	RATING	CHARACTERISTICS
	0	Normal, readily intelligible
MILD	1	Inconsistent intelligibility depending upon situation or topic. Parents and others usually have only slight difficulty understanding.
MODERATE	2	Intelligible if topic is known. Consistent difficulty with intelligibility with parents and other persons.
SEVERE	3	Intelligible only infrequently if topic is well known.
VERY SEVERE	4	Intelligible only with single words. Almost never intelligible.

Language

Language Severity Rating

	RATING	CHARACTERISTICS
	0	Normal
MILD	1	According to appropriate diagnostic tests used, the expressive or receptive, or both, skills indicate a difference from normal language behavior. May include dialect and bilingual differences.
MODERATE	2	Appropriate diagnostic tests indicate a noticeable delay from the norm. Conversational speech shows definite indications of language deficit. A twelve (12) to seventeen (17) month delay.
SEVERE	3	Appropriate diagnostic tests indicate a language problem that is interfering with communication and educational progress and is often accompanied by an articulation problem. An eighteen (18) to twenty-three (23) month delay.

| VERY SEVERE | 4 | Appropriate diagnostic tests indicate a significant gap from the norms. Communication is an effort. Could range from no usable language to unintelligible communication. Educational progress is extremely difficult. Usually accompanied by an articulation problem. Twenty-four (24) or more months delay. |

For any student whose intellectual functioning falls two (2) or more standard deviations below the mean, mental age rather than chronological age shall be utilized in determining severity.

Voice

Voice Severity Rating

	RATING	CHARACTERISTICS
	0	Normal
MILD	1	Inconsistent or slight deviation. Check periodically.
MODERATE	2	Voice difference is not noted by casual listener. Child may be aware of voice.
SEVERE	3	Voice difference is consistent and noted by casual listener. Child may be aware of voice. Medical referral is required.
VERY SEVERE	4	There is a significant difference in the voice. Voice difference is noted by casual listener. Parents are usually aware of the problem. Medical referral is required.

Fluency

Fluency Severity Rating

	RATING	CHARACTERISTICS
	0	Normal
MILD	1	Observable nonfluent speech behavior present. Child is not aware or concerned about the nonfluent speech. Normal speech periods reported or observable and predominant. Indirect services. Monitor.
MODERATE	2	One to three stuttered words per minute. Observable nonfluent speech behavior present and observable on a regular basis. Child is becoming aware of the problem, and parents, teachers, or peers are aware and concerned.
SEVERE	3	More than three stuttered words per minute or other stuttering behavior is noted on a regular basis. Child is aware of a problem in communicating. Struggle, avoidance or other coping behaviors are observed at times.
VERY SEVERE	4	More than ten stuttered words per minute. Communication is an effort. Avoidance and frustrations are obvious. Struggle behavior is predominant.

Speech and Language Impaired Categories

Four programs are described under the category of Speech and Language Impaired.

Each category reflects unique procedures for classifying students in relation to their degree (severity) of handicap, type of handicap, or age.

1. *Speech and Language I:* A part-time program for students with articulation, language, voice, and fluency disorders. Severity may range from moderate to very severe. Services are provided in the student's home school.
2. *Language II (Severe Language Disabilities):* Program for students with very severe language disabilities as a primary handicap. Services are often provided in a school other than the student's home school.
3. *Nonvocal Communication:* A program for students with very severe impairments in speech as well as expressive language. Students are provided with training in an alternative communication system. Services are often provided in a school other than the student's home school.
4. *Public Education Providing Preschool Education and Remediation (PEPPER):* A program for preschool (3–5 years old) students with speech and language disorders. Services are provided to students at a school site. Services may be provided in the student's home.

These categories are detailed in the following presentation.

1. SPEECH AND LANGUAGE I

Definition

One whose basic communication system, whether verbal, gestural, or vocal, evidences disorders, deviations, or general developmental needs in language, speech, fluency, or voice quality, which hinder academic learning, social adjustment, self-help skills, or communication skills.

A. *Criteria for Eligibility*

The Speech and Language Impaired Program consists of four

(4) categories, (speech, language, fluency and voice), each of which has separate eligibility criteria.
1. *Speech:* Nonmaturational articulation disorders characterized by substitutions, distortions, or omissions of speech sounds. (The presence of a myofunctional—tongue thrust—disorder in the absence of any measured articulation deficit shall not be used to determine eligibility). A student is eligible for Speech and Language I who—
   a. Demonstrates any delay from the expected age of developmental acquisition of one (1) or more separate phonemes in any word position as measured by standardized articulation assessments of (1) sound-in-word production and (2) a sound-in-sentence or conversational sample (Severity Rating 2, 3, or 4). *See* Figure 8-4.
   b. Does not meet criterion (a) above, but demonstrates less than 75% intelligibility in conversational speech and errors in more than four (4) separate phonemes in any word position (Severity Rating 2, 3, 4).
2. *Language:* Receptive or expressive problems or processing (perception, understanding) or disorders of syntax, semantics, morphology, or phonology. Eligible students include
   a. Any kindergarten to fifth grade student who demonstrates a language age of at least twelve (12) months below his/her chronological age, as measured by two (2) standardized language assessments.
   b. Any sixth to twelfth grade student who demonstrates a language age of at least twenty-four (24) months below his/her chronological age, as measured by two (2) standardized language assessments.

If language age cannot be obtained from the test score, language performance at or below tenth (10th) percentile may be used as an alternate scoring method under (a) and (b).

Note: For any student whose intellectual functioning falls between two (2) and three (3) standard deviations below the mean (Educable Mentally Retarded), mental age rather than chronological age shall be utilized in determining eligibil-

If student's chronological age is:

3	4		4½	5	6	7
Vowels	n	t	f	l	r	
p	ŋ		d		v	ʃ
b	w		k		j	tʃ
m	h		g			
					s	Consonant Blends
					z	

Figure 8-4. Broward County Phoneme Development Chart.

ity under (a) and (b) above. For any student whose intellectual functioning falls three (3) or more standard deviations below the mean (Trainable and Profoundly Mentally Retarded), developmental inventories of (pre) speech or language behaviors may be substituted for one or more standardized language assessments in determining eligibility under (a) and (b).

3. *Fluency:* Inappropriate rate of flow of speech characterized by any of the following: repetitions, prolongations, blocks, hesitations, interjections, broken words, revisions, incomplete phrases or ancillary movements that are indicative of stress or struggle.

   Any student is eligible who evidences more than one (1) stuttered word per minute on the Stuttering Evaluation form, which measures automatic, imitation, and conversational speech fluency *and* whose teacher and/or parent indicates the presence of stuttering behavior on the *Parent/Teacher Checklist for Voice and Fluency Problems* (Severity Rating 2, 3, or 4).

4. *Voice:* Disordered frequency, intensity, intonation, respiration, or resonance inappropriate to student's age and sex.

   Any student is eligible who evidences voice characteristics that consistently deviate from normal, as measured by the *Voice Evaluation,* and whose teacher and/or parent indicates the presence of deviant voice characteristics on the *Parent/Teacher Checklist for Voice and Fluency Problems* (Severity Rating 2, 3, or 4).

Note: Any student with a voice disorder that is consistently noted by listeners and the child or consistently poses an

extreme problem with speaking shall be referred for an otolaryngological evaluation prior to providing direct therapy, and the referral shall be documented on the I.E.P. (Severity Rating 3 or 4).
B. *Procedures for Screening*
All students being considered for a speech and language program shall be screened for hearing.
C. *Procedures for Student Evaluation*
1. Speech/language clinicians shall be responsible for implementing and conducting formal identification and diagnostic assessment procedures for students with a suspected disability in language, speech, fluency, or voice. Parent consent for formal individual evaluation is required prior to any speech and language evaluation that singles the student out from his/her regular or exceptional classmates.
2. At least two measures of communication ability shall be administered (and failed) to determine a student eligible for each category of the speech and language program.
3. Standardized test instruments or published normative data in speech and language pathology shall be used in the assessment of students evidencing a suspected disability in speech, language, fluency, or voice.
4. Medical and psychological examinations (optional) shall be requested by the speech-language clinician when deemed appropriate to the assessment of a suspected disability in speech, language, fluency, or voice.
5. Developmental and social histories (optional) shall be included when deemed necessary by the speech-language clinician.
6. Reevaluation must occur every three years and shall consist of at least an assessment in the disability area for which the student was originally determined eligible.
7. Parent(s) shall be notified of the results of an evaluation in which the student's performance on the assessments are within normal limits. This notification shall be documented on the Speech and Language Referral form and the form shall be sent to the parent(s).
D. *Procedures for Determining Eligibility and Educational Placement*
A speech/language clinician shall be a member of the eligi-

bility and placement staffing committee.
E. *Procedures for Providing an Individualized Education Plan*
   For students eligible for placement both in speech and language, and another exceptional student education program, it is necessary to develop only one I.E.P.
F. *Procedures for Dismissal or Reassignment*
   Dismissal is defined as removal from the program based on one of the following criteria:
   1. Satisfactory achievement of program goals resulting in acceptable speech, language, fluency and/or voice based on reevaluation and/or review of the I.E.P. by the speech/language clinician using any of the following criteria:
      a. At least 80 percent correct and acceptable use of speech (articulation), language, or voice skills in a conversational situation.
      b. Speech (articulation) or language skills within nine (9) months of the developmental age (M.A. or C.A.) utilized in determining eligibility.
   2. Maximum expected improvement in speech (articulation), language, fluency, or voice based on reevaluation and/or review of the I.E.P. by the speech/language clinician.
   3. The parent(s) or student requests dismissal before program goals are achieved and the staffing committee concurs. The speech/language clinician should counsel the parent(s) and student concerning possible effects of premature dismissal.
   4. A student dismissed, based on graduation or completion of school before program goals are achieved, shall be referred to agencies for continuation of services.
G. *Special Program Organization*
   The severity of the speech and/or language impairment will determine the type and amount of remedial services. Figure 8-5 is used as a guide for recommending appropriate indirect or direct services.
   1. *Indirect Services*
      a. The speech/language clinician may provide consultation services to parents and school personnel who may interact with or have the primary educational responsibility for a speech and/or language impaired student who may, or

SEVERITY RATINGS*

TYPE OF SERVICE	1 MILD	2 MODERATE		3 SEVERE		4 VERY SEVERE	
		IND.	GROUP	IND.	GROUP	IND.	GROUP
	Indirect Services Consultation	Up to 2 hrs/ week	Up to 3 hrs/ week	Up to 4 hrs/ week	Up to 5 hrs/ week	Up to 6 hrs/ week	Up to 6 hrs/ week
AMOUNT	In-service to teachers Parent counseling Classroom observations Monitoring students Classroom consultation Home Programs						

* Refer to the Criteria for Eligibility and the Appendix for definitions of severity for each disorder.

Key to terms:
- Type – Represents a continuum of appropriate service recommendations. Individual and group therapy may be combined with the total recommended hours/week not to exceed the maximum recommendation for group therapy with the severity rating category.
- Individual – One student (individual therapy is a recommended delivery model for students with very severe disorders).
- Group – Usually not more than 4 students/group except when students in group have moderate problems. Not more than 6 students/group.
- Very Severe – Students in this category may be eligible for Language II programs if the primary handicap is language.

Figure 8-5. Recommended guide for providing indirect or direct speech and language services.

may not, be receiving direct services. Consultation may include staff development activities, conferences to discuss strengths and weaknesses, and developing home or class speech and/or language remedial programs.
   b. The speech/language clinician may provide consultation services to students. Consultation may be provided on an occasional basis and may include monitoring students who are potential candidates for direct services, providing information about speech and/or language improvement, or monitoring students dismissed from direct services.
  2. *Direct Services*
    Part-time Speech and Language I
    Eligible students with moderate, severe, or very severe impairments may be provided with direct speech and/or language remedial services as part of the regular or exceptional student program.
H. *Instructional Program*
  1. *Philosophy:* Adequate communication skills commensurate with physical and mental abilities are essential to a student's overall academic, social, emotional, and career success. Speech and language services are provided to eligible students to insure that they may achieve their fullest communicative potential.
  2. *Curriculum:* A continuum of developmental skills in articulation, language, fluency and voice will be provided. Entry level skills are determined by the speech/language clinician for each student.
  3. *Methodology:* Remedial activities for eligible students are selected by the speech/language clinician to enable the student to achieve the goals specified in the I.E.P.
I. *Support Services*
  Use services available in the community.

2. LANGUAGE II

Severe Language Disabilities

Definition

One whose basic verbal communication system evidences very severe disorders or deviations in language which hinder acquisition of academic learning and communication skills.

A. *Criteria for Eligibility*
  1. Intellectual Function: A score which falls no lower than two (2) standard deviations below the mean on an individually administered, standardized test of intellectual functioning.
  2. Auditory acuity no greater than a 30dB loss in the better ear unaided *or* a statement from the Eligibility and Placement Committee that the student's inability to perform adequately on tasks which require auditory processing or language is not due to poor auditory acuity.
  3. Visual acuity of at least 20/70 in the better eye with best possible correction *or* a statement from the Eligibility and Placement Committee that the student's inability to perform adequately on tasks which require auditory processing or language is not due to poor visual acuity.
  4. A statement from a school psychologist indicating that inability to perform adequately on tasks which assess language skills is not due to emotional disturbance.
  5. Deficits and/or delays in communication abilities more than two (2) years below computed expectancy age in one or both of the following areas, as measured by at least two standardized assessments in each area:
     a. Receptive language (auditory skills, vocabulary, syntax, morphology, comprehension).
     b. Expressive language (morphology, syntax, semantics, pragmatics).
  6. Academic delay as measured by standardized tests of academic achievement such as the California Achievement Test, Stanford Achievement Test, Metropolitan Achievement Test, Shelquist Informed Reading Inventory.

B. *Procedures for Screening*
   The evaluation for eligibility in the Speech and Language I program shall be required for students suspected of demonstrating a severe language impairment.

C. *Procedures for Referral*
   Complete requirements for Speech and Language I.
   In addition, students who are being considered for the Language II program shall be referred to the Area Diagnostician. The

Area Diagnostician shall perform any additional assessment(s) if necessary. Referrals shall include the following information:
1. Speech and Language Referral form and case history.
2. A current (not older than one year) parent consent for speech and language evaluation.
3. A current (not older than one year) psychological report. If a current report is not available, a referral for Psychological Services is required.
4. Speech and Language folder.

D. *Procedures for Student Evaluation*
Each of the following areas shall be assessed:
1. General expressive communication abilities.
2. General receptive communication abilities.
3. Specific oral expressive communication abilities.
4. A transcribed conversational sample of at least 50 utterances, unless performed as part of (2) above.
5. Specific receptive communication abilities.
6. Speech Mechanism.
7. Auditory Skills, as appropriate
8. Articulation
9. Psychological Function
Psychological evaluations of students with a suspected language impairment should assess nonverbal performance as well as verbal abilities. Nonverbal performance abilities may be considered as a more valid indication of a language disabled student's potential.
10. Academic achievement scores or anecdotal records supplied by the student's classroom teacher.

E. *Procedures for Determining Eligibility and Educational Placement*
The eligibility and placement committee shall include the area speech/language diagnostician.
If the student does not meet all the eligibility criteria but the evaluation team feels the program may be appropriate, the Curriculum Supervisor for Speech and Language shall be notified to hold a prestaffing to discuss eligibility.

F. *Procedures for Providing an Individual Educational Program*
Refer to Speech and Language I.

G. *Procedures for Dismissal or Reassignment*
Dismissal is defined as removal from the program based on one or more of the following criteria:
1. Satisfactory academic achievement;
2. Communication skills within one (1) year of expectancy age.
Note: Dismissal may be made to the Speech and Language I program.

H. *Special Program Organization*
Eligible students with very severe language impairments may be provided with direct remedial services in a part-time program up to 12 hours per week.

Students may also receive articulation, voice, or fluency services in addition to the language disabilities program, although the combined services shall not exceed 12 hours/week.

I. *Instructional Program*
1. *Philosophy:* The Language II program is designed to provide eligible students with a continuum of services. Students recommended for placement in the Language II program have demonstrated their inability to perform acceptably or progress adequately in a less restrictive situation. They require daily intervention in language to develop skills to enable them to function adequately in the mainstream. The recommended program design should provide for the integration and modification of the academic curriculum within the language disabilities program and an inclusion of language experiences into the academic program. The severity of the language disability is such that eligible students would not be able to apply language skills in the academic program without a total integration of both curriculums.

A team-teaching model consisting of a speech/language clinician and basic or specific learning disabilities teacher is recommended.

2. *Curriculum:* A continuum of developmental skills in language that are used in academic and social situations will be provided. Articulation, voice, or fluency disabilities may be remediated by the Speech and Language I clinician or Language II clinician depending on severity.

3. *Methodology:* Since severely language disabled students have

poor communication/interaction skills, activities will be designed to remediate language structures as well as functions and will provide specific practice in interpersonal use of language skills.

Strengths as well as weaknesses will be used in planning instructional activities, such as role-playing, rehearsal, reenactment, and pantomime.

3. NONVOCAL COMMUNICATION

Definition

Defined as one who, because of a significant neuro-muscular, neurological, physical, or central processing disorder, cannot be expected to develop speech as a primary method of oral expression and who evidences normal or near normal receptive language abilities and nonverbal intelligence.

A. *Criteria for Eligibility*

In addition to the criteria 1–6, Language II (Severe Language Disabilities) have a:
1. Diagnosis of neuro-muscular, neurological, or physical problem affecting the ability of the student to use normal speech as a primary method of oral expression. Diagnosis may include, but not be limited to, the following: dysarthria, cerebral palsy, muscular tone or degenerative disorders, facial or oral deformities (excluding cleft palate) as a primary impairment, or
2. Diagnosis of a central processing disorder affecting the ability of the student to use normal speech as a primary method of oral expression. Diagnosis may include, but not be limited to, the following: apraxia, severe expressive aphasia.

B. *Procedures for Screening*

The evaluation for eligibility in the Speech and Language I program shall be required.

C. *Procedures for Referral*

Complete requirements for Speech and Language I.

In addition, students who are being considered for the nonvocal communication program shall be referred to the Area Diag-

nostician. The Area Diagnostician shall perform any additional assessment(s) if necessary. Referrals shall include the following information:
1. Speech and Language Referral form and case history;
2. A current (not older than one year) parent consent for speech and language evaluation;
3. A current (not older than one year) psychological report. If a current report is not available, a referral for Psychological Services is required.
4. Speech and Language folder.

D. *Procedures for Student Evaluation*

The same assessments as required by Language II. Articulation and Speech Mechanism assessment shall receive particular attention related to stimulability, conversational intelligibility, oral structure and function. Appropriate referrals should be made to physicians, neurologists, or physical therapists.

Particular attention shall be given to assessments of receptive vocabulary, syntax, morphology and semantics, nonverbal skills in perception and observations, and descriptions of the student's present level and method of expressive communication.

Progress in previous therapy should be reviewed.

E. *Procedures for Determining Eligibility and Educational Placement*

The eligibility and placement committee shall include the area speech/language diagnostician.

If the student does not meet all the criteria but the evaluation team feels the program may be appropriate, the Curriculum Supervisor shall hold a prestaffing to discuss eligibility.

F. *Procedures for Providing an Individual Educational Program*

Refer to Speech and Language I.

G. *Procedures for Dismissal or Reassignment*

Dismissal is defined as removal from the program based on one or more of the following criteria:
1. Satisfactory academic achievement;
2. Satisfactory use of alternative communication system;
3. Communication skills within one (1) year of expectancy age.

Note: Dismissal may be made to the Speech and Language I program.
H. *Special Program Organization*
Eligible students may be provided with direct remedial services in a part-time program up to 12 hours per week.
Students may also receive articulation, voice, or fluency services in addition to the program, although the combined services shall not exceed 12 hours per week.
I. *Instructional Program*
 1. *Philosophy:* The primary purpose is to provide the student with an alternative method of language expression as a means for social interaction, cognitive growth, and academic achievement within the regular classroom as soon as possible. A team teaching model consisting of a speech/language clinician and a basic or specific learning disabilities teacher is recommended.
 2. *Curriculum*
   Curriculum will include the following:
   a. Selection of initial communication methods such as
     1. Pictorial or orthographic systems.
     2. Symbol systems (BLISS).
     3. Gestural systems, if appropriate.
   b. Training in the use of systems.
   c. Articulation therapy, as appropriate.
 3. *Methodology*
   Methodology will include the following, as appropriate:
   a. Selection of a method for using the system, such as
     1. Communication boards.
     2. Electronic or mechanical devices.
     3. Synthetic voice systems.
     4. Typewriters.
     5. Writing.
   b. Training other personnel to provide support.

4. PRESCHOOL PROBLEMS

Statement of Philosophy

An I.E.P. will be developed for all preschool children verified as speech and language delayed or disordered. The speech and language clinician will participate in the development of all I.E.P.s that warrant a communication component. Speech and language problems may be evident in the child's articulation, language, voice, or fluency. Definitions of articulation, language, voice, or fluency problems are consistent with those specified for the school age population. However, in considering the extent of delay in relation to the child's age, a one year (rather than 18 month) delay in articulation or language development will be considered significant.

Federal guidelines and the state plan for P.L. 94-142 specify that children closest to school age with the most severe problems will be served first. Priority will be given to four and five year old children. Severity rating scales are available in articulation, language, voice, and fluency sections for the school age population.

Federal guidelines and the state plan for P.L. 94-142 specify that management in the home may be the least restrictive environment for three year old children. Class enrollment or direct therapy management may be considered as the least restrictive environment for four and five year old children. Information from parents, social worker, audiologist, physician, psychologist, optometrist, psychiatrist, and nursery school teachers should also be considered in determining the least restrictive environment.

Guidelines for Caseload Selection

I.E.P.s with a speech and language component will be developed for

1. children who demonstrate a speech and language delay or disorder in addition to delay in other area(s) of development. Children in this category are generally enrolled in classroom or homebound programs with supportive speech and language services.
2. children who have a speech and language delay or disorder only. Children in this category may be served through
    a. outpatient therapy program: a program of direct therapy in which the clinician implements the I.E.P. by working with the child during sessions at the Special Services Center. Children with severe articulation or language delays or disorders and voice problems other than those resulting from vocal abuse will be considered for direct therapy.

b. home-based program: a program in which the clinician implements the I.E.P. by working with the child and/or parents during visits in the child's home. The clinician may also implement the I.E.P. by working with a group of parents, e.g. clinician discusses and models techniques for use by a group of parents of children with fluency problems. Children with milder articulation delays or disorders, language delays or disorders, voice problems resulting from vocal abuse, and fluency problems will be considered for home-based programs. Also, those children who are more stimulable will be considered for home-based programs.

Some Program Comparisons

Some comparisons of the Montgomery County and Broward County program manuals regarding case load selection will be presented.

Montgomery County, Pennsylvania	Broward County, Florida
General Case load Selection	*Four Programs for Speech and Language Impaired*
1. Lists priorities for general selection	1. Does not generally delineate priorities for or exclusions from the therapeutic process.
2. Lists exclusions from the therapeutic process	2. Lists four programs, the first of which (Speech and Language I) is comparable to that of Montgomery County's; the other three programs are designed for more specific problems: a. Language II (Severe Language Disabilities) b. Nonvocal Communication c. Public Education Providing Preschool Education and Remediation
	3. Each program has its own specific eligibility criteria

Montgomery County, Pennsylvania | Broward County, Florida

Articulation

Disorder — 3 or more sounds in error or 7 years old with a single sound in error

Developmental Delay — normal sound sequence development delayed a year or more chronologically

Difference — dialect, bilingualism, production is an acceptable approximation, 70%–90% accuracy of error sound, or malingering

Nonmaturational articulation disorders characterized by substitutions, distortions or omissions (myofunctional disorder in absence of measured articulation deficit — not used to measure eligibility)

a. demonstrates delay from developmental acquisition of one or more separate phonemes in any word position as measured by sound-in-word production and sound-in-sentence or conversational sample
b. demonstrates less than 75 percent intelligibility in conversational speech and errors in more than four separate phonemes in any word position

Articulation Severity Rating

Normal — within developmental norms

Mild — inconsistent misarticulations, sounds stimulable, six months or less below developmental levels; consistent misarticulations not interfereing with communication, may have stimulability but age or other factors preclude self-correction

Moderate — interference with communication, frustration, some stimulability

Severe — unintelligible or interferes with communication, frustration, refusal to speak, limited stimulability

Articulation Severity Rating

0 *Normal*

1 *Mild* — inconsistent misarticulation of phonemes (substitutions, omissions, distortions); sounds stimulable and within expected developmental range

2 *Moderate* — consistent misarticulation of 1–4 phonemes, may interfere with intelligibility depending on number of misarticulations; phonemes stimulable but no correction expected due to age and other factors

3 *Severe* — interferes with communication, frustration, some phoneme stimulation, distracts listener, intelligibility often affected

4 *Very Severe* — unintelligible, interferes with communication; frustration; refusal to speak at times, stimulability is difficult, distracts listener

Fluency

Disorder — disruption due to repetitions, prolongations, hesitations, interjections, and/or struggle behaviors; 3 or more stuttered words per minute without secondaries, or 5 or more stuttered words per minute with secondaries, e.g. circumlocution and/or struggle.

Difference — irregular speech flow patterns, inappropriate rate, cluttering, nonsevere episodic stuttering, developmental dysfluency, or imitated dysfluency

Inappropriate rate of flow of speech characterized by repetitions, prolongations, blocks, hesitations, interjections, broken words, revisions, incomplete phrases, or ancillary movements indicating stress/struggle.

Eligibility: more than one stuttered word per minute or Stuttering Evaluation form measuring automatic, imitated, and conversational speech fluency *and* parent and/or teacher agreement to presence of stuttering behavior on *Parent/Teacher Checklist for Voice and Fluency Problems*

Montgomery County, Pennsylvania

Fluency Severity Rating

Normal—.5 or less stuttered words per minute with no secondaries.

Mild—observable nonfluency (.5–1 stuttered words per minute); child unaware; normal speech periods

Moderate—1–3 stuttered words per minute; regular nonfluent observable speech behavior; child becoming aware, others are aware

Severe—more than 3 stuttered words per minute or other regular stuttering behaviors; child aware; struggle, avoidance or coping behaviors

Broward County, Florida

Fluency Severity Rating

0 *Normal*

1 *Mild*—observable nonfluent speech behaviors; child not aware/concerned; many observed normal speech periods; indirect services—monitor

2 *Moderate*—1 to 3 stuttered words per minute; regularly observed nonfluent speech behavior; child and other becoming aware

3 *Severe*—more than 3 stuttered words per minute or other stuttering behavior on regular basis; child aware; struggle, avoidance, or other coping behaviors are observed

4 *Very Severe*—more than 10 stuttered words per minute; communication is an effort; obvious avoidance and frustration; predominance of struggle behavior

Voice

Disorder—abnormality in pitch, loudness, quality resulting from pathology or inappropriate use of the vocal mechanism producing communication interference or maladjustment

Difference—listing variance in pitch, loudness and quality, e.g. dialect, episodic pitch changes, acute laryngitis; check periodically

Disordered frequency, intensity, intonation, respiration, or resonance inappropriate to age and sex

Eligibility—deviation from normal on *Voice Evaluation* and parent/teacher agreement as to presence of deviant voice characteristics on *ParentTeacher Checklist for Voice and Fluency*

Note—voice disorder consistently noted by listeners and child or consistently poses an extreme problem with speaking—refer for an otolaryngological exam prior to direct therapy and noted on the I.E.P.

Voice Severity Rating

Normal—optimum pitch: male: $\frac{1}{3}$ from bottom of range; female: $\frac{1}{3}$ from bottom of range plus two to three notes
Loudness—70 dB

Mild—inconsistent/slight deviation not noted by casual listener but possibly by student

Moderate—inconsistent and noted by casual listener; student may be aware

Severe—significant voice deviation; noted by casual listener and usually parents

Voice Severity Rating

0 *Normal*

1 *Mild*—inconsistent/slight deviation; check periodically

2 *Moderate*—voice difference not noted by casual listener; child may be aware

3 *Severe*—voice difference consistent and noted by casual listener; child may be aware; medical referral required

4 *Very Severe*—significant voice difference; noted by casual listener; parents usually aware; medical referral required

Montgomery County, Pennsylvania

Broward County, Florida

Language

Disorder—deviant acquisition and use of receptive,* cognitive,* and/or expressive* systems—causing socially and/or educationally handicapping condition

Receptive/expressive problem or processing or syntax, semantics, morphology or phonology disorders

Delay—pattern of language acquisition that follows a developmental sequence but is delayed by one or more years chronologically

a. K–5th grade student with language of twelve months below chronological age—two tests

Differences—atypical language patterns that may not interfere with communication, e.g. ethnic and regional dialect

b. 6th–12th grade student with language of 24 months below chronological age—two tests

(or, if L.A. not obtainable, use language performance below 10th percentile)

Note—intellectual functioning two and three standard deviations below mean (EMR)—mental age rather than chronological age in determining eligibility; intellectual functioning more than three standard deviations below mean (TMR and PMR)—use developmental inventories of (pre) speech or language behavior substituted for formal asessments

Language Severity Rating

Normal—receptive and expressive language within normal limits

Mild—six to eight month delay in receptive and expressive language

Moderate—expressive/receptive language disorder limits or intereferes with student's ability to interact or respond appropriately in learning and/or social situations

Severe—expressive/receptive language disorder preventing student from appropriately interacting or responding in learning or social situations

Language Severity Rating

0 *Normal*

1 *Mild*—expressive and/or receptive skills different than normal; inconsistent; 0–11 months delay; dialect and bilingual differences

2 *Moderate*—noticeable difference delay from normal; conversational speech reflects deficit; 12–17 months delay

3 *Severe*—language problem interfering with communication and educational progress, often with an articulation problem; 18–23 months delay

*Receptive
   1. Discrimination

4 *Very Severe*—significant difference from norm; communication is an effort; range

Montgomery County, Pennsylvania	Broward County, Florida
2. Vocabulary 3. Syntax 4. Morphology 5. Semantics	from no usable language to unintelligible communication; educational progress is extremely difficult; usually articulation problems; 24 or more months delay
*Cognition 1. Sensori-motor 2. Sequencing and Memory 3. Classification 4. Concepts 5. Numbers 6. Problem solving	*intellectual functioning two more standard deviations below the mean, mental age rather than chronological used in determining severity

*Expressive
1. Phonology
2. Vocabulary
3. Syntax
4. Morphology
5. Semantics

CASE LOAD

A Quiet Revolution

The purpose of the survey completed by Sommers and Hatton (1979) was to update information concerning speech, language, and hearing programs provided by itinerate clinicians in the schools. Although previous survey information was available, the most comprehensive, the United States Office of Education–Purdue University study (Darley, 1961), was badly out of date, and a more recent study by Neal (1976) focused mostly on services provided to secondary students. Data presented here sought to identify a number of factors not studied in other surveys, particularly as they may relate to major changes in programs and services resulting from the impact of P.L. 94-142.

The present study was based on data obtained from 166 respondents as compared with Neal's fifty-nine and was not limited exclusively to ASHA members as was Neal's. The present investigation assessed the types of children served, types of service provided, therapy techniques used, and other aspects of public school programs. Although present results can be compared to advantage with the findings from Neal's study, we have information not previously studied by other investigators, and we compared programs and services in various parts of the country.

Results from the U.S. Office of Education–Purdue University survey showed that more than 80 percent of the typical public school clinician's case load consisted of elementary school children with articulation problems. The typical case load of 130 children contained few if any language disordered children and relatively small numbers of children with voice, stuttering, cleft palate, cerebral palsy, or other such disorders (Darley, 1961).

In 1971 O'Toole and Zaslow, writing about the changes in public school programs, postulated that a "quiet revolution" was taking place. Resulting basic areas of change included (a) reduction of case loads, (b) fewer articulatory defectives in case loads, (c) more language impaired children in case loads, (d) increased responsibilities for diagnostic and consultative services. Although O'Toole and Zaslow did not provide data to support their observations of a "quiet revolution" in the schools, some of Neal's findings did. Data from the present survey were also used to provide for a comprehensive check of the O'Toole and Zaslow hypothesis.

CASE LOAD INVESTIGATION
Questionnaire

A preliminary questionnaire was developed and submitted to a small group of speech, language, and hearing supervisors in schools for critical analysis and recommendations. The resulting thirty-nine item survey form, presented in Appendix A, was designed to obtain information about SLPs, school districts served, employment of ancillary personnel, case load size and makeup, services provided by the clinician, and the type of therapy (operant vs. traditional) used. Respondents were asked to complete the questionnaire using data from the 1976–77 school year.

Sampling

A national, regional sampling plan was used. The regions of the country as used by ASHA in its surveys consisted of East, Midwest, Southwest, West and Southeast. The regions, states sampled, and numbers of respondents by region are contained in

Regions	Number of Respondents	
EAST—Maine, New York, Ohio, Pennsylvania, Vermont.........	57	(34%)
MIDWEST—Indiana, Iowa, Nebraska, South Dakota............	25	(15%)
SOUTHWEST—Arkansas, Kansas, New Mexico, Texas..........	30	(19%)
WEST—Alaska, California, Hawaii, Idaho, Nevada, Washington...	32	(19%)
SOUTHEAST—Florida, Kentucky, South Carolina, Virginia, West Virginia.............................	22	(14%)
Total number of states—24	Total number of respondents—166	

Figure 8-6. States randomly selected to represent regions of the country and respondents.

Figure 8–6.

Random choice of participating SLPs from the selected states was made in two ways: first, letters were sent to state supervisors of speech, language, and hearing services or other responsible persons asking for a list of speech, language, and hearing clinicians in schools. Most states submitted such lists. In the case of a few states from which lists were not available, random selection of school clinicians was made using the ASHA *Directory.* More than 500 of the 600 persons sampled were selected from state lists. Although 180 persons returned questionnaires, fourteen either were not complete or appeared invalid and had to be discarded. Thus, 30 percent of those contacted returned questionnaires, a percentage essentially the same as Neal's but with twice as many respondents.

Questionnaires were mailed in the Fall of 1977. In February, 1978, returned questionnaires were analyzed.

Results—Schools and Personnel

The Clinicians

Figure 8–7 contains a summary of the degrees held, ASHA membership, and certification status of the respondents from each of the five regions. A total of 120 of the 160 respondents reported holding masters degrees (71%). The percentages of those holding masters degrees by region were rather consistent (from 67–77%). None of the respondents held the doctorate. Sixty-five percent across all regions were members of ASHA, and of the total number, 47 percent reported holding clinical certification. Respondents from the Midwest region reported the smallest percentage of ASHA certification. Perhaps this finding is related to the data in Figure 8–8. These data on the mean numbers of years of professional experience in speech pathology tended to show that respondents from the Midwest region were less experienced, particularly in contrast to those from the Southwest and Western regions. Ninety-two percent of the respondents were females. The range of male/female respondents by region was nonsignificant.

Ancillary Personnel

From 17 to 32 percent of respondents indicated that their school districts employed specially trained clinicians to work with language impaired children. The national mean was 25 percent. Differences by region were nonsignificant. Significant differences were obtained, however, for the employment of educational audiologists. Nationally, 30 percent of the respondents indicated that their school districts had the services of educational audiologists. The regional percentages, presented in Figure 8–9, show that Midwest region respondents reported having such services to a significantly greater degree than clinicians from the four other regions (mean for the four other regions = 23%).

School Districts Served

Respondents were asked to state whether their schools were located in rural, urban, or both rural and urban communities. Based upon a coding of 1–3 respectively, although the mean ratings of all five groups ranged from a low (more rural) for the East to a high (more urban) for the West, these differences were not statistically significant.

The numbers of schools served by a clinician did not differ significantly from region to region, ranging from a mean low of 3.58 for the Southeast to a high of 4.07 for the Southwest. The national mean was 3.83.

Establishing the Therapy Program 415

Accreditation	East		Midwest		Southwest		West		Southeast		National	
	N	%	N	%	N	%	N	%	N	%	N	%
B.A., B.S. Degree	13	23	10	40	7	23	10	31	8	33	46	29
M.A., M.S. Degree	44	77	15	60	23	77	22	69	16	67	120	71
Ph.D. Degree	0	0	0	0	0	0	0	0	0	0	0	0
ASHA Membership	38	73	14	56	23	77	21	66	14	58	110	65
CCC	29	51	9	36	16	53	16	50	9	37	79	47

Figure 8-7. Levels of training and accreditation of respondents.

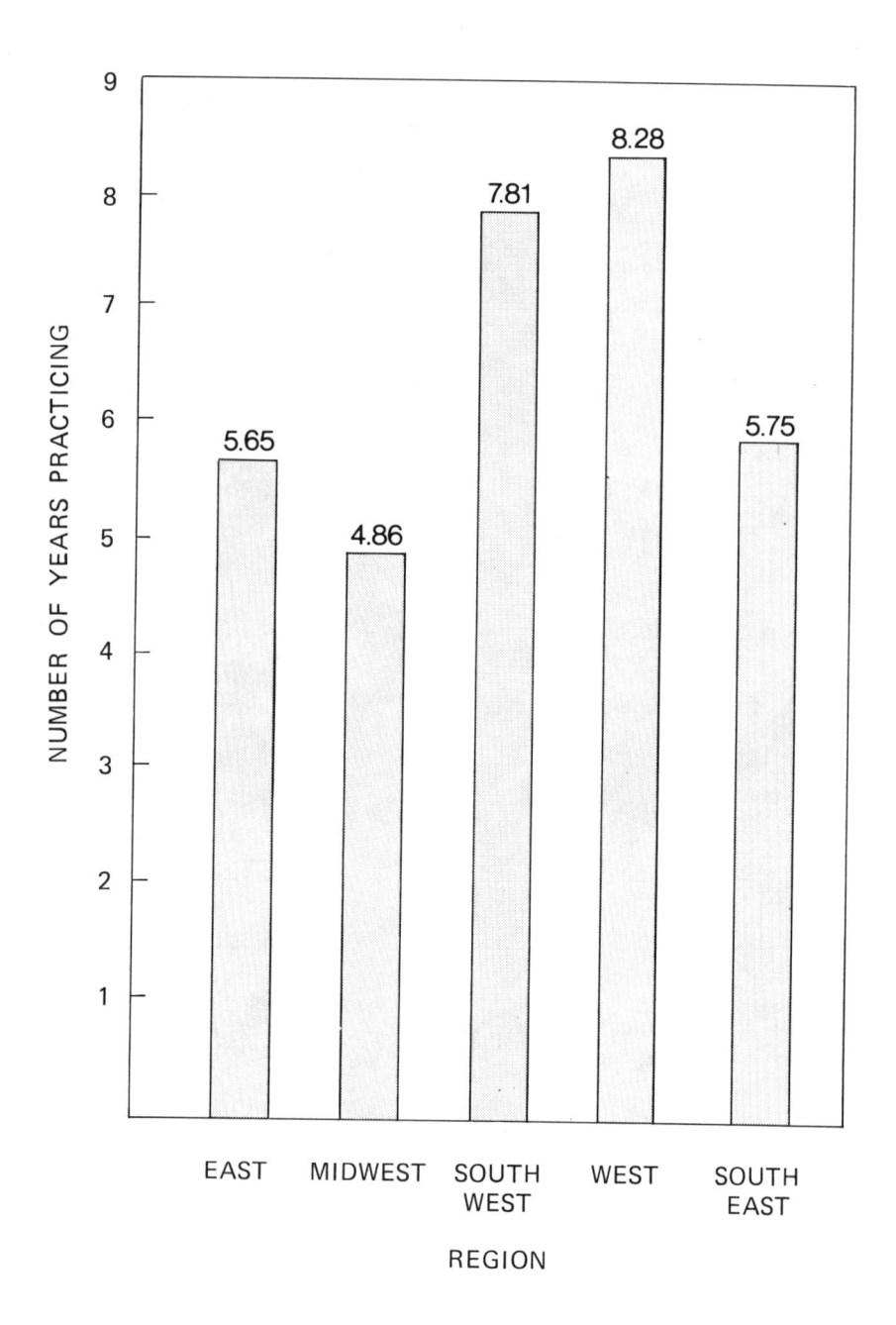

Figure 8-8. Number of years practicing per region.

PERCENTAGE OF SCHOOL DISTRICTS HAVING AN EDUCATIONAL AUDIOLOGIST

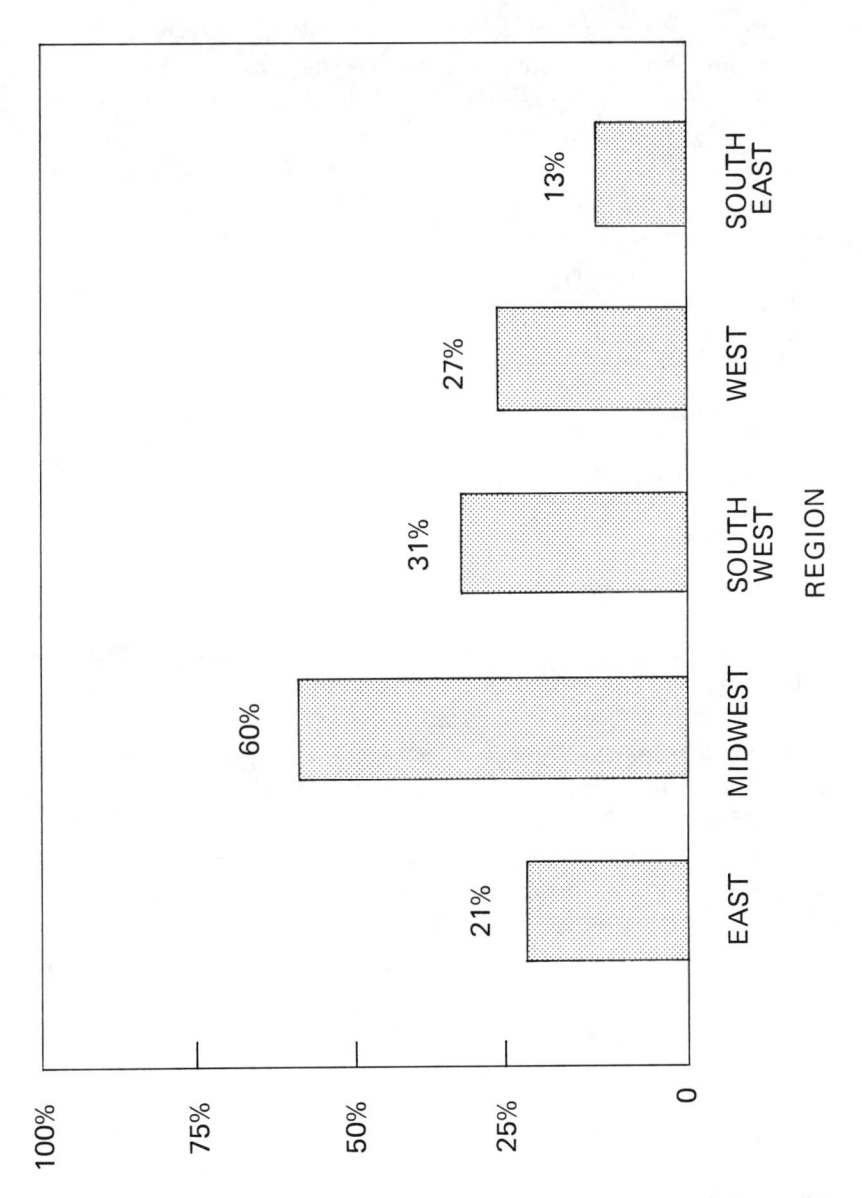

Figure 8-9. School districts having the services of educational audiologists by region.

Results—Case Loads

Case Load Size

Nationally, active case loads of SLPs averaged sixty-four children. Significant regional differences were found. The typical Midwest case load contained only forty-nine children, as compared with ninety-four in the Southeast. Significantly more voice disordered children received therapy in the Southwest (6.8 percent of the case load as compared to a national average of 2.4 percent.) The numbers of children receiving therapy for fluency disorders were also significantly lower in the Midwest than in the other four regions.

Case Load Composition: Communication Disorders

A description of the active case loads of the respondents is contained in Figure 8–10. The numbers and percentages of six categories of speech-language disorders are presented according to national and regional averages. In the first category, Language with Articulation, the children received language therapy but no specific correction for their articulation defects. Nationally, 14.9 percent of active school case loads contained such problems. In the second category, Language with No Articulation, children had only language problems, thus language therapy was provided. On the average, 9.6 percent of children from this category were in national case loads. These two categorizations accounted for the total language therapy emphasis in case loads, their combined percentage being 24.5. Thus, about one-fourth of the school SLPs' case loads nationally were children who received services for their language problems. Categories three and four consisted of the articulation therapy emphasis in case loads. In category three, Articulation with Language, children had both problems yet received therapy only for the articulatory component. This group constituted 19.1 percent of the typical national case load. The fourth category, that of Articulation and No Language, comprised by far the largest percentage (48.9%) of nationwide case loads containing such children. Category five, Fluency, and category six, Voice, accounted for the remaining 7.5 percent of average national case loads.

Establishing the Therapy Program

Region	Lang. w/Art.	Lang. no Art	Caseload Art. w/Lang.	Art. no Lang.	Fluency	Voice	Total # in Caseload	Mn. Caseload
East Number Percentage Mean	528 14.6 9.26	436 12.1 7.65	613 17.0 10.75	1829 50.6 32.08	110 3 11.93	96 2.7 1.68	3612	73.35
Midwest Number Percentage Mean	214 17.1 8.56	133 10.6 5.32	384 30.7 15.36	464 37.1 18.56	31 2.5 0.54	24 2 0.96	1250	49.30
Southwest Number Percentage Mean	313 15.5 10.43	151 7.5 5.03	432 21.4 14.4	836 41.4 27.90	82 4.1 2.73	204 10.1 6.8	2018	67.3
West Number Percentage Mean	259 15.4 8.09	130 7.7 4.06	335 19.9 10.47	801 47.6 25.03	117 6.9 3.65	42 2.5 1.31	1684	52.6
Southeast Number Percentage Mean	276 13.3 12.54	178 8.6 8.09	265 12.8 12.04	1269 61.1 57.68	50 2.4 2.27	38 1.8 1.72	2076	94.3
National Number Percentage Mean	1590 14.9 9.57	1028 9.6 6.19	2029 19.1 12.22	5199 48.9 31.32	390 3.7 2.35	404 3.8 2.43	10640	64.08

Figure 8-10. Numbers, types, and percentages of communication disorders in school case loads.

Inspection of the data summarized in Figure 8–10 will reflect a rather consistent regional pattern of case load composition. The percentages of each of the six categories are highly similar, except for categories three and four, the articulation therapy ones, in which the percentage of children in the Southwest was higher than the other regions.

A detailed breakdown of the six types of communication disorders existing in case loads is presented in Figure 8–10. Figure 8–11 contains this analysis by grade level for the category of Language Problems with Articulation. The national pattern of enrollment for these children was rather consistent across grade levels. The mean numbers of such children were greater in grades one through three in all regions except the Midwest. Generally, two or three secondary students were enrolled, except in the Midwest (mean of 1.2) and Southeast (mean of 4.5). Figure 8–12 contains similar information for children in case loads from the category of Language and No Articulation. As shown in the preceding analysis, the largest numbers of children in this category were from grades one through three. Few preschool children of this type appeared in most regional case loads (mean of 3.3 in the Midwest, 3.0 in the West, 11.0 in the Southeast and one or zero in the other two regions).

Children having Articulation with Language disorder, as shown in Figure 8–13, were most often served in grades one through three also. Larger mean numbers of kindergarten children of this type appeared in most regional case loads. A slight tendency for more secondary students of this type to be in case loads also appeared.

Figure 8–14 contains a summary for the Articulation with No Language type of disorder. National mean enrollments again reflect high variability. As seen in earlier analyses, regional returns show a rather consistent pattern of greater average numbers of children in case loads from grades one through three. However, the Midwest mean of 11.9 children from these grades is significantly smaller than the Southeast's mean of 56.6. The East showed a much larger mean preschool enrollment than the other regions.

Figure 8–15 contains the Fluency category summary. The national mean for the preschool group is spurious, because this statistic was inflated by the mean of 10 children reported from the West. A

Geographic Region

Grade Level	East Mn.	East Range	Midwest Mn.	Midwest Range	Southwest Mn.	Southwest Range	West Mn.	West Range	Southeast Mn.	Southeast Range	National Mn.	National Range
Preschool	4.8	1–21	4.8	1–16	4.5	3–6	2.5	1–5	4.7	1–10	4.2	1–21
Kindergarten	3.6	1–18	4.7	1–25	4.9	1–30	4.3	1–15	6.8	1–20	4.8	1–30
Grades 1–3	6.1	1–33	4.1	1–15	7.7	1–40	5.3	1–30	7.8	1–29	6.2	1–40
Grades 4–6	3.7	3–10	3.1	1–12	3.1	1–10	3.1	1–8	2.4	1–8	3.1	1–12
Grades 7–12	3.8	1–10	1.2	1–2	2.4	1–5	2.6	1–11	4.5	4–5	2.9	1–11

Figure 8-11. Mean and range of children having language and articulation disorders, nationally and by region.

	Geographic Region									
Grade Level	East		Midwest		Southwest		West		Southeast		National	
	Mn.	Range	Mn.	Range	Mn.	Range	Mn.	Range	Mn.	Range	Mn.	Range
Preschool	1.2	1–2	3.3	2–5	1.0	1–3	3.0	3–5	0	0	1.7	1–5
Kindergarten	4.2	1–11	2.9	1–6	2.7	2–3	4.1	1–20	5.7	2–9	3.9	1–20
Grades 1–3	7.2	1–36	5.2	1–19	6.2	1–18	3.6	1–8	6.8	1–16	5.8	1–36
Grades 4–6	2.8	1–10	2.3	1–5	6.3	1–15	3.3	1–8	7.3	2–20	4.4	1–20
Grades 7–12	2.8	1–6	0	0	1.0	1–3	2.0	1–3	11.0	3–19	3.4	1–19

Figure 8-12. Mean and range of children having language but no articulation disorders, nationally and regionally in case loads.

Establishing the Therapy Program

Grade Level	East Mn.	East Range	Midwest Mn.	Midwest Range	Southwest Mn.	Southwest Range	West Mn.	West Range	Southeast Mn.	Southeast Range	National Mn.	National Range
Preschool	2.6	1–6	4.4	1–16	1.0	1–3	1.0	1–4	5.5	1–10	2.9	1–16
Kindergarten	5.0	1–31	3.6	1–10	7.9	1–35	5.1	1–23	4.9	1–20	5.3	1–35
Grades 1–3	9.1	1–14	11.9	1–65	9.0	1–40	9.7	1–25	8.6	1–40	9.7	1–65
Grades 4–6	2.9	1–8	4.3	1–20	4.8	1–20	4.1	1–12	2.7	1–7	3.8	1–20
Grades 7–12	2.2	1–5	3.3	1–10	5.0	1–20	3.0	1–5	7.0	1–18	4.1	1–20

Geographic Region

Figure 8-13. Mean and range of children having articulation with language disorders in case loads, nationally and regionally.

424   Speech-Language Programming in the Schools

Grade Level	Geographic Region											National	
	East		Midwest		Southwest		West		Southeast			
	Mn.	Range	Mn.	Range	Mn.	Range	Mn.	Range	Mn.	Range	Mn.	Range
Preschool	10.8	1–60	1.8	1–3	3.0	1–5	2.0	1–4	0	0	3.5	1–60
Kindergarten	6.0	1–25	4.7	1–48	9.6	1–40	8.4	1–50	3.9	1–10	6.5	1–50
Grades 1–3	24.7	2–80	11.9	3–30	19.8	2–85	20.5	1–78	56.6	2–88	26.7	1–88
Grades 4–6	9.6	1–29	11.7	1–72	8.1	1–33	11.6	1–44	8.1	2–19	9.8	1–72
Grades 7–12	4.3	1–9	3.2	1–9	4.7	1–8	3.9	1–8	3.3	2–5	3.9	1–9

Figure 8-14. Mean and range of children having articulation but no language disorders in case loads, nationally and regionally.

Establishing the Therapy Program 425

Grade Level	East Mn.	East Range	Midwest Mn.	Midwest Range	Southwest Mn.	Southwest Range	West Mn.	West Range	Southeast Mn.	Southeast Range	National Mn.	National Range
Preschool	1.0	1–2	1.0	1–3	0	0	10	10	0	0	2.4	1–10
Kindergarten	1.2	1–2	1.0	1–2	2.3	1–5	1.8	1–4	1.0	1–2	1.5	1–5
Grades 1–3	1.5	1–4	1.3	1–3	2.5	1–7	3.0	1–11	2.1	1–5	2.1	1–11
Grades 4–6	1.9	1–8	1.7	1–3	2.3	1–6	2.1	1–5	1.3	1–2	1.9	1–8
Grades 7–12	1.5	1–4	1.5	1–2	2.0	1–6	7.8	1–30	1.8	1–4	2.9	1–30

Geographic Region

Figure 8-15. Mean and range of children with fluency disorders found in national and regional case loads by grade levels.

generally low incidence of children in case loads for fluency disorders appears rather evenly across the grade levels in all regions except the West, in which an average of 7.8 children were reported.

More voice disordered children were served in the Southwest, particularly in grades one through three and four through six. This pattern is not typical of case load compositions in the other four regions. Generally in the other four regions, almost identical numbers of voice defective children appeared across all grade levels, and few if any preschool voice defective children were reported.

Case Load Composition: Etiologies

An analysis was completed of the various types and numbers of children enrolled by etiological type as reported by grade level. The etiological types consisted of (1) cleft lip and/or cleft palate, (2) severe brain damage, (3) minimal brain dysfunction, (4) deafness, (5) hard-of-hearing, (6) emotionally disturbed, (7) autism, (8) mild mental retardation, (9) severe mental retardation, and (1) "other" (functional).

In the first of these, Cleft Lip and/or Cleft Palate, the regional patterns by numbers of children and grade levels served were almost identical. On the average, 1.2 to 1.3 children were in regional case loads, and most of them were in grades one through three. The national mean was 1.0, and regional means ranged from 0.20–2.0. Distribution of such problems across grade levels was random. No significant regional differences were found.

In the second etiological type, Severe Brain Damage, the East showed a mean of 2 children enrolled at the preschool and kindergarten levels. Other regions reported essentially no such children enrolled at the younger age levels. No significant regional differences in numbers and/or grade levels seemed to exist. In a national average case load of sixty-four students, approximately 0.84 severely brain damaged children were enrolled, mostly from grades one through three and four through six.

Children labelled minimal brain dysfunction comprised the third etiological type. All five regions of the country showed that the largest numbers of such children were in grades one through three, a mean of 4.5. A mean of 2.58 children appeared in case loads across all grades, preschool to twelve. A tendency for more children of this type to be enrolled in the East was observed, particularly in grades one through three and four through six in which the East's mean enrollments of 6.6 in grades one through three and 2.9 in grades four through six were above the national averages.

An average of 1.24 deaf children per case load was reported nationally. This average seemed to be affected by the mean of 4 in grades one through three in the Midwest region and mean of 5 in the Southeast, while the means from the East, Southwest, and West were 1, 1, and 2, respectively. In grades seven through twelve the West mean of three was more than twice as large as any of the other regions. Midwest respondents reported an average of two deaf children in their case loads; West and Southeast, 1.4; and the East and Southwest, 0.6 each across all grade levels.

On the average, 1.5 hard-of-hearing children were reported in national case loads. In the Southwest and West mean kindergarten enrollments of 2.3 and 3.0, respectively, were higher than the national mean of 1.8. The West region's average of 2.5 hard of hearing children was greater than all other regions. Generally, distribution of such children was relatively uniform across all grade levels from kindergarten to grade twelve.

A mean of 1.46 emotionally disturbed children appeared nationwide. Again, the largest numbers of such children were enrolled in grades one through three and four through six. All regions reported essentially the same mean numbers totally and by grade level. The mean numbers of emotionally disturbed preschool and junior/senior high school children reported were uniformly very low across the five regions (range of 0–2, mean = 0.8).

The average number of children diagnosed as autistic varied considerably by region. Respondents from the East, for example, reported a mean of three autistic children per clinician at the preschool level while respondents from the Southwest and Southeast regions reported none and the Midwest and West regions, one each. Reports from the West indicated a mean of five autistic children from grades seven through twelve, while the other regions reported few, if any. The national mean enrollment of autistic children was 0.94. The means of 1.4 in the East, 1.8 in the West, and 0.40 in the Southwest demonstrated some regional variability.

The range of mildly mentally retarded children in case loads across the nation appeared to be very large, suggesting that some clinicians may serve only mentally retarded children while others have more traditionally balanced case loads. The national mean enrollment of such children in case loads across all grades (preschool to 12) was 3.56. The mean numbers were almost identical nationally for grades one through three, four through six and seven through twelve, the mean being 4 children. Smaller average numbers of mildly mentally retarded preschool and kindergarten children were reported nationally. The regional range across all grade levels varied from a low of 2.4 in the Southwest to 4.4 in the Southeast. The national mean of preschool children of this type served seemed greater in the East (mean of 4.7) and the Southeast (mean of 5.0). The national mean for preschool enrollment was 2.6, and respondents from the Southwest reported no such children in their case loads.

For the severely retarded child, respondents nationally indicated that a wide range of services was being provided. The range of national case loads was large at each series of grade levels, perhaps indicating the specific assignments of some school clinicians to severely mentally handicapped children. On the average, 4.58 such children were reported per SLP.

The final etiological type of "other" consisted of many children for whom no specific diagnostic grouping according to etiology was possible. These appeared largely to be in the troublesome category of "functional," a descriptor considered by some (Powers, 1957, and Sommers and Kane, 1974) to be a diagnosis by default. At the preschool level the national mean enrollment in case loads was 4.8. The means for kindergarten, grades one through three, four through six, and seven through twelve were 9.5, 22.3, 9.1, and 3.7, respectively. Eighty-three percent of the enrollment of this type of child in national average case loads came at the traditional elementary level (kindergarten through sixth grade). Forty-five percent of the enrollment across all grade levels was in grades one through three. Preschool enrollment was 9.7 percent; for grades seven to twelve it was 7.5 percent.

Figure 8–16 contains mean numbers of individual sessions for each region. These differences are statistically significant. The East and Midwest means were significantly greater than those of the Southeast and Southwest regions.

The average length of individual sessions was not significantly different across regions, ranging from 18.5 minutes in the Midwest to 26.7 minutes in the West. The national average was 22.3 minutes.

The average length of group sessions was significantly different by region. These data are presented in Figure 8–17. The mean length of group sessions in the Southeast, Southwest, and East was significantly longer than that of the Midwest region. The average length of group therapy sessions nationally was twenty-three minutes.

No significant differences were found across regions for the numbers of children enrolled in group sessions. This figure ranged from a low of 3.4 in the Midwest to a high of 5.5 in the Southeast region. The national average enrollment was four children.

The mean number of weekly group therapy sessions per SLP was not significantly different across the regions, the range being from 14.7 in the Midwest to a high of 24.0 in the Southeast. The national mean was 19.4 sessions weekly.

Parent Involvement

Respondents replied to the request for information concerning parent training or counseling. The percentages of respondents by region who were actively involved in parent training and counseling were not significantly different, ranging from 80 percent in the West to 90 percent in the Southwest. The national mean was 83 percent.

Differences across regions for the amount of time weekly devoted to parent training and/or counseling were also not statistically significant. The Southwest respondents reported the least number of minutes weekly, 63, and the West the most, 81; the national mean was 74. Information concerning how parents were trained and counseled and the purposes of these efforts was not specifically obtained.

AVERAGE NUMBER OF INDIVIDUAL SESSIONS

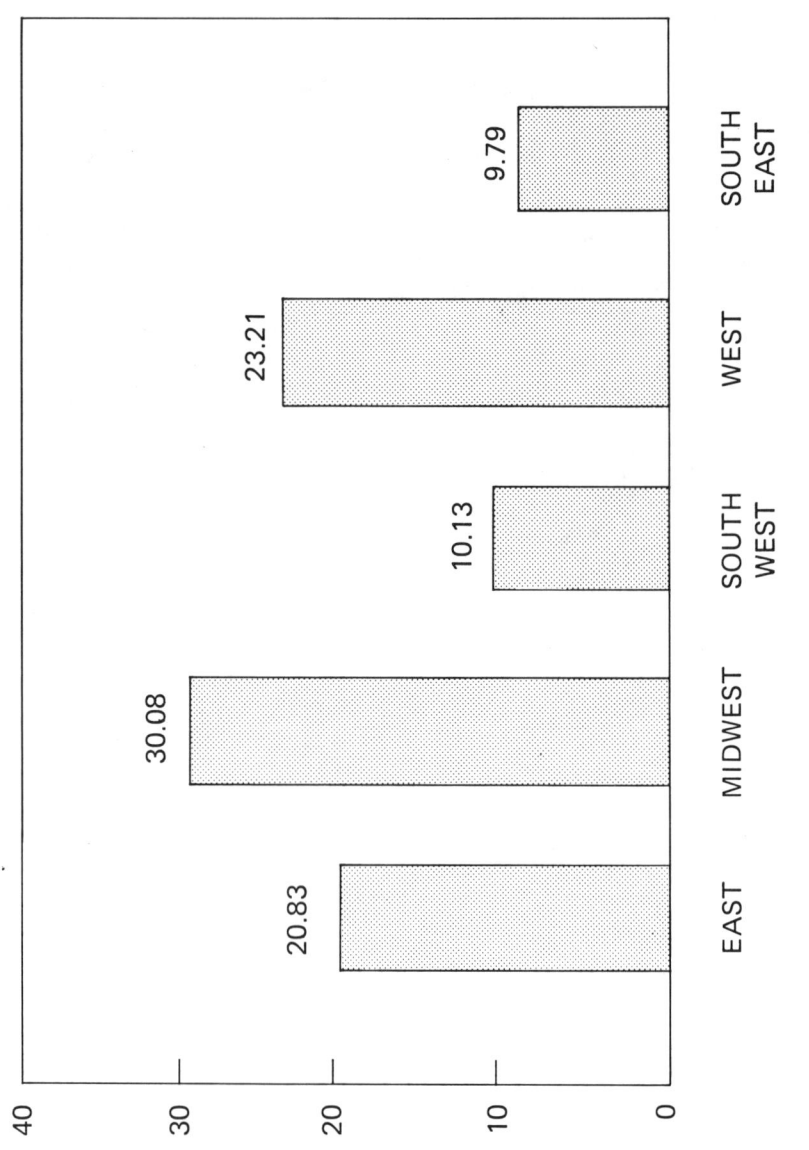

Figure 8-16. Average number of individual sessions per week, per region.

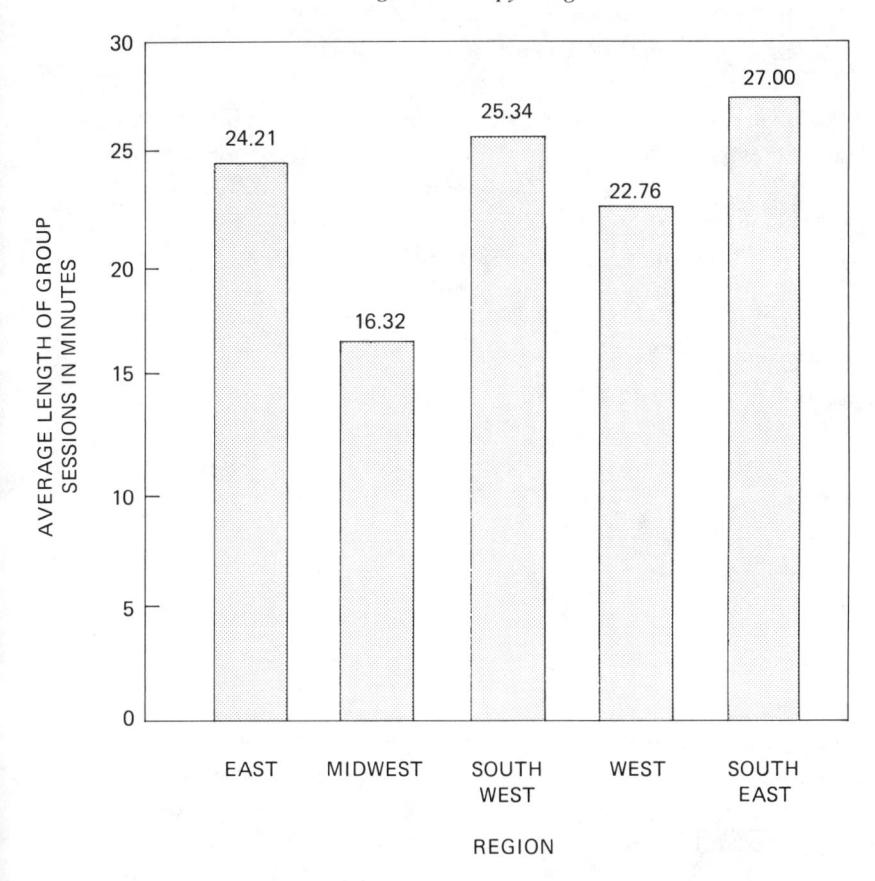

[Figure: Bar chart showing average length of group sessions in minutes per region: East 24.21, Midwest 16.32, Southwest 25.34, West 22.76, Southeast 27.00]

Figure 8-17. Average length of group sessions in minutes per region.

Therapy Schedules

Respondents were asked to indicate the scheduling plan that they followed in providing therapy under the categories "traditional" (itinerant or intermittent), "intensive" (block), or a combination of the two. All regions reflected greater use of traditional scheduling. These figures ranged from a low of 70 percent in the East to a high of 83 percent in the Southwest; the national mean was 77 percent. Generally the intensive, modified block or a combination of the two tended to be equally used across the regions and accounted for the remaining percentages.

Speech Improvement Classes

The average numbers of children served in speech improvement classes weekly showed significant differences across the regions. As revealed in Figure 8-18, the number of children enrolled in speech improvement classes varied from a low of 5.5 in the Southwest to a high of 14.4 in the Midwest. The national average was 9.4.

Therapy Approaches

Figure 8-19 contains a summary of information provided by respondents by grade level probing their use of either operant or traditional speech-language therapy approaches. These data show that traditional therapy approaches were popular in all regions with the national average preference across all grade levels being 58.7 percent vs. 41.3 percent favoring operant. However, since the majority of children in case loads regionally and nationally were enrolled in grade one through six, these percentages are probably less reflective of type of therapy used than the 53.2 percent for traditional and 46.8 percent for operant reported as national averages for these grades (also contained in Figure 8-19). All regions reported that twice as many secondary students, or more, received traditional therapy as operant except in the Midwest where the use of traditional and operant approaches was split almost equally. The East and Midwest respondents preferred traditional approaches with preschool and kindergarten children, while the Southwest, West, and Southeast preferred operant.

Therapy Supervision

The availability of speech, language, and hearing personnel certificated to supervise therapy varied considerably within many of the five regions. While regional differences were not statistically significant, 88 percent of the Midwest respondents reported that they had such services. The Southeast showed the smallest number, 45 percent. The national mean was 58 percent.

Summary

The national average length of group sessions was scarcely greater than averages shown for length of individual lessons, 23

AVERAGE NUMBER OF CHILDREN IN SPEECH IMPROVEMENT CLASSES

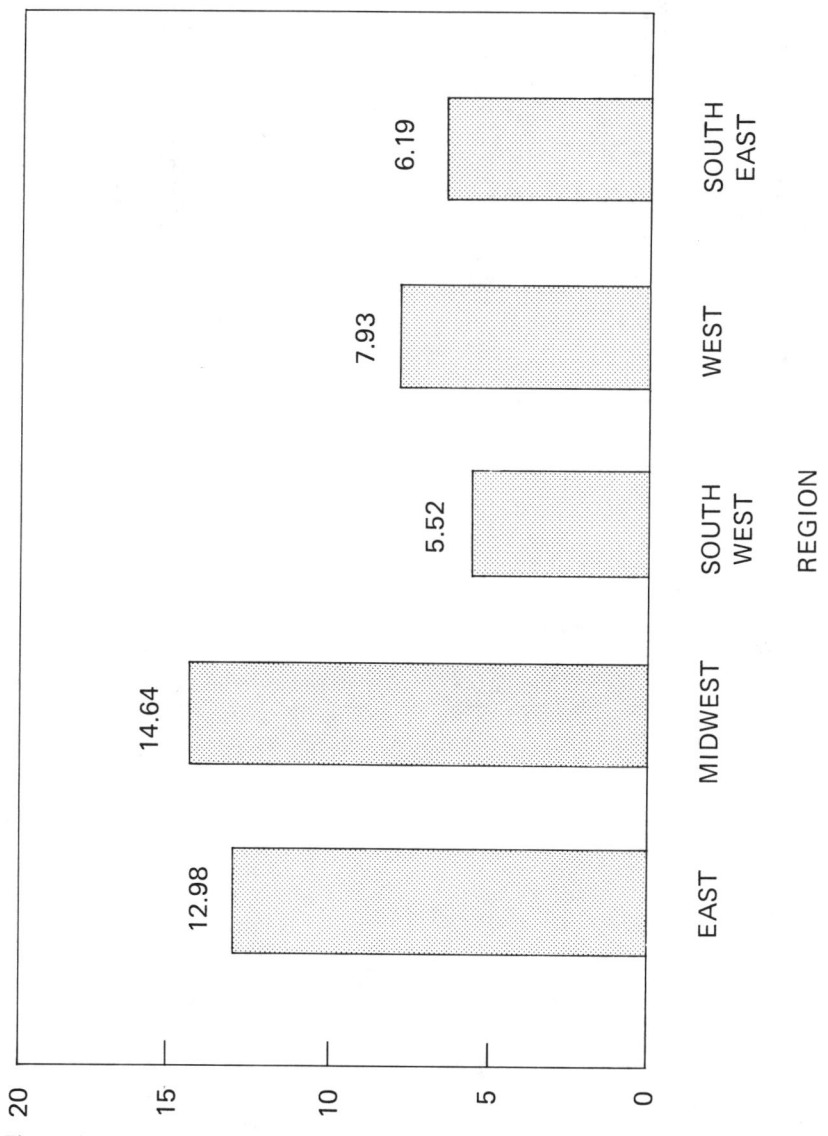

Figure 8-18. Average number of children seen in speech improvement classes per region.

434   Speech-Language Programming in the Schools

GEOGRAPHIC REGIONS

Therapy Type	East P/K	East E	East S	Midwest P/K	Midwest E	Midwest S	Southwest P/K	Southwest E	Southwest S	West P/K	West E	West S	Southeast P/K	Southeast E	Southeast S	Overall P/K	Overall E	Overall S	Mean
Operant	28.9	48.6	33.2	27.9	51.4	49.1	54.1	41.2	33.7	51.4	39.6	31.4	65.7	53.2	11	45.6	46.8	31.6	41.3
Mean		36.9			42.8			43.0			40.8			43.3					
Traditional	71.1	51.4	66.8	72.1	48.6	50.9	45.9	58.8	66.3	48.6	60.4	68.6	34.3	46.8	89	54.4	53.2	68.4	58.7
Mean		63.1			57.2			57.0			59.2			56.7					

P/K - Preschool, Kindergarten
E - Elementary (1–6)
S - Secondary (7–12)

Figure 8-19. Percentage of usage of operant versus traditional therapy by grade level, regions, and for regions combined.

and 22 minutes, respectively, although the average enrollment per group nationally was four children. Length of therapy sessions, both individual and group, averaged lowest in the Midwest, 15.5 minutes and 16.32 minutes, respectively. The Midwest reported the lowest average number of weekly group sessions, 14.7 per clinician, as compared with the 19.4 national average and the high of 24.00 in the Southwest.

In the Southwest, West, and Southeast operant methods were apparently favored for use in preschool and kindergarten, but traditional therapy was more widely used in elementary and secondary grades; whereas in the East and Midwest traditional methods were favored for preschool and kindergarten with no strong preference shown for elementary and secondary grades. There would appear, then, to be no strong preference nationally or regionally for either approach to therapy. A substantial majority of respondents from all regions indicated that they provided some type of parental counseling and/or parent training.

Discussion

Although many of the country's school programs are similar in administration, organization, and personnel, the Midwest and Southeast regions appear to be different from some of the others in a number of ways. First of all, respondents appear younger in experience, probably reflecting more recent training. Second, the mean case loads in the Midwest are considerably below those of some of the other regions. Third, Midwest SLPs appear to receive more technical supervision and are more frequently provided with the assistance of educational audiologists. Fourth, Midwest respondents reported significantly larger numbers of individual therapy sessions than respondents from other regions. Midwest clinicians appeared to have case loads distributed more evenly across the grade levels than clinicians from the other regions. This information should not be construed by readers as either suggesting superior services or otherwise. Most of these characteristics are basically inadequate indices of "superior service."

In contrast to some of the characteristics of school programs of the Midwest region are those of the Southeast. This region reported the highest mean case loads. Typically, SLPs from this region reported much larger numbers of children enrolled for articulation therapy, particularly from grades one through three. Southeast and Midwest respondents' years of professional experience means were not significantly different from those of respondents from the East, yet their percentages holding masters degrees and clinical certification were lower.

The patterns of clinician experience, certification, case load size, case load composition, and other factors, while clearly not consistently the same, were found to be more alike than different in the Southwest and West regions. Their total case loads approximated the national mean of 64 students. Their enrollment of children for language and articulation therapy patterns were somewhat similar across grade levels. Their clinicians were found to have more professional experience. Their use of operant and traditional therapy methods was also similar overall and by grade levels.

Comparison with Earlier Surveys

Some of the findings from the present investigation can be related to both the Purdue University–Office of Education study (Darley, 1961) and the Neal (1976) survey. The Neal (1976) survey data were gathered using only ASHA members; the Purdue University–Office of Education (1961) survey used a large variety of sources to identify respondents; the present effort depended largely upon lists of school personnel supplied by state departments of education personnel. Thus, it is not surprising to note that Neal (1976) reported that 89 percent of his respondents held masters degrees, and we found this figure to be 71 percent. Neal (1976) also reported that 81 percent of his respondents held ASHA CCC certification, and we found this national percentage to be 47 percent. Our findings show regional differences on some of these statistics; however, on the average, about three out of four reported having masters degrees.

Neal (1976) compared the numbers of schools served by clinicians in his sample with the number reported in the Purdue–Office of Education study (Darley, 1961) and concluded that a sizeable reduction had taken place. Our data support this conclusion also; the typical SLP in our sample provided services in three or four school buildings.

Case load size averaged 130 in the 1959 national survey (Darley, 1961). Further evidence of the high case loads that characterized early years came from the a study by Coates, Garbee, and Herbert (1963). Case loads ranged from 24 to 400 children, and the mean for California SLPs was 139. Neal (1976) reported a drastic reduction; his mean case load size was reported to be 72.7. We found the national average case load size to be even lower, the mean being 64.1. This may suggest that national average case load sizes have diminished even further since the time of Neal's report.

Figure 8–20 contains a comparison of the case load composition reported in the 1959 Purdue study (Darley, 1961), Neal's (1976) survey, and the data from the present investigation. Since each study differed in items that comprised each questionnaire, not all comparisons were possible. This is particularly true in the inci-

Type of Disorder	1959 Purdue Survey ($N = 1462$) (%)	Neal (1976) Survey ($N = 47$) (%)	Present Survey ($N = 166$) (%)
Articulation	81	65.6	64.1
Language	4.5	21.4	24.5
Fluency	6.5	3.2	3.7
Voice	2.3	2.6	3.8
Etiologies			
Cleft palate	1.5	1.2	1.0
Cerebral palsy	1.0	0.9	0.8*
Min. Brain Dysfunction	—	—	2.6
Hard of Hearing	2.5	3.0	1.5**
Deaf	—	—	1.2
Emotionally Disturbed	—	—	1.5
Autistic	—	—	0.9
Mildly Retarded	—	—	3.6
Severely Retarded	—	—	4.6

*The number of cerebral palsied children in caseloads was not requested in the present investigation. Information gathered on the severely brain damaged probably includes the cerebral palsied.

**Numbers of deaf children per se were not included in the Purdue and Neal studies. It is possible that the present data showing 1.5% for the hard of hearing and 1.2% for the deaf may be comparable to the 2.5% from the Purdue study and the 3.0% from the Neal study.

Figure 8-20. A comparison of the results from the 1959 Purdue–U.S. Office of Education survey, the 1976 Survey by Neal, and the 1979 Sommers and Hatton investigation.

dence data related to etiologies where data from the present information were more specific concerning the types of etiologies within case loads. It can be seen that Neal's (1976) results are very similar to those from the present investigation when case load composition is determined by types of disorders. Neal's findings related to the percentages of cleft palate and cerebral palsy are almost identical.

Other comparisons with Neal's results are difficult to make; however, some of the organization factors of school therapy programs can be contrasted. Neal reported that the average length of an individual therapy session at the elementary level was 24.5 minutes in comparison with 22.3 minutes in the Sommers-Hatton investigation. He also reported group therapy sessions at the elementary level to average 27.6 minutes compared to 23.0, but significant differences were found across the five regions of the country.

Neal (1976) gathered data concerning the clinicians' use of traditional and intensive (block) scheduling and reported that 68.4 percent of his respondents used traditional scheduling at the elementary level and 75 percent at the secondary level. Data from the Sommers-Hatton investigation across all grade levels were variable by region studied but average 77 percent use of traditional scheduling; the remaining percentages were intensive, modified block scheduling or a combination of the two. Thus, the data from the Neal (1976) survey and the present one tend to show a favorable degree of agreement.

Zaslow and O'Toole, referring in 1971 to the "quiet revolution" that they were beginning to observe, sensed the beginnings of developments that those who participated in the Purdue-U.S. Office of Education Study, even as recently as 1961, could not foretell. Impelled by P.L. 94-142 and attendant state legislation, continued and rapid changes can be expected. Very telling findings of this investigation are the data showing that of the average case load of 64, 18, or 28 percent came under the heading of severely impaired. This puts to death, if indeed it still breathed, the myth that the SLP works only with /r/ and /s/ disorders.

Some of the findings from the present investigation may have implications for the training of speech-language clinicians. SLPs, on the average nationwide, see four children in group therapy, twice weekly for periods of thirty minutes. They average nineteen group therapy sessions weekly. This suggests that training institutions should provide more group therapy experiences and instruction to students to prepare them for the school environment.

Present findings show that 80 percent of clinicians either do some parent training or counseling or both. More emphasis seems warranted in training programs on parental counseling and training techniques. It is likely that few clinicians have received meaningful amounts of such experiences prior to entering into school programs.

Present findings point out areas for further study. With information on numbers and makeup of case loads as they are, we need to determine optimum conditions for implementing the most effective and efficient delivery of services: What are the advantages of true group therapy (using group interaction) versus individual therapy? the operant or precision approach versus the so-called traditional? a primarily language-oriented approach versus more direct work on articulation? How can the more severely handicapped child best be treated in the school setting? It would appear that, in no small way, the future of our profession lies in the schools. Surveys such as this, national and regional, should probably be done and results reported at intervals of no less than five years to keep abreast of these important developments.

Case loads of clinicians working in schools are uniquely tied to the types of problems that are encountered in schools. Depending upon the clinics, institutions, private programs, private practitioners, and special schools for exceptional children that exist in the area, the SLP may find varying degrees of speech defectiveness and various types of organic speech problems in his case load. For the most part, however, 1977 information shows that 43 percent or more of the problems encountered and scheduled for therapy are articulation disorders. It is also probably true that most clinicians have some children who are either "speech deviant" or only mildly speech defective, not enrolled in therapy, and they tend to be from grades kindergarten through third. Finally, it should be observed that the case load composition reflects all that has preceded it. If case finding and case selection have been done with diligence and thoughtfulness, the case load will be well constituted.

SUMMARY

The soundness of the judgements of the speech-language pathologist is a prime determinant in the success of the program. The foundation for therapy to be provided rests upon the axes of case finding, case selection, and case load practices. It follows logically that without well-supported and thoughtful judgements concerning the "what" and "how" of these pillars of the program, little meaningful success will be attained by even the most dedicated speech-language pathologist.

It sometimes happens that an SLP will be presented with an opportunity to establish a new therapy program in a school area. At this time, the clinician is in the best position to develop his rationale and ultimate decisions about which procedures to incorporate as basic tenets of his total program. Many clinicians will be fortunate enough to be able to make these decisions themselves; others, less fortunate, will embark upon a road of trying to convince and cajole others that such measures are of vital concern to the overall success of the program. In most instances, the persevering SLP will achieve her purposes.

It frequently happens that a speech-language pathologist enters a school system in which a history of practice has been developed concerning case finding, case selection, and case load. The logical next question them may become, "How do I manage to change these methods which appear ineffective and inefficient?" The answers are not easily forthcoming, since they are highly dependent upon the uniqueness of every situation and the personalities of those involved. However, it probably holds true that all professionals are "selling" something during the time of their careers; the SLP in this setting must "sell" also if she is going to prevail. Data often speak louder than words. Data gathered from local programs may tend to be more impressive to some school administrators than published data from research reports. Both types of data can be obtained to bolster the arguments of the clinician concerning a need for a change in methods of case finding, case selection, or case load. Under most conditions, the chief problem would appear to be one of being able to demonstrate and convince others that either or both effectiveness or efficiency of the services will improve as a result of the proposed changes in doing things.

Finally, it should be said that attempts to fractionate a corrective program and view case finding, for example, as a discrete factor may be misleading in judging the worth of the service. The inextricable nature of case finding, case selection, and case load makes it difficult to appraise the effectiveness and efficiencies of a school program unless all three of these factors are studied, one to another. Regardless of the quality of the therapy provided by the clinician, these ingredients of the program stand as basic and vital determinants of success in a school setting.

STUDY ACTIVITIES

1. What are some ways in which the teacher referral technique of case finding might be improved?
2. Are there some instances not presented in this chapter in which others besides the clinician should influence the choice of a case-finding technique?
3. What types of forms or records could be developed by a clinician as archives of his case-finding technique? Where should these records be stored?
4. What are some possible explanations for the finding that secondary school teachers have been inefficient in locating students with speech or voice problems?
5. What are some other ways of accomplishing case finding at the secondary school level? How could you evaluate the effectiveness of such methods?
6. Should elementary and secondary students be required to receive speech therapy?
7. What are other factors besides those mentioned that might be important in case selection?
8. What are some basically unanswered questions regarding case-selection techniques? What types of investigations might be necessary to answer these questions?
9. In your own opinion, what constitutes the most desirable type

of case load for an SLP? Who should be included and what should be the case load size?

10. What are the implications of decisions about case finding, case selection, and case load upon actual therapy techniques used by the clinician?

REFERENCES

Alpiner, J., Ogden, J., and Wiggins, J. The Utilization of Supportive Personnel in Speech Correction in the Public Schools: A Pilot Project. *Asha, 12,* 599–604, December, 1970.

Baynes, R. An Incidence Study of Chronic Hoarseness Among Children. *Journal of Speech and Hearing Disorders, 31,* 172–176, May, 1966.

Berry, M. *Language Disorders of Children.* New York: Appleton-Century-Crofts, 1969.

Carrow, E. *Test for Auditory Comprehension of Language.* Austin, Texas: Learning Concepts, 1973.

Clase, J. Ethical Implications of Screening. *Language, Speech and Hearing Services in Schools, 7,* 50–56, January, 1976.

Coates, N., Garbee, F., and Herbert, E. California's Public School Programs for Speech and Hearing Handicapped Children: Dilemmas and Horizons. *Voice: Journal of the California Speech and Hearing Association (Monogr Suppl),* 1963.

Darley, F. (Ed). Public School Speech and Hearing Services. *Journal of Speech and Hearing Disorders (Monogr Suppl), 8,* 1961.

Deal R., McClain, B., and Sudderth, J. Identification, Evaluation, Therapy, and Follow-up for Children with Vocal Nodules in a Public School Setting. *Journal of Speech and Hearing Disorders, 41,* 390–394, August, 1976.

Dell, C. *Treating the School Age Stutterer.* Memphis: Speech Foundations of America, 1980.

DesRoches, C. Speech Therapy Services in a Large School System: A Six-Year Overview. *Language Speech and Hearing Services in Schools, 7,* 207–219, October, 1976.

Diehl, C. and Stinnett, L. Efficiency of Teacher Referrals in a School Testing Program. *Journal of Speech and Hearing Disorders, 22,* 113–117, March, 1956.

Dublinske, S. and Healey, W. PL 94-142: Questions and Answers for the Speech-Language Pathologist and Audiologist. *Asha, 20,* 188–205, March, 1978.

Dunn, L. Peabody Picture Articulation Test. Circle Pines, Minnesota: American Guidance Service, 1965.

Emerick, L. and Hatten, J. *Diagnosis and Evaluation in Speech Pathology.* Englewood Cliffs: Prentice-Hall, 1974.

Faircloth, M. and Faircloth, S. An Analysis of the Articulatory Behavior of a Speech-Defective Child in Connected Speech and in Isolated-Word Responses. *Journal of Speech and Hearing Disorders, 35,* 51–61, 1970.

Freeman, G. *Speech and Language Services and the Classroom Teacher.* Reston, Virginia: Council for Exceptional Children, 1977.
Fudala, J. Arizona Proficiency Scale. Los Angeles: Western Psychological Services, 1970.
Goldman, R. and Fristoe, M. Goldman-Fristoe Test of Articulation. Circle Pines, Minnesota: American Guidance Service, 1969.
Irwin, R. B. *Speech and Hearing Therapy.* Englewood Cliffs: Prentice-Hall, 1953.
James, H. P. and Cooper, E. B. Accuracy of Teacher Referrals of Speech Handicapped Children. *Exceptional Children, 33,* 29–33, 1966.
Johnson, W. et al. *Speech Handicapped School Children,* rev. ed. New York: Harper and Brothers, 1956.
Joint Committee on Dentistry and Speech Pathology-Audiology. *Position Statement of Tongue Thrust.* American Speech and Hearing Association, 1977.
King, R. and Berger, K. *Diagnostic Assessment and Counseling Techniques for Speech Pathologists and Audiologists,* Pittsburgh: Stanwix House, Inc, 1971.
Kirk, S., McCarthy, J., and Kirk, W. The Illinois Test of Psycholinguistics Abilities. Urbana, Illinois: University of Illinois Press, 1968.
Lee, L. The Northwestern Syntax Screening Test. Evanston, Illinois: Northwestern University Press, 1969.
Lee, L. Developmental Sentence Analysis. Evanston, Illinois: Northwestern University Press, 1974.
Mason, R. and Proffit, W. The Tongue Thrust Controversy: Background and Recommendation. *Journal of Speech and Hearing Disorders, 39,* 115–132, May, 1974.
McCarthy, D. *The Language Development of the Preschool Child.* Minneapolis: University of Minnesota Press, 1930.
McCoy, P. Seider, R., and Hyman, M. Efficiency of Teacher Identification and Referral of Children with Voice Disorders. *Ohio Journal of Speech and Hearing, 14,* 178–183, 1970.
McDonald, E. and McDonald, J. Comparison of the Longitudinal and Cross-sectional Norms of the Screening Deep Test of Articulation. Research Project No. 73024H, Report Number Three, Department of Special Education, Appalachia Intermediate Unit 08, 1976b.
Menyuk, P. *Sentences Children Use.* Cambridge, Massachussetts: MIT Press, 1969.
Mullen, P. and Whitehead, R. Stimulus Picture Identification in Articulation Testing. *Journal of Speech and Hearing Disorders, 42,* 113–117, February, 1977.
Neal, W. Speech Pathology Services in Secondary Schools. *Language, Speech and Hearing Services in Schools, 7,* 6–16, January, 1976.
O'Toole, T. J. and Zaslow, E. L. Public School Speech and Hearing Programs: Things Are Changing. *Language, Speech and Hearing Services in Schools, 1,* 3–9, 1971.
Pendergast, K., Dickey, S., Selmar, J., and Soder, A. Photo Articulation Test. Danville, Illinois: The Interstate Printers and Publishers, 1966.
Pickering, M. and Dopheide, W. Training Aides to Screen Children for Speech and Language Problems. *Language, Speech and Hearing Services in Schools, 7,* 236–241, October, 1970.
Powers, M. H. Functional Disorders of Articulation—Symptomatology and Eti-

ology. In L. E. Travis (Ed.), *Handbook of Speech Pathology*. New York: Appleton-Century-Crofts, 1957.

Provonost, W. Case Selection in the Schools: Articulatory Disorders. *Speech and Hearing Services in Schools, 1,* 17–23, 1970.

Roe, V. and Milisen, R. The Effect of Maturation upon Defective Articulation in Elementary Grades. *Journal of Speech and Hearing Disorders, 7,* 37–50, February, 1942.

Sommers, R. et al. Factors Related to the Effectiveness of Articulation Therapy for Kindergarten, First, and Second Grade Children. *Journal of Speech and Hearing Research, 10,* 428–437, September, 1961.

Sommers, R. et al. How Valid Are Children's Language Tests? *The Journal of Special Education, 12,* 393–407, 1978.

Sommers, R. and Hatton, M. School Speech, Language and Hearing Programs: A Survey of Clinicians, Programs and Services. *Ohio Journal of Speech and Hearing, 14,* 274–293, Fall, 1979.

Sommers, R. K. and Kane, A. R. Nature and Remediation of Functional Articulation Disorders. In S. Dickson (ed.), *Communication Disorders, Remedial Principles and Practices.* Glenview, Illinois: Scott, Foresman and Company, 1974.

Sommers, R. and Sitler, S. Correlation between Spontaneous and Imitative Speech Tests in Five and Six Year Old Children and their Relationship to Connected Spontaneous Speech. Unpublished research report, 1980.

Task Force Report on School Speech, Hearing and Language Screening Procedures. *Language, Speech and Hearing Services in Schools, 4,* 109–119, July, 1973.

Templin, M. and Darley, F. Templin-Darley Tests of Articulation, 2nd ed. Iowa City: Bureau of Educational Research and Services, 1969.

Van Hattum, R. J. Speech and Language Services in Schools: More than Remediation Procedures. In L. Bradford (Ed.), *Communicative Disorders: An Audio Journal for Continuing Education.* New York: Grune and Stratton, 1977.

Van Hattum, R. J. (Ed.). Screening in School Programs. In J. Northern (Ed.), *Seminars in Speech, Language and Hearing.* New York: Brian C. Decker, Thieme-Stratton, 1981.

Van Riper, C. *Speech Correction Principles and Methods,* 4th ed. Englewood Cliffs, Prentice-Hall, 1963.

Van Riper C. and Erickson, R. Predictive Screening Test of Articulation, 3rd ed. Kalamazoo: Continuing Education Office, Western Michigan University, 1973.

Van Riper, C. and Irwin, J. Voice and Articulation. Englewood Cliffs: Prentice-Hall, 1964.

Wertz, R. and Mead, M. Classroom Teacher and Speech Clinician Severity Ratings of Different Speech Disorders. *Language, Speech and Hearing Services in Schools, 6,* 119–124, July, 1975.

Wilson, F. The Voice-Disordered Child: A Descriptive Approach. *Language, Speech Hearing Services in Schools, 1,* 14–22, 1970.

Wilson, F. and Rice, V. *Programmed Approach to Voice Therapy.* Austin, Texas; Learning Concepts, Inc., 1977.

Zemmol, S. A Priority System of Caseload Selection. *Language, Speech and Hearing Services in Schools, 8,* 85–98, April, 1977.

APPENDIX 8A
SPEECH AND LANGUAGE THERAPY IN THE SCHOOLS
(Please base all data on '76–'77 school year)

CLINICIAN

Name (optional) _____ Address (optional) _____ Phone _____

Male or female _____ Member of ASHA? _____ CCC? _____

Number of years in Speech and Hearing _____ Highest degree earned _____

Are you employed full-time? _____ If not, how many hours per week? _____

LOCALE

Name of school district _____ Location (State) _____

Rural or urban? _____ Number of schools you service _____

What grades does district serve— K thru 12? _____ What ages—3 thru 21? _____

Total number of children enrolled in the schools you serve _____

Does the district employ a specially trained therapist to work with language? _____

Does the district employ an educational audiologist? _____

CASE LOAD

Average number of children for whom you provide therapy each week _____
(excluding children seen in classrooms for speech improvement programs)

Average number of children for whom you provide diagnostic services each week? _____

Average number of group sessions each week _____
  Length of session: maximum _____, minimum _____, average _____.
  Number in group: maximum _____, minimum _____, average _____.

Average number of individual sessions per week _____
  Length of session: maximum _____, minimum _____, average _____.

Average number of children seen each week in speech improvement classes _____

Do you follow intermittent (traditional) or intensive (block) type scheduling? _____

Does your system provide technically trained speech and hearing supervision? _____

Are you doing parental training or counseling? _____
  Average time each week devoted to such activities? _____

Do you serve children enrolled in special classes for the emotionally disturbed? _____

  What services do you provide? _____

  Average number of these children seen per week _____

  Individually or in groups? _____

  Average length of lesson _____

APPENDIX 8B

CASE LOAD BREAKDOWN AS TO PRIMARY DIAGNOSIS
(numbers of clients)

Primary Diagnosis	Pre-School	Kinder-garten	Grades 1 – 3	Grades 4 – 6	Grades 7 – 12	Post-High
Language – severe with articulation components						
with no artic components						
Articulation – with language problems						
with no language problems						
Fluency						
Voice						

CASE LOAD BREAKDOWN AS TO ETIOLOGY
(numbers of clients)

Primary Diagnosis	Pre-School	Kinder-garten	Grades 1 – 3	Grades 4 – 6	Grades 7 – 12	Post-High
Severe Mental Retardation						
Mild Mental Retardation						
Emotionally Disturbed						
Hard of Hearing						
Deaf						
Cleft lip – cleft palate						
Autistic or autistic-like						
Severely brain damaged						
Minimal brain dysfunction						
Other						

APPENDIX 8C

Type of Therapy: Operant (Precision, etc.) or Traditional (Van Riper, Sensori-Motor, etc.) Indicate the percentage within each category applicable to your program, e.g. 25% preschool is operant, 75%, traditional.

	Operant	Traditional
Preschool, Individual		
Preschool, Group		
Kindergarten, Individual		
Kindergarten, Group		
Grades 1 3, Individual		
Grades 1 3, Group		
Grades 4 6, Individual		
Grades 4 6, Group		
Grades 7 12, Individual		
Grades 7 12, Group		
Post-high, Individual		
Post-high, Group		

Chapter 9

SCHEDULING

Dolores E. Battle and Rolland J. Van Hattum

According to the dictionary, a schedule is a plan, a timetable (Thorndike-Barnhardt, 1973). To develop a schedule effectively, one must consider many factors. What has to be accomplished? When does it have to be done? What resources and facilities are available? How much flexibility is there? How much time is available? An important determinant of the success of the school speech-language program is the effective and efficient management of the time available and the manner in which the program is planned.

Time is a precious commodity to all of us. It is not unusual to see the slogan "Time is money" posted conspicuously in manufacturing plants or business offices. Time may not be money to the school speech-language pathologist directly, but it certainly is an important aspect of total program planning and the total cost of operation of the school program. The efficient management of time may be of greater importance to school personnel than to business or industry because of the limitations on the school day, the school year, and other mandates. Each school day is usually no longer than six hours in duration, and each school year is usually approximately 180 school days, or a potential of 1,080 school hours. Not only is this lack of time alarming to one attempting to provide services to children in school environments, but mandated curricula and other demands on the time available subtract from the potential time available for speech-language programming (Van Hattum, 1969).

There are three important aspects of the use of time facing the speech-language pathologist working in the schools: planning and scheduling the program for the year, scheduling services for each week, and scheduling the clinical day. The three aspects are interrelated. One cannot rationally schedule the year without consideration of how each week and day will be planned. Each decision that is made affects all three aspects, and any attempt to view them separately is, at best, artificial. In spite of this limitation, this chapter will discuss those factors which must be considered in scheduling the speech-language program for the year, the week, and the day. The impact of P.L. 94-142 on scheduling will be presented throughout the chapter as relevant. Several possible basic formats for scheduling will be discussed. The factors that must be considered in selecting and designing a schedule will be presented. Application of these factors will be presented through sample programs. Effects of the factors on scheduling the week and the clinical day will be discussed.

SCHEDULING THE YEAR

The Impact of P.L. 94-142

As detailed in Chapter 3, in November, 1975, The Education for All Handicapped Children Act, P.L. 94-142, was passed as the result of several years of civil rights legislation, which initially began as a movement to provide equal protection under the law and due processes for the blacks of this nation and led to the extension and interpretation of the constitutional rights guaranteed in the Fifth and Fourteenth Amendments to the handicapped in the area of education. The legislation has had the most significant impact in the history of special education and related services to the handicapped of the nation, including the communication handicapped. The essence of the law assures handicapped children the rights to a free, appropriate public education and necessitates many changes in the educational roles and in planning, coordinating, and scheduling of special educational services. The law requires that children be identified and placed in appropriate programs on the basis of individual need from the time the need is identified until it no longer exists.

The relevancy of P.L. 94-142 to the communication handicapped lies in the provision that the failure to provide appropriate services to the communication handicapped is a violation of federal law. Many changes and modifications in traditional speech-language programs and the examination of the appropriateness of traditional practices have become necessary, especially with regard to scheduling.

Scheduling is the professional responsibility of the speech-language pathologist and is based on the needs of the persons to be served. Prior to P.L. 94-142, other persons often made decisions or instituted policies that dictated the schedule to be used. As Irwin (1953) pointed out, some boards of education and supervisors were most anxious that speech-language pathologists see all children with speech-language disorders in the district. The schedule was intended to make certain that all children had equal access to the services. However, children were placed on waiting lists, often never receiving the services they required. In other cases minimal services were provided in large and/or scheduled infrequently in an attempt to accommodate all the children needing assistance.

As of September 1, 1978, all children identified and evaluated as being handicapped and in need of special education were required to have appropriate education available to them. It has been since 1974 (P.L. 93-380) (*Federal Register,* August 21, 1974) that school districts receiving federal funds have been required to develop plans to eliminate waiting lists and to provide appropriate services to all handicapped children. In addition, districts that required staff to accommodate those on waiting lists by scheduling all children fewer times per week than is considered appropriate, thus increasing case load, or who increased class size, were required to be prepared to defend their decision as one that satisfies the needs of the children in terms of appropriate education (Healy and Dublinske, 1978).

Thus, before the implementation of P.L. 94-142, scheduling systems often represented a compromise between meeting the needs of as many children as possible and establishing the pattern that best accommodated other school personnel. School SLPs often scheduled children one or two times each week throughout the school year, or for three or more days each week, often for a relatively short period of time. Since many children were enrolled in the programs, and resulting case loads were large, the service provided was often inadequate to meet the needs of children, particularly those more severe cases. Parents of more severely impaired children often had to supplement school services with private speech-language sessions at local hospitals or speech and hearing clinics.

The implementation of P.L. 94-142 has also mandated that children who traditionally were often excluded from speech-language programs in the schools (such as the mentally retarded, the emotionally disturbed, and the physically disabled) received appropriate educational services including, where appropriate, speech-language services. This has resulted in greater need for program alternatives and for flexibility in speech-language programming to meet their individual needs. The flexibility extends to the area of program scheduling to meet the mandate of excellence and quality of services to the communication handicapped.

While necessitating flexibility, P.L. 94-142 has placed several restrictions and requirements on the administration of speech-language programs. These restrictions apply not only to scheduling the year but also to scheduling the week and the day. The law has had a major impact on the concept of the "school year." The implementation of the law necessitates that the speech-language program operate on the basis of "I.E.P. years" (Individual Education Program), which vary for individual students, depending on their original placement dates. For example, if an I.E.P. was developed in April, the I.E.P. is applicable for one year unless the needs of the child change significantly. The child's I.E.P. would then be in effect until the following April, and thus be in effect at the beginning of the next school year, including the first day of school. The law requires that handicapped children have an I.E.P. in effect the first day of school and be receiving service the first day of school. The majority of the speech-language program case load in the fall would be that which was carried over from the previous spring *(Federal Register,* 121a.342). The traditional practice of scheduling the year to allow screening, evaluation, and placement to fill the first several weeks of the school year followed by establishing a schedule to provide direct service in each school for the majority of the school year, and of concluding the year with reevaluation and dismissals may no longer be appropriate and may require modification (Healy and Dublinske, 1978).

The Regulations for P.L. 94-142 address this issue as follows:

> 121a.342 When individualized programs must be in effect. (a) on October 1977, and at the beginning of each school year thereafter, each public agency shall have in effect an individualized educational program for every handicapped child who is receiving special education from that agency.

In addition, the COMMENT that appears under 121a.342 is pertinent to scheduling the speech-language program.

> COMMENT: Under paragraph (b) (2) it is expected that a handicapped child's individual educational program (IEP) will be implemented immediately following the meeting under p.121a.343. An exception to this would be (1) when the meeting occurs during the summer or a vacation period, or (2) when there are circumstances which would require a short delay (e.g. working out transportation arrangements). However, there can be no undue delay in providing special education and related services to the child.

Both of these statements lead to the conclusion that although it may not be possible to have the speech-language schedule ready the first day of school, the SLP cannot afford the four to six week period of screening and evaluation that traditionally has preceeded actual implementation of the speech-language schedule.

In the traditional speech-language program, time was allotted for reevaluation and report writing at the end of the school year. While program evaluation and reporting continue to be necessary, report writing and reevaluation for individual cases must be an ongoing process throughout the school year. P.L. 94-142 requires that agencies "initiate and conduct meetings to periodically review each child's individualized program and, if appropriate revise, its provisions. A meeting for this purpose must be held at least once a year" *(Federal Register,* August 23, 1977, Sect.121a.343).

> COMMENT:... meeting may be held anytime throughout the year, as long as IEP's are in effect at the beginning of the school year.... The timing of these meetings could be on the anniversary date of the last IEP meeting on the child, but this is left to the discretion of the agency.

Although it is entirely possible that a school may decide to hold its annual review meetings for each child at the end of the year, many schools are finding that it is physically impossible to manage in this fashion. Review meetings that are scheduled to coincide with the child's birthdate, with the letters of the last name, or according to some other scheme that distributes the review meetings throughout the school year may be more efficient to manage.

While P.L. 94-142 necessitates that speech-language programs operate on the basis of "I.E.P. years" rather than on the basis of the traditional "school year," each school year must be planned to allow identification and placement of children who are either new to the school or who are referred for service by either parents or teachers. Once the schedule is fixed, it may need to be altered to accommodate newly identified children or changes in individual needs.

The impact of P.L. 94-142 on speech-language program scheduling is significant. Any schedule that is planned for the speech-language program must be *flexible* to allow time for the full range of activities and role functions of the speech-language pathologist throughout the school year. It must be *efficient* to allow for added responsibility without impairing appropriate direct service. It must be *effective* in providing appropriate speech-language services to the communicatively handicapped.

Research Relating to Scheduling Systems

The first of the previously mentioned variables in scheduling refers to the number of *weeks* the SLP spends in a school consecutively or the total number of weeks a client or school is scheduled to participate in the speech-language program. This may vary from as few as two weeks to the entire school year. It may refer to a number of weeks of service separated by a number of weeks with no service or limited service. The second variable refers to the number of *days* per week of service each client or each school participates in the program. This might vary from one day per week to as many as five days per week. The third variable refers to scheduling hours within each school day. The various combinations of these variables, which in themselves vary, result in a possible infinite variety of scheduling systems.

Prior to 1966, research investigating the effects of scheduling in the schools had not been extensive. However, changing roles of the speech-language pathologist stimulated interest in determining the conditions under which programs were more effective.

Much of the resulting research regarding scheduling involved study of the variables concerning scheduling the year and the week. The studies were often comparisons between the *intensive* or *"block" system* and *traditional* systems of scheduling known variously as the "regular," "itinerant," or "intermittent."

Discussions of intensive or "block" systems usually refer to schedules in which the cases are seen for more than three days a week in a variety of patterns across weeks. The traditional itinerant systems usually refer to those systems of scheduling in which cases are scheduled three or fewer days each week whether or not the speech-language pathologist travels to one or more schools. Discussion in the literature also refers to systems in which the traditional intermittent system is combined with an intensive system. According to these systems, the same children receive intensive service during one module or set of weeks followed by traditional intermittent service in another module. Chapter 8 describes the frequency of use of various systems.

Much of the literature describing scheduling systems is not consistent in the use of these terms, which makes comparison of systems rather confusing. Rather than rely on labels, it is more productive to rely on the function of the systems. For purposes of discussion, the following terms will be used in discussing scheduling systems; the modular or block system, the intensive system, the traditional-intermittent system, and the combination system.

The Modular or Block System

The modular or block system of scheduling is focused along the first variable in scheduling, the number of weeks a school receives service. In the modular or block system, the speech-language service is not provided for the entire school year to a particular school. Rather, periods or modules of *several weeks*, from as few as two weeks to an entire semester, are repeated throughout the year. For example, School A may be served for six weeks while School B receives no service. The programs are then alternated such that School B receives service and School A receives no service. The pattern is repeated throughout the year such that each school receives service for one-half the school year with the time distributed throughout the school year.

There is considerable variation in the use of the term "block" in the literature. For example, Van Hattum (1961) described twenty-six variations of block scheduling. Van Hattum conducted a study in which some school speech-language pathologists described the "block" system as a "concentrated or intensive program varying in length from two weeks to a full semester." Others reporting stated that the system involves therapy sessions four or five times per week, while some described it as involving a period of therapy in one group of schools with two sessions per week followed by a shift to another group of schools. One SLP described his program as a block program by saying that he went to one block of sixteen schools during the first semester and saw children either once or twice a week. Then, during the second semester, he went to a second block of fifteen schools. This would hardly meet the criteria of intensive therapy usually associated with the block or modular system.

In selecting the block or modular system of scheduling, the speech-language pathologist must use caution not to violate the availability of speech-language programs to handicapped children. As stated previously, according to the regulations for P.L. 94-142, there can be no interruption in the service that is provided to speech-language handicapped children until the need for service no longer exists *(Federal Register,* August 23, 1977, Sect.121a.343). In addition, no children identified as in need of service may be unserved or waiting for service except during those times when school is not in session. In the block or modular system there are groups of children waiting for service. In addition, classroom teachers faced with a child with a severe communication disorder, such as unintelligible speech or severe stuttering, are often impatient in having to wait several weeks or months before help can be provided the child.

The Intensive System versus Traditional-Intermittent System

The intensive system is focused on the number of *days* per week a child is scheduled for therapy. The term is usually reserved for speech-language programs that provide service to individual children four or five times per week. There is some confusion in the literature in the use of the term "intensive" because it is often confused with the term "block" system, which refers to the number of *weeks* a child receives consecutive therapy.

The traditional intermittent system refers to speech-language programs that provide service on a basis of three or fewer days per week, whether or not the SLP is itinerant, travels among schools.

An early study reported by Backus and Dunn (1947) showed that more progress was obtained during six weeks of daily therapy than was possible during an entire school year of twice a week therapy.

Although there is some evidence to the contrary, the literature generally supports that schedules which allow for direct service on an intensive basis of four or more sessions per week yield greater benefits than service provided on the traditional intermittent basis of three or fewer sessions per week.

A survey by Bingham (1962) revealed that most speech-language pathologists provided individual therapy at intervals of once (29%) or twice weekly (49%). Groups met twice a week 52 percent of the time and once a week 33 percent of the time. Only 6 percent of the persons reporting met individuals or groups three, four, or five times weekly, and none reported seeing children more than once daily. There are only a few studies that have reported the effects of frequency of providing services upon progress in therapy. Even these data are questionable because of the lack of control on the type of therapy given, on the type of disorder, and on the expertise or personality of the person administering the therapy.

Van Hattum (1959) reports that five years of records were available for the Rochester, New York schools using the twice a week method of scheduling. Dismissal rates under the system were from 18 to 21 percent. A similar period of time, using an intensive system of daily sessions during two six-week modules per school year, yielded dismissal figures ranging from 38 to 41 percent. In addition the speech-language pathologists reported that they preferred the intensive system and that there were administrative advantages. Both the children and the classroom teachers found that it was easier to remember when therapy was scheduled. The speech-language room was in daily use during the module. The materials and supplies were concentrated in a few schools. The speech-language pathologist became better acquainted with the school personnel. Finally, in therapy, the SLPs found it easier to plan and execute a program of therapy when the children were seen daily. They reported better remembering of planning, of goals, of techniques on their part and of homework on the part of the children.

MacLearie and Gross (1966) reported on five studies conducted in Ohio that attempted to determine the effectiveness of intensive versus intermittent scheduling on the remediation of speech disorders and on various factors related to their success. The East Cleveland study (Holderman 1966) examined the relative effectiveness of the traditional and intensive modular plan of scheduling with defective sibilant sounds in grades two through six. In this study the traditional plan was defined as two thirty-minute sessions, two days a week for twelve weeks. The intensive plan was defined as therapy received for four half-hour sessions, four days a week for six weeks. The total number of sessions in each plan was twenty-four. The researchers commented that the data appeared to indicate a decided difference in the rate and degree of progress. The judges' evaluation showed improvement in the intensive group twice as large as in the traditional group. Thus, within the limits set forth in the study, a favorable result was found for the short-term intensive therapy schedule.

The second study reported by MacLearie and Gross (1966) was conducted by Wiedner (1966) in Brecksville, Ohio. Children received speech therapy either under the traditional intermittent system, defined as two one-half hour sessions each week throughout the school year for a total of eighty sessions, or under the intensive modular system, defined as four times per week for six consecutive weeks in two separate six-week modules during the school year, for a total of forty-eight sessions. The results indicated that more children received help under the intensive modular plan. More children were dismissed as corrected, although the percentage was only slightly higher, and it appeared that there was less remission of improvement among the intensive group when examined again in September following the June dismissal even though they had had fewer sessions.

As a corollary to his study, Weidner (1966) surveyed the classroom teachers as to their preference for either the intermittent or the intensive program. Of the thirty-five teachers surveyed, thirty preferred the intensive system, two had no opinion, and three preferred the traditional system.

Ervin (1965) reported on a study in which the suitability of intensive and traditional intermittent therapy for second and third grade articulation cases was studied. The traditional intermittent program was defined as two days a week therapy for twenty weeks. The intensive program consisted of therapy four days a week for two five-week periods, one in the fall and one in the spring. The intensive therapy schedule was found to be more effective in terms of improvement for functional disorders of articulation. Ervin cautioned that further generalizations concerning other types of speech disorders of organic etiology and higher grade levels required further investigation.

Bietzel (1966) followed up on Ervin's research in a study in Dayton, Ohio from 1961 to 1964, in which he compared the traditional intermittent system, defined as two thirty-minute sessions each week throughout the school year, and the intensive system, defined as four thirty-minute sessions per week, as to (1) the age at which children best respond to intensive scheduling, (2) the type of speech problem for which intensive scheduling seems most effective, (3) the optimum length of time for a period of intensive scheduling, and (4) the feasibility of scheduling both systems concurrently in the same building. The results indicated that the best results were obtained under the intensive therapy system. Best results were obtained with articulation problems of children in grades four, five, and six, while children in grades seven and eight showed the least improvement. Intensive scheduling was least effective with organic problems. A greater number of children received speech therapy with the intensive program.

Bietzel (1966) further reported that the intensive therapy scheduling system was preferred for a number of administrative reasons. There was better integration of the speech-language program with the total school program. There were more frequent contacts between the speech-language pathologists and other school personnel. There was reduction in the effect of absenteeism on speech progress. The time allotted to speech screening was shortened. There was an increase in the number of conferences with parents and teachers. There were fewer problems in scheduling upper elementary children, since they could be seen at times that best suited their programs.

Ausenheimer and Irwin (1971) studied the effects of providing articulation therapy twice a week (64 sessions), three times a week (96 sessions), and four-times a week (40 sessions). Progress in each group of ten children was assessed three times, at the end of eight, sixteen, and thirty-two weeks. At the end of the eight weeks, the intensive group (four times a week) scored significantly higher than the other two groups. However, after thirty-two weeks, the twice a week group made the largest gains. This finding supports the finding of an earlier study (Irwin 1966) that greater gains are made when sessions are held over a longer period of time. One would have expected that the three times a week group would have made the largest gains because of the increase in the number of sessions and the increased frequency of those sessions. Although the children were randomly assigned to groups, controlling factors such as severity or type of error in each group, the type of therapy, abilities of the speech-language pathologist, or motivational factors were not mentioned.

Weston and Harber (1975) reported the results of a study comparing the effectiveness of five different scheduling systems in which the type of therapy was controlled. Their results support those of Ausenheimer and Irwin (1971) in that over a longer period of time children receiving therapy for two days each week made more significant gains in the speech-language program than children scheduled for three or four days per week. Seventy children with articulation disorders in grades one through six participated in a three-year project in which the paired stimuli technique for a modification of articulation behavior was used (Weston and Irwin 1971). The subjects were divided into five groups of fourteen subjects each. Subjects in Group 1 had therapy on Monday, Wednesday, and Friday; those in Group 2 attended on Tuesday and Thursday; subjects in Group 3 attended Monday and Wednesday; subjects in Group 4 attended Monday, Tuesday, Thursday, and Friday; and those in Group 5 attended Monday, Tuesday, and Friday. Sessions were scheduled for thirty minutes. The time required for each subject to meet criterion of 80 percent or more in words in which the target sound appeared in two fifteen-minute probes was considered to be an objective measure of progress. The two times a week groups required two sessions to reach criterion, whereas the three to four times per week groups required three to five sessions.

The results showed that, according to this study, therapy two times per week (Monday and Wednesday or Tuesday and Thursday) was more effective in terms of time to reach criterion than therapy scheduled in the three remaining combinations (three and four times per week). The differences were significant. The suggestion was made that children enrolled in less intensive operant therapy schedules are better able to integrate what was learned in therapy while removed from the actual therapy session. Although the findings are in contrast to research cited earlier concerning the benefits of intensive scheduling, it is difficult to determine whether the results can be applied to more traditional therapy. In this study the children scheduled for four sessions of articulation therapy per week made the slowest progress.

The effect of intensive and intermittent scheduling systems on the mentally retarded has been studied. These studies become important as increasing numbers of speech-language pathologists are expected to provide speech-language programs for the mentally retarded under the provisions of P.L. 94-142. The results of the study conducted by Wilson (1971) on the effect of frequency of session on error reduction among the mentally retarded further supports the appropriateness of intensive therapy for the mentally retarded. Seven hundred seventy-seven educable mentally retarded children, six to sixteen years of age, were subdivided into three groups. Group 1 had two thirty-minute therapy sessions each week. Group 2, a placebo group, met for two half-hour periods each week but received no instruction in sound correction. Group 3, the control group, did not have any therapy or any special treatment. Therapy using the Van Riper method was given by three speech-language pathologists to both individuals and groups of not more than four for a three-year period. The amount of progress was determined by judges who evaluated responses to an articulation test. An analysis of variance showed no significant difference among the amounts of progress made by the three treatment groups. The conclusion was drawn that speech-language therapy provided on a traditional intermittent basis of two sessions per week to educable mentally retarded students has no more effect than maturation on sound error reduction among the educable mentally retarded.

Sommers (1970) conducted a study to determine the effect of frequency of practice as governed by scheduling among the educable mentally retarded. One hundred twenty children with an average IQ of 70 were given the Carter-Buck Articulation Test (1958) and the McDonald Deep Screening Test (1964) and were then divided into four groups. The control group received no therapy. One experimental group received one thirty-minute speech therapy session each week for thirty weeks, for a total of thirty sessions. The other experimental group received intensive therapy of four thirty-minute sessions each week for thirty weeks for a total of 119 sessions. As one might expect from the greater number of sessions, the subjects who received intensive articulation therapy of four sessions each week significantly improved their articulation as measured by the Deep Test when compared to the controls. The subjects who received the traditional intermittent therapy of one session per week did not improve significantly as compared to the controls. The results of the study, however, rather than support the notion of superiority of intensive therapy over intermittent therapy for the mentally retarded suggest that greater progress is made with greater amounts of therapy. Had both groups received the same amount of instruction, more could have been learned about the effects of scheduling for the mentally retarded.

Much of the study of the effects of traditional intermittent versus intensive therapy yields inconclusive results because of poor control of such variables as the total number of sessions, types of disorders, types of therapy techniques, and the motivation of the speech-language pathologist and of the students. On the basis of controlled learning experiments from psychology, it could be recommended that increased progress could be obtained from providing more frequent instruction as in intensive therapy, but there are virtually no data available from speech research to support this conclusively.

The ASHA Task Force on Traditional Scheduling (1973) reported the following advantages of intensive scheduling: (1) children have better carry-over from session to session, (2) speech-language pathologists have better opportunities to function as members of the school staff, and (3) travel time and need to transport materials and equipment are reduced. The following disadvantages of the intensive modular block cycle system were listed: (1) many organic speech disorders, language disorders, and some functional speech disorders require therapy for a longer period of time in the school year than may be scheduled in the block plan; (2) some schools may not receive services until late in the school year, and these services might not come in the stage of the child's rehabilitation program when they would be most beneficial.

This lack of well-controlled studies in support of either the modular, intensive, or intermittent systems over the other, when viewed with the advantages and disadvantages of each system as cited, has led some speech-language pathologists to reject the exclusive use of either of the three systems of scheduling in favor of a combination of the three.

Combination of Intensive and Traditional-Intermittent Scheduling Systems and Modular Systems

In the attempt to obtain the advantages of both the intensive and the intermittent scheduling systems of scheduling, speech-language pathologists have used both systems in their programs. Work et al. (1973), for example, described a speech-language program in Broward County, Florida, in which a modular schedule of three successive blocks of therapy was used during the 1971–72 school year. Elementary School A was scheduled for four mornings per week and Elementary Schools B and C two afternoons per week. At the end of ten weeks the elementary schools were rotated. By the end of the school year each elementary school had been scheduled for intensive four days a week therapy for ten weeks and intermittent two days a week therapy for twenty weeks. Using this system, the children were served for the entire school year, although the amount of therapy which they received during a particular period varied. In addition, the speech-language program was in the school for the entire year, and the speech-language pathologist was available to participate with other school personnel during the entire year.

The fourth and fifth Ohio studies on scheduling reported by MacLearie and Gross (1966), previously cited, studied the combination scheduling system as compared to traditional and intensive systems used alone. In the Crawford County study, Irwin et al. (1966) compared three groups on the basis of intensiveness of scheduling. Group I used the traditional intermittent system of scheduling of two thirty-minute sessions each week for the school year. Group II used a more intensive schedule of three thirty-minute sessions for one school year. Group III used a combination of both intensive and intermittent scheduling. Four thirty-minute sessions were held for an eight-week module followed by a once a week intermittent schedule for the second eight-week module. The findings indicated that there were no significant differences among the three groups following eight weeks of therapy. A connected speech sample score, which was used as one measure, was the only measure to show a significant difference among the groups. Although all groups showed gains, the amount of gain increasing with the number of sessions held each week, the differences between the gains for each group were not significant. The greatest gain was found in Group III, which used the combination of intensive followed by intermittent scheduling. The results also indicated that greater gain was made when sessions were held over a longer period of time. Although each had thirty-two sessions, twice-weekly scheduling for sixteen weeks resulted in more improvement on total speech scores than four times per week for eight weeks. Following sixteen weeks of therapy, no significant differences existed between Group I (two times a week) and Group II (three times a week). Irwin concluded that all groups showed improvement on all test measures from module to module and that all groups made the greater gains early in therapy, i.e. during the first eight-week module. The author concluded that the gains shown by the group scheduled four times per week were slightly greater than the gains of the other groups, but not significantly so. Also, twice a week scheduling was shown to be as effective as three times a week scheduling, but not significantly so. The lack of significant gain between the eight-week period and the sixteen-week period was thought to be the result of a plateau of learning rather than a factor of scheduling.

Weaver and Wollersheim (1963) conducted a study in the Champaign, Illinois schools that compared a system which combined intensive and traditional-intermittent scheduling to one that used traditional scheduling system used alone. After three weeks of screening the intermittent system proceeded in the "usual manner," according to the authors. The combination system consisted of three five-week modules—two intermittent and one intensive. In the intensive module, service was provided four days per week. When the school was not in the intensive module, service was provided one day per week. Results indicated greater improvement under the combination system than under the traditional-intermittent system. A questionnaire submitted to teachers and administrators revealed that administrators preferred the combination system and commented on such factors as ease of scheduling, improved working relationships between the speech-language pathologist and other school personnel, and improved motivation on the part of the children. Of the forty classroom teachers who reported, two stated no preference, and thirty-four of the remaining thirty-eight preferred the combination system. They, too, referred to such factors as ease of scheduling, increased speech benefits, and better motivation. Even some of the teachers who preferred the intermittent system pointed out these factors but were more concerned about the disruption of classes, which they felt was more noticeable during the intensive module of the combination system.

Norris (1966) conducted a study in Cleveland, Ohio using the combination system in scheduling to determine if the order in which the two systems were used had an effect on progress in therapy. In this study, traditional-intermittent therapy was defined as two thirty-minute sessions per week over five weeks for a total of ten sessions. Intensive therapy was defined as daily thirty-minute therapy sessions for two weeks for a total of ten sessions. Under the traditional-intermittent scheduling system notebook lessons were taken home to be reviewed by the child and his parent. Under the intensive scheduling system the notebooks were kept in school. There was no reason stated for this procedure. The differences in parental support may account for some of the differences reported in the study. Two program sequences were used. In program A intensive scheduling was followed by traditional-intermittent scheduling. In program B traditional-intermittent scheduling was followed by intensive scheduling. The researchers reported that the difference in average gain, while favoring the intensive method, was not statistically significant. Children showed significant improvement under each program. All groups made their greatest gain in their first therapy program regardless of the scheduling method used. Although the results were not statistically significant, the intensive-therapy-first program had a greater average gain than the traditional-therapy-first program. However, the traditional-therapy-second program had a better average gain than the intensive-therapy-second program. The researchers concluded that the optimum program may be a period of intensive therapy followed by a period of traditional-intermittent therapy.

The research reports relating to scheduling are usually confusing and seldom conclusive. There is a lack of consistency in the use of terminology. Further, the research methodology used, due to the complexity of the problem, often appears not to control adequately the great number of variables necessary for good research. In fact, one of the major problems may be that too many variables are altered in a single study with few controls that would allow one to make conclusive statements. Indeed there was no study reported that attempted to determine the effects of scheduling on the long-term effects of therapy, i.e. the amount of retention of skills after therapy had been terminated. Any speech-language pathologist who has dismissed a case in June as corrected only to find regression toward the old pattern in September realizes the importance of this factor. Mowrer (1977) suggests that one possible way to determine the effects of frequency of practice session is to provide five twenty-minute therapy sessions daily to one group (100 minute total) and five sessions to another group, one session each week (100 minute total). Assessment of progress could be given one week, four weeks, and eight weeks after the final therapy session. In this way the long-term effects of frequency of session could be accurately measured.

On the basis of the available information, it would seem that the following observations are defensible:

1. Systems of scheduling that provide speech-language ther-

apy four or five days a week appear to yield higher dismissal rates than systems that provide therapy three or fewer days per week.

2. There appears to be little difference between systems that provide service two and three days per week.

3. Service scheduled two day per week yields little gain over service scheduled one day.

4. Intensive therapy appears to be more productive with articulation disorders than with disorders associated with organic conditions.

5. Although kindergarten and first grade children were not studied, intensive therapy appears to be effective with elementary children in grades two through six.

6. Because of higher dismissal rates, more children receive therapy in intensive systems of scheduling.

7. Speech-language pathologists report administrative advantages of intensive scheduling such as reduced forgetting of time, reduced forgetting of appropriate techniques, increased interaction with school personnel, and children not forgetting therapy content.

8. Administrators and teachers report that intensive scheduling is easier administratively, and they are impressed with the increased opportunity for the speech-language pathologist to function as a member of the school staff and multidisciplinary team.

9. The exclusive use of the block or modular system is no longer appropriate for most speech-language programs because of the requirements of P.L. 94-142.

10. The greater gains appear to take place early in therapy regardless of the system of scheduling used.

11. There is evidence to support that greater gains are made when therapy is conducted over a period of time.

12. The available evidence supports that an intensive module of therapy to teach a new skill followed by traditional-intermittent schedule to support practice of the skill over time may be the optimal scheduling pattern.

Although the available evidence appears to favor intensive systems of scheduling, the lack of solid evidence to support any single system paired with the number of factors that are unique to any given situation which may govern the system established mandates careful consideration of the selection of a scheduling system or combination of systems as a viable alternative for individual children in the speech-language program.

Within any given program there may be need to provide a self-contained full day class for children with severe speech-language disorders. There also may be need to provide daily support services for children having severe hearing losses, severe to moderate language disorders, and severe stuttering, articulation, or voice problems. Itinerant program services or a combined intensive-itinerant program providing regularly scheduled intermittent support services for children who have moderate hearing losses, mild language problems, or problems of articulation, fluency, and voice not requiring an intensive program may be necessary. In addition, there is need to provide classroom assistance for integrating the objectives of all pupils receiving direct services into the classroom curricula and for consulting with teachers about children who have less severe speech differences that may not require direct service (Garrard, 1979).

Providing appropriate schedule alternatives for all communication handicapped children through flexible scheduling patterns will contribute to quality speech language programs for all.

SCHEDULING THE WEEK

A study reported in 1961 (Knight, Hahn et al., 1961) indicated that the school speech-language pathologist worked an average of 35.20 hours per week. Time was divided as follows: therapy 23.09 hours, travel 2.68 hours, conferences 2.53 hours, report writing 2.12 hours, preparation of lessons 3.23 hours, and other duties 1.55 hours. Chapter 8 provides updated material dealing with these data.

Since the implementation of P.L. 94-142 and other legislation not only has the speech-language pathologist become more involved with general education, but she also has become involved in preparing individualized educational programs, meeting with multidisciplinary teams, participating in in-service training, meeting with parents, conducting identification and evaluation programs, and expanding the availability of habilitation services to children aged three to twenty-one years.

The rules and regulations for P.L. 94-142 *(Federal Register,* August 23, 1977) outline the major responsibilities and role functions of the speech-language program in the schools as follows:

121a.13 (12) "speech pathology" includes
   (i) identification of children with speech or language disorders.
   (ii) diagnosis and appraisal of specific speech or language disorders.
   (iii) referral for medical or other professional attention necessary for the habilitation of speech or language disorders.
   (iv) provision of speech and language services for habilitation or prevention of communication disorders
   (v) counseling and guidance of parents, children and teachers regarding speech and language disorders.

Although these functions are not entirely new to the definition of speech-language services in the schools, the law makes it clear that functions which often were neglected or given minimal importance in relation to the provision of direct service to children are recognized to be important components of the program and are indeed mandated by the provisions of the law.

Blanchard and Nober (1978) reported the effects of Massachusetts special education reform law, Chapter 766, on 211 public school SLPs fourteen months after its September, 1974, implementation and made implications on a national scale to the anticipated effects of P.L. 94-142. The Massachusetts school speech-language pathologists reported increased involvement in interaction with other specialists, formal parent education, general parental involvement, formal teacher in-service education, supervision, preschool screening, case load hearing threshold testing, preparation of resource room materials, and increased paperwork and report writing. The reporting personnel placed significant emphasis on increase in interaction with other specialists and increased paperwork. The personnel were required to be more accountable in their program management and had increased their interaction with other specialists, parents, and teachers, both in verbal and written activities, such as the preparation of individualized programs. In spite of these many added responsibilities, the speech-language pathologists reporting did not indicate a significant difference in the actual amount of treatment time with pupils.

If the school speech-language pathologist is to be accountable for the broadened scope of providing appropriate education to the communication handicapped, it is essential that the program be planned and scheduled so that effective and efficient use is made of available time to fulfill the various role responsibilities.

Time For Identification, Diagnosis, and Appraisal

P.L. 94-142 requires that (1) all children who are handicapped regardless of the severity of their handicap, and who are in need of special education and related services are identified, located, and evaluated and, (2) a practical method is developed and implemented to determine which children are currently receiving needed services, special education and related services [*Federal Register,* August 23, 1977, 121a.128(1)(2)]. This assessment is, where appropriate, to include assessment of communicative status (121a.532). The amount of time that is used for testing will depend on the identification and diagnostic procedures that are used and the number of children who are involved in the assessment program. Whereas it may take only five minutes to identify that a child is in need of further diagnostic services, a complete diagnostic evaluation of communication status may require several hours, depending on the severity of the problem. Adequate time must be reserved for testing at the beginning of the school year and in new programs. In addition, because referrals for testing and reevaluation can be made at any time during the school year, time for diagnosis should be made available throughout the school year. The demand for testing time will fluctuate throughout the year; however, sufficient time should be reserved because the testing must be completed within thirty days of identification of need for testing for the purpose of determining that the child is handicapped and may require special education and related services.

Time for Consulting and Referral

According to the rules and regulations of P.L. 94-142, children who have a speech impairment as their primary handicap may not need a complete battery of assessments, e.g. psychological, physical, or adaptive behavior. However, a qualified speech-language pathologist would (1) evaluate each speech impaired child using procedures that are appropriate for the diagnosis and appraisal of speech and language disorders and (2), where necessary, make referrals for additional assessments needed to make an appropriate placement decision (121a.532 Comment). This does not relieve the speech-language pathologist from the responsibility of consulting with parents and teachers. Indeed it gives increased responsibility to the speech-language pathologist for consulting and making adequate referrals. Sufficient time should be allowed in the planning of the week to allow for this process.

When the child has a handicapping condition in addition to or other than a speech-language impairment, the speech-language pathologist will be involved in the assessment of his communication status. Thus, the role functions of the speech-language pathologist include consulting with other staff members in planning school programs to meet the needs of the children as indicated by the diagnostic tests, interviews, and evaluations.

When the diagnostic assessment on a child is complete there must be a meeting with members of the multidisciplinary team to determine whether the child is handicapped and in need of special education and related services (121a.532all,12a.540). There must then be a meeting with the parents to explain the results of the testing and, if necessary, to develop an individualized educational program.

Each school district is also responsible for reviewing and revising a handicapped child's individualized program at least once each year *(Federal Register,* August 23, 1977, 121a.343).

As mentioned previously, each child in the speech-language program must receive an annual review for the purpose of revising the individualized educational program. These responsibilities place demands on the speech-language pathologist, who must not only make time available but must also make time available when other personnel are able to meet. Sufficient time must be allowed to complete the consulting process during the time limits imposed by the legislation (121a.3401).

Time for Habilitation Service

The major portion of the speech-language program is the providing of habilitative service to the communication handicapped. According to the continuum of services concept (Healey and Jones, 1972) this may take the form of direct service to children in need or the form of indirect service provided through consultation and demonstration lessons with classroom teachers (*see* Figure 6-5). Usually four days each week are used for therapy, with one day reserved for the remaining role functions.

Once a child has been placed in the speech-language program on the basis of the individualized educational program, the service must be continued until there is no longer need or until the program has been revised. Every effort must be made to provide the service as outlined, in the attempt to reach the annual goals provided. This will require all the professional expertise of the speech-language pathologist and sound clinical judgment. The speech-language program becomes an important part of the child's curriculum. However, because the child is usually missing portions of other classroom instruction, therapy time should be used in an effective and profitable manner to reach the objectives as quickly and as efficiently as possible.

Time for Counseling and In-service

An important part of the speech-language program is holding conferences throughout the year with administrators, teachers, and parents. Time should be allowed for consulting with administrators regarding facilities, reports, procedures being used, and the overall objectives of the speech-language program. Conferences with teachers are essential to coordinate and integrate the activities and goals of the speech-language program with those of the regular classroom. Conferences include making suggestions for carry-over activities into the classroom and for helping the teacher understand the limits of the child's speech-language ability and how these limitations affect the child's ability to function in the classroom. It may involve making suggestions to the teacher on how to modify the classroom instruction to assist the child in profiting from instruction. Although conferences with teachers are frequently brief, they can extend to one-half hour or more. Sufficient time should be allowed for this function to increase the overall effectiveness of the speech-language program.

Conferences with parents are equally important. The parents of communication handicapped children are becoming increasingly aware of the need for their involvement in the speech-language program. Their involvement in the individualized educational program development and annual review makes them aware of the importance of their contribution to the speech-language program. Many of them are willing to help at home to increase the progress of their child. Although finding a time to meet with parents that is convenient to all may sometimes be difficult, especially when both parents are employed outside the home, time for this essential function should not be avoided because of inconvenience. Telephone conferences may supplement face-to-face conferences when additional information is desired or when the speech-language pathologist wishes to provide information to the parents.

Time should be reserved for in-service training. Public Law 94-142 regulations require that each state and local education agency provide a system of personnel development for general and special education, related service, and support personnel (121a.380–121a.387).

Many school districts have in-service education programs throughout the year and frequently ask the speech-language pathologist to participate in these general training sessions. The participation may last for a few minutes in which the SLP explains certain aspects of the program to full sessions or series of sessions for the general education of the staff in understanding certain aspects of communication disorders. In-service training leads to increased cooperation with classroom teachers, administrators, and parents. The time that may be involved is good investment in terms of increased cooperation and understanding by the classroom teachers and administrators.

The many responsibilities and role functions of the speech-language pathologist require considerable organization and careful management of time. Each is important. There must be time provided each week for each function according to the respective needs of the speech-language program.

Factors to the Examined in Scheduling

From results of research available and from reports of the speech-language pathologists working in the schools, there are several factors to be considered in determining the weekly program schedule. Several of these factors can be related to efficient management of administrative aspects of the program, while others are more directly related to effective clinical management of cases in the program. All of the factors do not carry equal weight; the relative importance of each factor can be expected to vary with each individual circumstance. Indeed the speech-language pathologist must remain flexible to establish an order of priority for each of the factors for each given circumstance at any given time. The priority system may alter at any time during the school year to accommodate the situation that presents itself at each particular moment.

Administrative Factors

The administrative factors are those factors which are related to the overall management of the speech-language program. They are related to the program schedule for the day, the week, and the year. The administrative factors in scheduling are as follows:
1. State and federal laws, rules, regulations, and guidelines
2. Tradition
3. Number of schools and distances between/among schools
4. Appropriate proportion of time
5. Travel time between/among schools
6. Coordination/office time
7. Availability of adequate space and facilities
8. Ability to see half day children
9. Ability to schedule secondary school students
10. Public relations

State and Federal Laws, Rules, Regulations and Guidelines

Public Law 94-142 requires that speech-language therapy be appropriate to the needs of the child as defined in the individualized educational program. It does not make specific program requirements for what is to be considered "appropriate"; this is left to the professional opinion of those providing the service. State laws and regulations of state departments of education often dictate requirements that affect schedules used in programs. For example, the state regulations may regulate the number of times per week a child with a particular handicapping condition may be served, the number of minutes per week or per session the child may be served, or the number of weeks throughout the school year the child may be served.

For example, the Regulations of the Commissioner of Education in New York State[1] require that severely speech-language impaired children (those with unintelligible speech or unable to communicate verbally) be provided speech-language therapy for thirty minutes each day, five days per week in individual or groups, not to exceed two children. Groups of five severely speech-language impaired children are to be provided service for sixty minutes, five days per week. Other speech-language impaired children, those with reduced ability to acquire, use, or comprehend speech or language, mild stuttering, or vocal disorders must be served for at least two thirty-minute periods per week in groups not to exceed two.

Other factors such as case load requirements may indirectly have a bearing on the type of scheduling that the speech-language pathologist may use. Providing appropriate service using flexible scheduling patterns results in a decrease in case load. For example, in reporting the impact of the Massachusetts Special Education Reform Act, Chapter 766, Blanchard and Nober (1978) indicated a 38 percent reduction in case load and a mandated maximum case load of fifty children per clinician.

Again using an example from New York State, the Regulations of the Commissioner limit the case load to twenty severely speech language impaired children. "When severely speech-language impaired pupils are provided service by teachers of the speech and hearing handicapped also serving other speech-language impaired pupils, the total caseload for each teacher shall not exceed 75 children" (Sect. 200.4-3). It would be administratively unwieldy to schedule some children for daily service while sched-

---

[1]Regulations of the Commissioner effective July 1, 1980 Sect. 2002.2 (b) #30 and Sect. 200.4 4-3.

uling seventy-four others on a twice a week basis.

In some cooperative programs where speech-language services are shared between several school districts, either written or verbal agreements or contractural agreements may exist that restrict the speech-language pathologist's expenditure of time to the number of pupils in each cooperating district or to the proportionate share of monies expended by each school district in support of the program.

When the scheduling system is dictated by rules and regulations and local guidelines or practices, little can be done to vary from them except that professional speech-language-hearing organizations on the local, state, and national levels should work toward the elimination of restrictions that limit professional options. Rules and regulations should allow flexibility to schedule according to the needs of the individual cases. No one would imagine legislation similar to that controlling speech-language programs that would require physicians to spend a required amount of time treating an illness or to spend as much time treating pneumonia as in treating the common cold or as much time ministering to a cut finger as to a heart attack! Yet this is frequently the situation confronting the speech-language pathologist.

Tradition

In spite of the many laws, rules, and regulations affecting scheduling practices, the factor of tradition as a controlling force in policy making in the local educational agency should never be underestimated. In fact it is often the most difficult factor to change. It is not unusual for the speech-language pathologist to be confronted by an administrator who has used a particular model for scheduling and prefers it for no reason other than that it has always been used.

It must be recognized that many persons are hesitant to depart from the scheduling methods that they have used and with which they are most comfortable. It is only after clear alternatives can be shown that may be more appropriate to the needs of the children and to the broader functioning of the speech-language program that change is accepted and promoted.

We are usually more willing to accept change when it is on

a trial basis because this implies a possible return to the known and to the comfortable. Thus, a speech-language pathologist contemplating program changes would do well to establish the need for change and to promote it through in-service meetings and documented reports before attempting to implement it. Even then it is wise to initiate change on an experimental basis. Change for change alone is not only valueless but can be needlessly disrupting. Change and the disruption that it may cause must be justified in terms of providing the most appropriate service possible to the speech-language handicapped, although it may be at the expense of the comfort of many teachers and other school personnel initially.

Where tradition is so strong that a change to alternate scheduling models is not feasible, the speech-language pathologist has the choice of informing parents so they are aware that appropriate speech-language service requires alternate scheduling models, leaving the due process procedure option to parents' actions, or to operate as efficiently as possible under existing conditions. With the weight of the federal laws to support the need for appropriate scheduling and service to the speech-language handicapped, there will seldom be situations where solid evidence to justify the need will fail to gain support.

Number of Schools and Distances Between/Among Schools

The smaller the number of schools assigned to the speech-language pathologist, the more flexibility in scheduling is possible. As the number of schools increases, the difficulty in scheduling increases and the likelihood that the program will provide significant help to the children decreases.

Work (1971) has provided recommendations regarding the number of speech-language pathologists who should be assigned to a school according to school enrollment; however, she cautions that professional interpretation of the need for service by children within a school must take precedence over decisions for assignment and scheduling that are based on population size and projected incidence of problems. The recommendation is for one full-time speech-language pathologist for every 750–1500 students in an elementary school. However, when there are special education classes the need to provide service will increase accordingly. Work (1971) recommends that where there are four or more classes for children in special education in a school, a full-time speech-language pathologist should be assigned.

A survey conducted by Neal (1976) indicated that the average number of schools served by a speech-language pathologist was 2.89. However, the information obtained indicated a wide range in the number of schools served. A study conducted in 1959 (Darley, 1961) revealed that approximately one-half of the speech-language pathologists served from three to six schools. However, a trend was seen toward the reduction in the number of schools served. Between 1959 and 1976 there was a fourfold increase in the percentage of clinicians serving only one school, from 10 percent to 39 percent. Since the enactment of P.L. 94-142 and the subsequent reduction in case load, there is every reason to believe that the average number of schools served by the school speech-language pathologist has continued to decline since the Neal Study, and will continue to decline. Sommers and Hatton discuss this in Chapter 8.

The number of schools that are assigned to the speech-language pathologist relates not only to the number of children in the school but also to the number of professional personnel to whom the speech-language pathologist must relate. This is especially true as a result of the increased involvement with school personnel in developing individualized educational programs and serving on multidisciplinary assessment teams. Perhaps one reason for increased gain under the intensive scheduling model is the increase in professional interaction. As the number of schools increases, the number of professional staff to relate to increases and the overall effectiveness of the program decreases. To provide appropriate education to the speech-language handicapped is not only a professional obligation but is a legal requirement. Even if it is more readily accomplished when fewer schools are assigned, the goal of appropriate service must be met regardless of the number of schools assigned. Providing services in all the facets required by P.L. 94-142 appears manageable for a speech-language pathologist who has a case load of forty to fifty students in a single school. If it is necessary to serve two or more schools, responsibilities will require a reduction in case load (Garrard, 1979).

Appropriate Proportion of Time

The provision of proportionate amounts of time when more than one school is assigned is another factor that must be considered in scheduling. However, it can not be used as a greater factor than the needs of the children being served, regardless of the school that they attend.

Where a school has a population of 2,000, for example, it is not necessarily true that the number of children will be equally be distributed among four schools of 500 pupils each. It is more likely that one school will have an enrollment of 1,000, one of 500, one of 300 and one of 200 or a similar disproportionate distribution. In addition, there is no need to assume that the number of speech-language handicapped children will be equally distributed among the buildings. It does not seem defensible to distribute time among the buildings based on enrollment alone. Rather it seems defensible to provide the time for each school dependent on the needs of the speech-language handicapped children who require service in each building.

Suppose that the speech-language pathologist used a half-day for office time and devoted the remaining twenty-seven hours of school time to therapy. The following example illustrates differences in the number of hours assigned to a school based on need for service versus enrollment.

If School A with an enrollment of 1,000 had 53 speech-language handicapped children; School B, enrollment 500, 18 speech-language handicapped children; School C, enrollment 300, 12 speech-language handicapped children; and School D, enrollment 200, 11 speech-language handicapped children requiring service. Dividing this number by the total number of hours available for therapy, 27, yields an approximate ratio of one hour of therapy to every 3.5 children. Thus, the school with 1,000 pupils would receive 15 hours; School B, 5 hours; School C and D 3.5 hours of service.

If the total school enrollment were used as the basis for the number of therapy hours available, there would be one hour of service for each 75 pupils. Under this system School A would receive 13.5 hours of therapy; School B, 6.75; School C, 12; School

D, 4; and School E, 2.75 hours of service. In view of the apparent disparity in time available to serve the speech-language handicapped according to need, it does not seem appropriate to use total enrollment as a basis for distributing time among buildings assigned. The needs of the children to be served must be paramount in the distribution of time between or among buildings.

Travel Time Between or Among Schools

The itinerant speech-language pathologist who travels between or among schools during the professional day must consider the time needed for traveling in planning a schedule. According to Knight, Hahn et al. (1961), the itinerant speech-language pathologist usually spends two to three hours per week traveling or 8 percent of the time available. This figure can vary either way depending on the number of schools visited each day and the distance between the schools and several other related factors. Time spent traveling among schools to provide service will necessarily reduce the case load, especially if services are to be provided on an intensive basis in several schools.

Anyone who has had driving experience in urban, suburban, and rural areas will recognize the importance of travel time. Although not always the case, urban schools may be a matter of a few blocks apart and thus a few minutes apart. On the other hand, suburban schools are frequently several miles apart, while rural schools can be many miles apart, especially in situations where the speech-language program is shared by several school districts.

Distance alone, however, may not be important. The actual time that it takes to travel between schools is the more important factor. It may be possible to travel twenty miles in a rural school district more quickly than a few blocks in urban districts, especially if travel involves a commercial district or must be made during heavy traffic hours.

The time to travel under less than ideal conditions must be considered. A trip that may require ten minutes on a sunny day in September, may require twice that amount on a snowy or rainy day in January.

In the attempt to reduce travel time, many supervisors assign speech-language pathologists to schools in one geographic region.

However, some systems attempt to provide the speech-language pathologist with a variety of experiences by assigning schools from varying socioeconomic areas. This practice prevents one speech-language pathologist from having all children from one socioeconomic class while another has all children in another socioeconomic class. For example, one may be assigned to one inner city school and one school in the outer periphery of the city to provide balance in case load, the result being increased travel time.

In planning travel time, one must not only consider the actual time to travel from door to door, but one must also consider the time involved in gathering materials, signing out of the building (if that is the local practice), getting to one's car, including removing ice and snow from the windows in Northern climates in the winter months, driving to the other school, and reversing the procedure upon arrival at the next school. Time must be planned such that the speech-language pathologist is ready to assume responsibilities at the second school without appearing harried but also without appearing to have taken more time than necessary to go from place to place.

The time for travel must be reasonable but must not be so long as to allow personal business to be done enroute. Many classroom teachers are already suspicious of the apparent freedom and flexibility of intinerant personnel and would look askance if told that the itinerant specialist was seen at the supermarket or at the local drive-in restaurant during school hours, even if this were the SLP's lunch period.

Finally, all the careful scheduling in the world may not be sufficient to eliminate the need for an occasional increase in the amount of time to travel between schools. An urgent telephone call from a concerned parent, inclement weather, unanticipated traffic problems, or automobile trouble may cause late arrival at the second school. If the delay will be long enough to cause a delay in the start of the program, the school and affected classroom teachers should be notified. This, coupled with a verbal explanation to persons affected, will reduce the amount of ill feeling generated by failure to adhere to the schedule.

Coordination/Office Time

Coordination or office time is that time designated for those components of the program that are not involved in the direct services for speech-language disorders. Adequate time must be reserved for coordinating activities. This time involves preparation of lessons; preparing of records and reports; correspondence, conferring with office personnel, administrators, and parents; preparation of reports from assessments; preparation of individualized educational programs and reviews; and providing consultation to teachers regarding prevention of communication disorders and children with minor speech-language differences.

P.L. 94-142 has placed a major responsibility on the SLP for those components of the speech-language program that are not involved in direct service to children. In addition to the role functions of identification, diagnosis, referral, and counseling parents, children, and teachers [Federal Register, August 23, 1977, 121a 13 (b) (12)] the speech-language pathologist may be expected to serve on special services teams that oversee the implementation of programs for the handicapped.

According to the survey of school speech-language pathologists conducted in 1961, (Knight, Hahn et al., 1961), 13 percent reported the use of one full day each week for coordination, 52 percent reported using one-half day each week, and 18 percent reported that they did not have work time for coordination activities. A similar survey conducted in Massachusetts after the implementation of Chapter 766 (Blanchard and Nober 1978) indicated that the increase in the amount of reports and paperwork represented the greatest change in professional activity as a result of the new law which, in many respects, is similar to P.L. 94-142 and preceded its implementation. Significant increased responsibility for developing individualized educational programs; preparing written reports from speech-language assessment; consulting with teachers, administrators, and parents; observing cases in classroom settings; and preparing or holding in-service meetings were cited as integral components of the speech-language program, while actual treatment time with pupils did not change.

To meet the challenge of providing appropriate education to

the handicapped, many school districts are developing resource or instructional materials centers for supplies and materials. The speech-language pathologist must allow time to use these facilities if techniques and methods are to respond to change. Time consideration should also be given for assisting with preparation of grant requests and the preparation of statistical reports required for state and federally funded programs.

Many administrators have been concerned with the failure of the professional staff to profitably use unscheduled time for coordination activities. That the SLPs reported in the Blanchard and Nober (1976) report were able to document significant increases in coordination activities, without a significant decline in the actual amount of direct service time, provides support to this concern. However, the challenge of meeting the requirements of P.L. 94-142 precludes the professional staff from using coordination time for personal business or social contacts.

The effective use of coordination time often determines whether a speech-language pathologist is able to conduct a program that is professionally satisfying as well as educationally appropriate for the communication handicapped in the school. Coordination time must not be viewed as a luxury that can be reduced by pressure to allow increased time for direct habilitative service. Coordination activities must be viewed as essential components of an effective program. Usually the equivalent of at least one full day of coordination time per week is necessary to allow the speech-language program to serve fully the needs of the speech-language handicapped in the school.

Availability of Adequate Space and Facility

One of the major concerns of the speech-language pathologist is the facility or room in which she must work. When speech-language programs were considered to be a "frill" in many school systems, personnel worked in any room or space available in the school including the teachers' room, the book room, or even the gym locker room. Many SLPs did not have a room to call their own but, rather, had to share the facility with the nurse, the psychologist, the music teacher, or the reading teacher. In many cases, the importance placed on the speech-language program in the school was reflected in the space or room assigned.

In recent years the importance of speech-language services has been recognized by administrators and other school personnel. With this increased importance has come the recognition of need for adequate space and facility. Recognition of the need for specialized equipment such as tape recorders, amplification systems, mirrors, and acoustic treatment has led to more permanent facilities being made available to speech-language personnel, although in many cases these facilities must be shared with other personnel.

The availability of space for the speech-language program varies throughout the country. Declining school populations due to the declining birth rate, population migrations from urban to suburban communities, and migrations from the northern to the southern regions of the country combine to make space more readily available in some schools. These same factors, however, have contributed to a lack of adequate space in other school districts. In addition, the addition of various resource personnel to the school staff has made increased demands on the space that may be available. This may include the addition of learning disabilities specialists, reading consultants, psychologists, guidance counselors, school social workers, school nurses, and a number of other persons who serve the school. Because of space demands, facilities for speech-language programs may have to be shared with other resource personnel. A complicated schedule can make sharing satisfactory work space difficult. Some administrators, especially those pressed for space, are reluctant to leave a room vacant for several weeks or even days while the speech language pathologist serves another school. Use of a room for brief periods scattered throughout the week, e.g. Tuesday morning, Wednesday from 10:00 to 11:00 and Friday from 2:00 to 2:30, usually makes the sharing of space difficult. Seeing the room occupied regularly is also reassuring to teachers and administrators that the speech-language program is a vital part of the program and the SLP is on hand to assist and consult with school personnel as necessary.

The speech-language program is best scheduled when the space assigned is used regularly throughout the school year. Although a room may be used for a same number of hours during the year in an intensive modular program as in an intermittent program, it may not seem so to administrators and other personnel who view a vacant room for several weeks or months. Upon return to the building after a lengthy absence, the speech-language pathologist may find the room occupied by other personnel who were "using" the facility in her absence. It may be difficult and place a strain on public relations to request that the facility be vacated by the "visitor." "Squatter's rights" often prevail in situations where space is limited.

All the evidence in the world can be gathered to indicate that one system of scheduling is superior to another, but if the room is not available to accommodate the system, it will probably not be possible to use it. If need be, a compromise can usually be worked out with other school personnel for space in another part of the building. Careful communication and good working relationships with other school personnel can usually deter problems that arise from conflicts in scheduling shared facilities and result in use of facilities that meet the needs of the children being served.

Ability to See Half-Day Children

Children in preschool and kindergarten classes who are in school only a half day or for fewer than five days per week can create scheduling problems. In many school districts the younger kindergarten children attend school in the morning, while the older children attend in the afternoon. In others, in the attempt to accommodate the bussing schedule, children in one portion of the school district attend school in the morning, while the others attend in the afternoon. To complicate the situation further, often the two groups will switch sessions at mid-year so that all children can experience both morning and afternoon sessions.

With the incentive of preschool grants provided under P.L. 94-142 (part 121 ml and 121 mq), many school districts have added programs for preschool children who often attend school only two or three days per week.

In the past, because of the many problems in scheduling, half-day children were excluded from the program. P.L. 94-142, however, requires that handicapped children five years old be provided appropriate education (121a.300). The speech-language program must be scheduled to allow kindergarten children to be served, as well as the three to five year olds who may be in special programs for the preschool handicapped.

In some cases scheduling may be facilitated by placing all half-day children who require service in the same session so that the children can be at the school when the service is available. This may not be in the child's best interest, because he may be placed in a grouping that does not meet his academic or social needs.

With the cooperation of parents it may be possible to schedule children either before the kindergarten session begins or to schedule them after the session. This plan has the advantages of allowing frequent contact with the parent and not removing the child from the kindergarten program. Although desirable, this situation may not be possible because of transportation—the parents may not be willing or able to transport the child to school early, and the school district may not be willing to provide transportation either early or late to accommodate scheduling. However, with planning, transportation to obtain appropriate services can be included in the child's individualized education program.

A scheduling system that allows the SLP to be at the school during each half-day session at different days during the week can resolve the problem of half-day children, in part. Alternating the schedule between morning and afternoon sessions for modular periods can also be effective in accommodating half-day children. Whatever system is established, five year old kindergarten children and preschool handicapped children must be provided an appropriate education based on their individual needs. These needs cannot be dictated by the schedule established but, rather, must dictate the schedule that is established.

Ability to Schedule Secondary School Students

As with kindergarten, middle school, junior high school, and senior high school schedules present unique problems in scheduling. Secondary schools are less able to tolerate the various systems of scheduling because their class schedules are more complicated and less flexible.

Neal (1976) reported that at the secondary level, the itinerant-intermittent method of scheduling was used by 75 percent of secondary school speech-language pathologists. The intensive modular system was used by 15.9 percent and other patterns by 9.3 percent. In addition, 77.8 percent of the respondents to the survey indicated that itinerant methods were most effective at the secondary level; 14.8 percent indicated the intensive method, while 7.4 percent indicated other systems.

Fifty-six percent of the respondents to the survey indicated that following a daily schedule or weekly schedule consistently in secondary schools is more difficult than in elementary schools. Sixty-two percent of the respondents indicated that extracurricular activities affected class attendance. In addition, 73 percent of the respondents indicated that the speech-language program at the secondary level was no more readily accepted by administrators than it was in the elementary schools, and 87 percent of those responding reported the same regarding teachers.

Problems in scheduling in the secondary school include the students' unwillingness to miss classes that they find interesting or that may be mandated by the state department of education. Further, students may not wish to miss classes that are difficult for them. The length of the school class period often creates problems. Secondary schools often schedule seven forty-five minute periods each day. Speech-language sessions are usually twenty to thirty minutes. This means that the student will have to miss half the regular academic subject and be subject to question from his peers about where he goes and why. This problem can be alleviated by scheduling the speech-language sessions to coincide with the regular periods in the school.

The time of the school day may also be a problem in scheduling in the secondary school. Often secondary schools begin the school day an hour or more before the elementary schools. In one suburban town, for example, the high school began its day at 7:20, the middle school at 8:20, and the elementary schools at 9:20 with similarly staggered dismissal time to facilitate use of school buses. Intinerant personnel assigned to both the high school and to the elementary school could conceivably have a school day that extended from the 7:20 beginning time for the high school to 3:30, the elementary school dismissal time. This significantly lengthens the SLP's work day.

The Task Force of Traditional Scheduling Procedures in the

Schools (1979) recommended the following concerning scheduling in the secondary schools: (1) the speech-language pathologist discuss scheduling periods with school administrators prior to the beginning of the school year or when the decision is made to enroll the student in the speech-language program; (2) the schools provide consideration to regularly scheduled speech-language classes with credit as part of the academic curriculum for those pupils in need of these services. (This may be possible and more readily accepted since the Elementary and Secondary Education Act, as amended, November, 1978, identifies oral communication as a basic skill on par with reading, mathematics, and written communication); (3) persons responsible for scheduling classes establish a rotational system so that the student does not miss the same class each time; and/or (4) scheduling during the regular academic year be omitted completely and intensive services be provided during a six-week summer period.

It is appropriate for secondary students to be involved in the development of the individualized education program. Such participation will allow the students to provide input as to the schedule that they find most accommodating. Fellows (1976) recommends that, in the course of counseling and conferring, the student's best and worst subjects should be determined and the schedule established so that the classes missed will have the least affect on academic grades and on state mandated courses.

Because of the many difficulties in scheduling, many secondary students traditionally have not been provided appropriate speech-language services. The federal laws now assure appropriate services to students through the age of twenty-one years. Students who continue to require speech-language services through the secondary school are generally of a more severe nature. They will require at least as much therapy time as the elementary schools. Schedules that provide service to secondary schools on a once-a-week basis because of scheduling difficulties are not justifiable in terms of the needs of the students. The schedule must be established that allows appropriate service to be provided to all students through the age of twenty-one years.

Public Relations

Although not the determining factor to be considered in scheduling, it is important that not only the school personnel but also the community understand and be satisfied with the scheduling system that is established. Taxpayers are becoming increasingly more concerned and interested in the way their tax dollars are being expended. The community may feel that service twice a week is sufficient for all children. Teachers, administrators, and other parents in the community may also benefit from an explanation as to the rationale of the schedule that is established. One system may seem to be more efficient to teachers and administrators. For example, some teachers feel that intensive scheduling causes children to miss certain aspects of the program every day and causes the children to fall behind. They would prefer the child to miss the classroom program only once or twice a week, even though over a longer period of time. Sometimes the "ease" factor is secondary to the previously mentioned tradition. One principal continually complained that the modular program in his school seemed less efficient to him although he was never able to explain why. It just "seemed less efficient." Conferences and multidisciplinary team assessment meetings can have the effect of educating school personnel regarding all aspects of the speech-language program including rationale for scheduling. Several years ago one PTA member worked diligently to have a program using the intensive modular system of scheduling changed back to an intermittent system because she was convinced that it was better for her son. Careful explanation with the parents during preparation of the individualized education program concerning the speech-language program as a whole and the reasons for recommending a particular schedule for the child could avoid such problems.

The participation of the parents, classroom teacher, and other school personnel in the I.E.P. conference and I.E.P. development elicits not only cooperation in establishing an effective schedule for the child but also an understanding of the speech-language schedule as a whole. Teachers, administrators, and parents are more cooperative when they understand.

Finally, perhaps the greatest aid to public relations and support by school personnel and community is the number of children served by the program and the number of children who are dismissed as no longer requiring service. A successful program is the guarantee of good public relations. A carefully planned weekly schedule is a significant factor in the development of a successful speech-language program.

Clinical Factors in Scheduling the Week

The clinical factors in scheduling the week are those factors which directly relate to providing effective and efficient management of each case. They are related to the basic principles of learning in changing and developing speech-language behavior.

Needs of Various Problems

The single most important factor to be considered in determining scheduling for speech-language programs is the need to provide all communication handicapped children a free, appropriate public education. It is the professional responsibility of the speech-language pathologist to determine the appropriate service for each case based on individual need as defined in the individualized education program. The schedule that is developed must function to allow the needs of each speech-language handicapped child to be met.

As there is a wide range of characteristics that constitute a particular problem, there must be a wide range of options available to provide appropriate service to assist these problems. As mentioned previously, there has been no research or professional agreement that clearly indicates the ideal scheduling system for a particular speech-language problem. Indeed, the variety of factors such as intelligence level, age, and the nature of the problem itself would make this nearly an impossible task. It is not surprising that there is some evidence that, regardless of the nature of the problem, the more therapy and the more intensive the therapy an individual receives, the sooner the problem will be alleviated.

Previously cited research supports that there may be advantages to scheduling articulation problems using an intensive mode of scheduling. However, schedules that accompany certain organic conditions may best be served by intermittent service over a longer period of time. Beyond this there is little research evidence to identify clearly which problems respond best to which type of scheduling. It is certain that scheduling models that allow the same pattern for each case are not justified in communication disorders any more than in the medical profession.

Time allotted and the treatment planned must depend on the individual problem as presented with its many associated factors and conditions. To meet the needs of various problems the schedule established must be, above all, flexible and able to accommodate individual need.

Amount of Help Throughout the Year in Relation to Extent of Gain

In considering various systems of scheduling it is helpful to compare programs not only on the basis of the amount of time each child receives during a total school year but also on the basis of the amount of time allotted to each child at any given time during the year. For example, under the traditional method of scheduling each child receives service two times a week for thirty-two weeks, totaling thirty-two hours of service for the year. If, on the other hand, using an intensive scheduling model the child were served for four half hours each week he would receive an equivalent amount of therapy in sixteen weeks. Several studies previously cited have indicated that children appeared to achieve greater gains under intensive programming, although the actual number of therapy hours was fewer. The factors of spaced learning versus paced learning explain this phenomenon. Available data from experiments in learning by psychologists show that learning of skills occurs more rapidly when the tasks are learned during massed learning than when the same task is learned with the same amount of practice time divided into shorter periods and spread over a longer period of time. Students who "cram" for an examination can learn the same material in as short a period of time as their more conscientious peers who studied regularly over the course of the semester. Unfortunately, data also indicate that forgetting occurs more rapidly as the result of massed practice (Mowrer, 1977).

It is less important in the long run to consider the number of hours of service provided to a child than to consider selecting the appropriate scheduling pattern to maximize progress for each child. Lauder (1966) states that improvement is more related to the competency of the speech-language pathologist than to the schedule system used. Or, it may be that children make greater progress when the SLP is using the system of scheduling with which she has the most confidence.

The amount of help provided throughout the year may not be the critical factor in producing gains by the children scheduled. If a child is making slow progress, assistance may be increased to provide daily service. However, if the techniques that are being used are inappropriate, if motivation by the child or by the speech-language pathologist is insufficient, if there is a personality conflict or if some other factor related to rate of learning, but not to frequency of service, is operative, increasing the amount of help available through the year will not yield proportionate gains. Frequency of service throughout the year or during a particular period during the year is only one factor of many that may affect the extent of gain in the speech-language program. There is a professional responsibility to examine all factors involved in the learning process to determine the most appropriate schedule for a particular child.

Forgetting and Retention

Perhaps two of the more important clinical factors to be considered in developing a schedule are forgetting and retention. These factors apply equally to the speech-language pathologist, to the classroom teacher and other school personnel, and to children enrolled in the program.

Although the factors of forgetting and its corollary, retention, are important aspects of the learning process, a search of literature in speech-language pathology yields little information other than global, pragmatic suggestions (Mowrer, 1977).

With regard to the speech-language pathologist, forgetting pertains to the goals of therapy for each child, the techniques that seem to be most effective, the stimulus materials that are to be used, the point at which the previous session ended, and where the next session should begin. In delivering individualized service to as many as seventy-five children in one week, there is little wonder that the speech-language pathologist would have difficulty remembering the details of specific programs for each child. As the number of cases increases, the time available for writing daily progress notes and for referring to these notes decreases, increasing the effects of forgetting.

Forgetting by the classroom teacher and other school personnel also needs to be considered in scheduling. The classroom teacher must be able to remember the speech-language schedule so as to send the child to "speech class" on time. The SLP who waits for a child to come only to have to go searching for the child who has failed to appear or the SLP who must send another child to get the missing children before sessions can begin is well aware of the problems created when the teacher cannot remember therapy time.

Generally, the more frequent the sessions and the more consistent the time that the speech-language class is scheduled the better will the teacher be able to remember. Certainly it is easier to remember that Johnny goes to speech-language every day at 9:00 than to remember that he goes Monday at 9:00, Tuesday at 10:00, Wednesday at 11:45, and Thursday at 1:20. Frequency of scheduling also helps the teacher to assist in carry-over activities.

Because other school personnel can forget that the school does have the services of a speech-language pathologist, in many respects it is better for the speech-language pathologist to be present in each school assigned on a periodic and frequent basis. Spending part of each week in each school assigned helps the school personnel feel that someone is at hand to assist and advise them.

Having to wait for several days or weeks or even months until the speech-language pathologist returns can be very frustrating. What may be an important question or an important observation may be set aside or forgotten while the SLP is out of the building.

Forgetting and retention are primarily important in regard to the learning accomplished by the child. For the child, the opportunity for forgetting may result from infrequency of weekly sessions or, in the case of a modular scheduling system, length of time between modules. If a child has therapy once a week, he has six days to forget what has been learned. With therapy every day, forgetting will be reduced.

A number of studies conducted in the field of psychology indicate that frequent review of learned material retards forgetting significantly. Frequent review has the effect of limiting the effects of interference from previous learning. Mower (1977) gives a hypothetical example in which the effect of daily review of material that was learned at 100 percent criterion was retained with 100 percent accuracy six days later with daily review. When no such review was provided during the six-day interval, retention dropped to 10 percent. Every speech-language pathologist who has experienced the incredible amount of forgetting that may occur after holiday periods, over the summer months, or after a lengthy absence can appreciate the meaning of this example.

Much of the research previously cited in support of various systems of scheduling has been inconclusive where the effects of scheduling have been concerned. Not only have previously mentioned factors not been controlled, but also the research has not demonstrated the effect of scheduling on long-term retention of gains. The relationship between the amount of progress achieved before therapy was suspended, or before there was an interruption in the therapy program, and retention needs to be examined with respect to scheduling. For example, how much progress is necessary before long-term retention of skills following suspension of therapy can be assured? Mowrer (1977) suggests that the effects of scheduling on long-term forgetting and retention could be determined by providing five twenty-minute therapy sessions daily to one group (100 minutes total) and five twenty-minute sessions to another group one session each week (100 minutes total). Retention tests could be given one week, four weeks, and eight weeks after the final instruction period so that the effects of scheduling on retention could be accurately measured.

Many factors need to be considered when planning a schedule for the week. Some are related to the needs of the child, and many are related to basic administrative necessity. Which factors or combination of factors apply to a given situation can only be determined by the persons directly involved. In any case the need to provide appropriate speech-language service to each communication handicapped child must remain paramount. Flexibility, then, becomes the key word in scheduling the week. The speech-language program must be flexible to provide appropriate alternatives to communication handicapped children based on individual need.

PLANNING THE DAY

Many variations of the daily schedule are possible, depending on the number of children to be scheduled, the pattern of scheduling, and the length of therapy sessions. Every program is dependent on the number of hours children are available and the variety of tasks that must be completed within the day. There are a variety of administrative and clinical factors that must be considered in planning the schedule for the day.

Administrative Factors in Planning the Day

Policies and Contracts

The basic rule for the SLP to follow is to be in school during school hours, performing school-related activities. Speech-language pathologists are school personnel subject to the same rights and benefits as other teachers in the school system. The major policies pertaining to the overall responsibilities are established by administrators, including the starting and ending of the school day. The speech-language pathologist who arrives at the school with the other teachers and leaves with the others is much more readily perceived to be a part of the regular educational program than one who arrives in time to see the first case and leaves as soon as the last case leaves.

Informing School Personnel

Teachers, administrators, and other school personnel, including office staff and paraprofessional workers, frequently note the work habits of itinerant personnel. The activities of the speech-language pathologist during the day are a concern to others who may not fully understand the diverse responsibilities of the position.

Staff may be resentful of what may appear to be relative freedom from the confining nature of classroom assignments. Therefore, it is important that the speech-language pathologist inform administrators and teachers fully of the activities of the day. Every member of the school staff should be provided a copy of the schedule that the speech-language pathologist follows. Any significant changes in the schedule should be made in writing and distributed to all school personnel. When other school personnel are able to see in writing the busy schedule and the diverse activities of the SLP, not only will they have a greater understanding of the nature of the speech-language program, but they will be less inclined to question the activities of itinerant personnel.

Following the Schedule

Once the schedule is prepared and distributed, it is essential that the schedule be followed. Prompt arrival at school and prompt initiation of therapy sessions aid the image of a program that is organized and efficient. There are many classroom teachers who expect Johnny to be taken for speech-language class exactly at the time scheduled. Any departure, even for as short a time as one minute, can result in a call to the office asking the whereabouts of the speech-language specialist.

Many classroom teachers begin and end classroom activity around the time that children are to attend speech-language therapy. If therapy is five minutes late, the teacher either has a child who is unoccupied for five minutes or twenty-nine children who are delayed in starting an activity. Returning children to the classroom on schedule is also essential for the same reasons. In addition, the children may be scheduled to go to special subject areas, to lunch, or home. Delay in return can result in the entire class being late.

Not abiding by the daily schedule can be cumulative. Five minutes late in getting started either means that the session is shortened or that sessions throughout the day will all be five minutes late, causing undue problems for classroom teachers. When unanticipated delays occur, such as a telephone call, a visit by a parent, or any number of difficulties associated with an itinerant schedule, teachers should be notified as soon as possible. Such delays should be as infrequent as possible.

Perhaps the major cause for delay in following the schedule is the impromptu conference or telephone call. Where possible, such conferences should be kept brief. If there is indication of need for a longer conference, the need to adhere to the schedule should be explained with assurance that the call will be returned or the discussion held later when more time is available to address the concern adequately. Social calls or conferences, of course, should not interfere with the therapy schedule.

The daily speech-language schedule should be developed in conjunction with the total school program so that it is not administratively unwieldy and articulates well with other special resource personnel and programs in the school. Once established, in order for the entire school program to run smoothly, the schedule must be followed.

Clinical Factors in Planning the Day

The clinical factors in planning the day relate to creating the optimal conditions for learning.

Scheduling the Most Appropriate Time

Classroom teachers usually prefer to have all the children remain in the classroom at the start of the school day. Such activities as opening exercises, attendance, and lunch count are important administrative functions, which the teacher must conduct with all the children present. In addition, many teachers use this time for announcements and for a general discussion of the plan for the day. Speech-language therapy sessions should not begin until this daily orientation period in the classroom has been completed.

In elementary schools, teachers generally consider the beginning of the school day to be the most productive for learning by young children. Many feel that young children are best able to profit from reading instruction early in the day. They would prefer that children not be scheduled for speech-language until after the daily reading class. This does not seem to be a crucial factor with older children. In many speech-language programs, the children in the upper elementary grades are scheduled for service in the early part of the day, leaving the younger children in the classroom for much of the morning activity. The time period when the morning instructional period has been completed and the children are scheduled for small group or independent seatwork is usually the best time to schedule younger children. In developing the schedule, the speech-language pathologist must not, however, allow the classroom teacher to retain the child in the classroom during optimal learning times and allow the child to go to speech-language when the child is exhausted. Developing communication competence is a vital part of the child's curriculum. The importance of improving communication as vital to improving educational performance needs to be a primary consideration in developing the child's schedule (Dublinske, 1980).

In developing a schedule it is sometimes wise to avoid scheduling a child for therapy immediately after physical education. Not only are the children often too tired to concentrate fully on the demands for improving communication, they are often too excited to settle into the demands of the program. It is also inadvisable to attempt to schedule a child at a time when he would miss special subject area classes such as physical education, art, or music, unless there is a reason why the child should not participate in the activity with his regular class. Resentment and hostility related to missing favorite subjects do not facilitate proper attitudes and motivation for improving communication skills. When it is not possible to schedule a child to avoid special subject areas, an attempt should be made to allow the child to participate in that class with another group.

Scheduling speech-language sessions to provide the least amount of disruption in the child's academic programming requires considerable planning and consultation with classroom teachers. Compromise may be necessary; however, it is usually possible to develop a schedule that meets the needs of all concerned.

Scheduling Group versus Individual

Speech-language pathologists usually schedule speech-language services in groups of two to six children. Bingham et al. (1961) reported that greater than 90 percent of all school therapy was provided in groups. Reduced case loads since P.L. 94-142 have likely increased the amount of individual therapy scheduled.

There has been considerable investigation of the relative

effectiveness of group versus individual therapy, including work by Pfeifer (1958), Sokolof (1959), Sommers (1964), and Sommers (1966). All four investigations have found that group therapy is as effective as individual therapy independent of grade level or of degree of articulatory defect. Schedules that provide for groups have been considered to be as effective and as efficient as schedules that allow individual therapy. The assumption is that the goals and activities provided for each member of the group are designed to meet unique needs and that the therapy program provided makes effective use of the time scheduled for all the children in the group.

Group therapy must be more than a round robin series of individual therapy interactions between individuals in the group and the speech-language pathologist. Mowrer (1972) provides an illustration that leads one to question the appropriateness of group scheduling where serial therapy is provided. Suppose fifty-two children are scheduled in groups of four children to a group. Each group is seen twice weekly for a total of forty-eight minutes of therapy. If the forty-eight minutes is divided equally, each child receives twelve minutes of direct therapy each week. During the other thirty-six minutes, the child would be waiting to respond, listening to others, evaluating their responses, and watching the other children in the group. Earlier Mowrer (1964) studied the effects of listening and watching activities in speech therapy. He found that children who watched and listened continued to misarticulate target phonemes, while children who actively participated by responding aloud learned to articulate properly. Although this is not in itself an indictment against group therapy, it does provide justification for caution to provide group interaction that is continuous and is not serial in group sessions. Individual therapy to each of several children in a group is not an efficient use of time and often leads to boredom and/or misbehavior by students.

There are classroom teachers who would prefer that all children who require speech-language services in their classroom be scheduled at the same time (for the sake of ease in their classroom schedule). While this may be possible and even desirable, in some cases the needs of the children involved must be considered. It is usually not justifiable to schedule a stutterer in the same time period as a cleft palate child. Indeed it is difficult to justify scheduling heterogeneous articulation groups, i.e. where there are different phonemes being corrected or in which children are at different stages in the correction process. Although Beasley (1950) advocated the inclusion of all types of speech-language disorders in groups for therapy to improve socialization and interaction with peers, heterogeneous grouping may not be justifiable as the appropriate form for scheduling to meet the unique needs of the communication handicapped.

Every effort should be made to keep scheduled groups small and homogeneous in terms of need, age, and anticipated rate of progress to maximize group interaction and continual responding within the group. Flexibility should be allowed to schedule both individual and group therapy as indicated by individual need, not by convenience or by the ability to see more children.

Length of Session

The length of the therapy session should also be determined by the needs of the children being served. Because the communication handicapped have different needs, there is need for considerable flexibility in scheduling the length of sessions. Although most sessions are scheduled for twenty-five to thirty minutes, there are occasions when longer or shorter sessions may be necessary. Therapy sessions in the secondary schools are generally as long as the usual school periods. Kindergarten and preschool sessions often are shorter.

It may be advantageous to schedule a child for two fifteen-minute periods during the day rather than one half-hour period. Such a scheduling pattern increases the frequency of the sessions and may have the effect of intensive therapy, since the child scheduled twice a day two times a week has been scheduled four times per week. MacDonald and Frick (1960) suggested that this pattern of scheduling may be beneficial in the initial skill-learning stages of therapy. It could also be useful as a child enters carry-over stages. A child could be scheduled for both group and individual therapy. A shorter individual therapy session could be used to meet unique needs and a longer group therapy session on the same day or in the same week to reinforce those skills in a more social setting.

The length of time of each scheduled therapy session, then, needs to remain flexible to provide alternatives for appropriate scheduling to meet the needs of the children. Finally, it is helpful to schedule a five-minute interval between sessions to allow children to return to their classroom and allow preparation for the next session.

Time to Consult With Teachers

The need to consult with teachers who have responsibility for children throughout the school day often necessitates that the speech-language pathologist arrive at school early and stay late to talk to the teachers when they do not have responsibility for children. Although classroom teachers usually have a preparation period, there is no guarantee that the SLP will be available at the same time as the teacher during the school day. This becomes particularly crucial when the classroom teacher is required to meet with the multidisciplinary team for discussion of children who have been referred for special services and with the I.E.P. planning committee. Although there are some administrators who release classroom teachers for this responsibility during the school day, it is more often the case that meetings take place either before or after school. Consequently, it is more likely that the SLP will find it necessary to arrive at school earlier than the classroom teacher and remain later than most.

Some itinerant speech-language pathologists are required to go to a central office before and/or after the school day. The practice is usually a good time for correspondence, conferences with office personnel, changing and preparation of therapy materials, and similar duties. When the practice then requires the speech-language pathologist to travel to another building to begin the therapy program, the available time for direct service and teacher consultation is reduced.

SAMPLE PROGRAMS

Although, as previously stated, infinite varieties of possible scheduling alternatives exist, it should be helpful to examine several representative systems. Some comments on the strengths and weaknesses are presented; however, no attempt is made to exhaust all possible comments for each one. For each program presented, three considerations have been stated: (1) the number of consecutive weeks that the speech-language pathologist serves a particular school; (2) the number of modules of therapy a school receives throughout the year; and (3) the number of times per week children are seen or, similarly, the number of times a school is scheduled each week.

One representative program for each of the scheduling models discussed earlier will be illustrated, i.e. (1) a traditional intermittent system, (2) an intensive system, (3) a modular system and (4) a combined intermittent-modular system. The number of schools used in each example is four, because this is close to the national average number of schools assigned. Speech-language pathologists will have to make adjustments in the samples provided to reflect their own unique circumstances. No attempt was made to provide samples of daily scheduling, because the alternatives are too numerous to warrant a single sample.

In the following samples the top line represents the yearly schedule with the number of modules and the length of modules expressed in weeks below the line. The bottom box shows a typical weekly schedule with the five days of the week. The letters A, B, C, and D represent the four schools, and O designates office time.

1. *Itinerant-Intermittent Schedule*

YEARLY SCHEDULE

September _____ June

Same Schedule

WEEKLY SCHEDULE

	Mon.	Tues.	Wed.	Thurs.	Fri.
A.M.	A	C	A	C	O
P.M.	B	D	B	D	O

Advantages. Each school receives an equal amount of time. Children receive help throughout the school year. There is sufficient office time. Facilities can be used on a regular basis throughout the year as well as be shared with other personnel. The schools are provided with service throughout the year.

Disadvantages. There is no provision for the varying needs of the children in the schools. Half-day children cannot be scheduled. There is considerable time for forgetting, i.e. from Wednesday to Monday. Consultation time is concentrated into a single day, which may not allow flexibility in meeting with teachers and other school personnel in all four schools.

2. *Intensive Yearly Schedule*

YEARLY SCHEDULE

September _____ June

Same Schedule

WEEKLY SCHEDULE

	Mon.	Tues.	Wed.	Thurs.	Fri.
A.M.	AO	D	A	DO	AO
	B	CO	B	C	BO
P.M.	C	B	C	B	C
	D	A	D	A	D

Advantages. Children receive help throughout the school year. Half-day children are able to be scheduled. Rooms are used on a regular basis throughout the school year. Forgetting is minimized. Unique needs of individual children can be accommodated. Office coordination time is provided for each school. Caseload is probably small.

Disadvantages. Increase in travel time will result in loss of time available for therapy. Large number of staff to whom to relate.

3. *Intensive-Modular Schedule*

YEARLY SCHEDULE

September __1__ __2__ __3__ __4__ June
           10 wks 10 wks 10 wks 10 wks

WEEKLY SCHEDULE FOR PERIODS 1 AND 3

	Mon.	Tues.	Wed.	Thurs.	Fri.
A.M.	A	A	A	A	BO
P.M.	B	B	B	AO	B

WEEKLY SCHEDULE FOR PERIODS 2 AND 4

	Mon.	Tues.	Wed.	Thurs.	Fri.
A.M.	C	C	C	C	DO
P.M.	D	D	D	CO	D

Advantages. Children receive intensive therapy for twenty weeks. Teachers become familiar with the schedule. Speech-language pathologist becomes acquainted with the staff. There is less forgetting by the children and the speech-language pathologist. Dismissal rate for articulation cases is high. Various scheduling needs of the children can be accommodated. Equal time is provided to each school. Travel time is minimized. Some half-day children can be scheduled. For twenty weeks the academic program is not disturbed.

Disadvantages. The room is vacant for half the year. Considerable forgetting may occur between periods. Academic program is interrupted daily for twenty weeks. Severe problems do not receive help throughout the school year. Half of the half-day children do not receive service.

4. *Combined Intensive Modular and Intermittent System*

YEARLY SCHEDULE

September___1_____2_____3_____4_____June
             10 wks   10 wks   10 wks   10 wks

WEEKLY SCHEDULE FOR MODULE 1

	Mon.	Tues.	Wed.	Thurs.	Fri.
A.M.	A	A	A	A	A
P.M.	AO	B	C	D	O

WEEKLY SCHEDULE FOR MODULE 2

	Mon.	Tues.	Wed.	Thurs.	Fri.
A.M.	B	B	B	B	B
P.M.	A	BO	C	D	O

WEEKLY SCHEDULE FOR MODULE 3

	Mon.	Tues.	Wed.	Thurs.	Fri.
A.M.	C	C	C	C	C
P.M.	A	B	CO	D	O

WEEKLY SCHEDULE FOR MODULE 4

	Mon.	Tues.	Wed.	Thurs.	Fri.
A.M.	D	D	D	D	D
P.M.	A	B	C	DO	O

Advantages. Children are seen throughout the school year and receive both intensive and intermittent help. Each school receives equal service. Speech-language pathologist is able to function as a member of the school staff throughout the school year. Office time is provided for each school throughout the year. One-half of half-day children can receive service. Some flexibility of scheduling is available during at least part of the year. Travel time is limited.

Disadvantages. The needs of the children may not be met throughout the school year. Intensive therapy may not be available to the child at the time when it would be most beneficial to him. Rooms must be available in varying schedules. One-half of the half-day children cannot receive service throughout the year.

Designing the Most Appropriate System

These are only a few of the infinite variety of ways in which the school week and the school year can be arranged. Each has its advantages and disadvantages. The systems presented here can be combined in a number of ways or other systems designed. Add to this the infinite ways in which the individual day can be arranged and the importance of the decisions of the speech-language pathologist become evident. The speech-language pathologist should examine his particular situation from all aspects, considering all of the factors, and design the system that best meets the unique needs of the children in the program. It is not an easy process. There is no single correct system. The many alternatives may be the reason that so many SLPs decide to use the traditional system. The need to provide appropriate service to an increasing variety of communication handicapped children will encourage and support the use of alternate scheduling systems. It is hoped that in the future research will provide more definitive answers about the effects of the various scheduling systems to provide more definitive answers, which will aid speech-language pathologists in the creative design of appropriate scheduling systems that will lead to the implementation of quality speech-language programs.

SUMMARY

The Education for Handicapped Children Act of 1975, P.L. 94-142, has given the speech-language pathologist an important role in the assurance of quality educational services to the communication handicapped. The manner in which the speech-language pathologist manages the time available is referred to as program scheduling. Program scheduling involves the effective and efficient management of time throughout the school year, during the school week, and within each school day, with the goal of appropriate service delivery to each communication handicapped child.

Comparisons are often made of the scheduling systems that are considered basic. The actual functioning of these systems can be classified by the number of consecutive weeks a particular school is served during the school year, the number of days per week a particular school is served during the week, and scheduling within each school day.

In designing the scheduling system to be used, the speech-language pathologist must consider the administrative and clinical factors that influence the effectiveness of the program. None of these factors deserves more importance than the need to provide appropriate service to the communication handicapped based on individual need. To meet the demand of appropriate individualized education there can be no single appropriate scheduling system. Any system that is designed must be *flexible* to meet the needs of each child. The flexibility must extend to various scheduling models within each day, during the week, and throughout the year. At any given time within any speech-language program, any and all of the basic systems or combinations of those systems could be functioning. Realistically, the system that is finally adopted should be administratively manageable, while meeting the diverse clinical needs of the communication handicapped in the schools.

STUDY ACTIVITIES

1. Rank the factors pertaining to scheduling the week in the order of importance you feel appropriate.
2. Are there factors included that you consider to be unworthy of inclusion in this list? Why? Are there factors omitted that should have been included? Why?
3. Do other professions have to contend with some of the restrictions in planning that the speech-language-learning profession does? If you can think of similar problems, discuss them.
4. How can the speech-language-hearing profession as it functions in the schools have more freedom to plan and execute programs in the way it considers most efficient and effective? What barriers do you see to this?
5. Is there any justification for operating programs to please school administrators, boards of education, and state department personnel?
6. Under each of the systems presented, add to the list of advantages and disadvantages.
7. Plan several additional programs. Schedule four schools using eight-week periods. Schedule three schools and a junior-senior high school using a combined method and five-week periods. Schedule five elementary schools with the following enrollments and approximately equal prevalence of speech problems: 1200, 250, 500, 300, 300.
8. What criticisms can you see in the studies on scheduling?
9. Set up a research study on scheduling that would add to our knowledge of the relative effectiveness with functional articulation problems and problems related to organic factors.
10. Give advantages and disadvantages of office or coordinating time always falling on the same half day, of this time being distributed throughout the week. How important do you consider this time to be? Why?

REFERENCES

ASHA Task Force Report on Traditional Scheduling Procedures in the School. *Language, Speech and Hearing Services in Schools, 4,* 100–109, 1973.

Ausenheimer, B. and Irwin, R. B. Effect of Frequency in Speech Therapy on Several Measures of Articulation Proficiency. *Language, Speech and Hearing Services in the Schools, 2,* 43–51, 1971.

Backus, O. and Dunn, M. M. Intensive Group Therapy in Speech Rehabilitation. *Journal of Speech and Hearing Disorders, 12,* 36–60, 1947.

Beasley, J. Group Therapy in the Field of Speech Correction. *Journal of Exceptional Children, 27,* 102–107, 1950.

Beitzel, B. East Cleveland Study. In *Experimental Programs for Intensive Cycle Scheduling of Speech and Hearing Therapy Classes.* Columbus, Ohio: Ohio Department of Education, 1966.

Bingham, D. J. *Program Organization in Public School Speech Therapy.* Des Moines, Iowa: Department of Public Instruction, State of Iowa, 1962.

Bingham, D. S. et al. Public School Speech and Hearing Services. In Program Organization and Management. *Journal of Speech and Hearing Disorders (Monogr Suppl 8),* 1961.

Blanchard, M. and Nober, E. H. The Impact of State and Federal Legislation On Public School Speech, Language and Hearing Clinicians. *Language, Speech and Hearing Services in Schools, 9(2),* 77–84, 1978.

Carter, E. T. and Buck, M. W. Prognostic Testing for Functional Articulation Disorders among Children in the First Grade. *Jounral of Speech and Hearing Disorders, 32,* 124–133, 1958.

DesRoches, C. P. Speech Therapy Services in a Large School System: A Six Year Overview. *Language, Speech and Hearing Services in Schools, 7(4),* 207–219, 1976.

Darley, F. (Ed.). Public School Speech and Hearing Services. *Journal of Speech and Hearing Disorders (Monograph Supplement),* 1961.

Dublinske, S. and Healey, W. C. P. L. 94-142 Questions and Answers for Speech Language Pathologists and Audiologist. *Asha, 20,* 188–205, 1978.

Dublinske, S. Advocacy Role for the School Services Program. *Language Speech and Hearing Services in Schools, 11(3),* 131–132, 1980.

Ervin, J. E. A Study of the Effectiveness of Block Scheduling Versus Cycle Scheduling for Articulation Therapy for Grades Two and Three in the Public Schools. *Journal of the Speech and Hearing Association of Virginia, 6(2),* 1965.

Federal Register. Education of Handicapped Children, *42(163),* August 23, 1977.

Fellows, J. B. The Speech Pathologist in the High School Setting. *Language, Speech and Hearing Services in Schools, 7,* 61–63, 1976.

Garrard, K. The Changing Role of Speech and Hearing Professionals in Public Education. *Asha, 21(2),* 91–98, 1979.

Healey, W. C. and Dublinske, S. Notes from the School Services Program: Waiting Lists No Longer Appropriate. *Language, Speech and Hearing Services in Schools, 9(4),* 203, 1978.

Healey, W. C. and Jones S. *Essentials of Program Planning, Development, Management and Evaluation: A Manual for School Speech and Hearing and Language Programs.* Washington, D.C.: American Speech and Hearing Association, 1973.

Holderman, B. East Cleveland Study. In *Experimental Programs for Intensive Cycle Scheduling of Speech and Hearing Therapy Classes.* Columbus, Ohio: Ohio Department of Education, 1966.

Irwin, R. B. *Speech and Hearing Therapy.* Englewood Cliffs: Prentice-Hall, 1953.

Irwin, R. B. Crawford County Study. In *Experimental Programs for Intensive Cycle Scheduling of Speech and Hearing Therapy Classes.* Columbus, Ohio: Ohio Department of Education, 1966.

Jones, S. and Healey, W. C. *Project Upgrade: Model Regulations for School Language, Speech and Hearing Programs and Services — Phase I, Recommendations for State Departments of Education in Implementing Comprehensive Regulations for Language Speech and Hearing Services in Schools.* Washington D.C.: American Speech and Hearing Association, 1973.

Knight, H., Hahn, E., et al. The Public School Clinician: Professional Definition and Relationships in Public School Speech and Hearing Services. *Journal of Speech and Hearing Disorders (Monogr Suppl 8),* 1961.

Lauder, C. Speech and Hearing Services in Schools: Organization and Administration of Programs. Paper presented to Council for Exceptional Children Convention. Toronto: Ontario, 1964.

MacDonald E. T. *Articulation Testing and Treatment A Sensory Motor Approach.* Pittsburgh: Stanwix House, 1964.

MacDonald E. T. and Frick. Some Factors which Influence the Frequency and Duration of Treatment Sessions. *Journal of Speech and Hearing Disorders, 22,* 724–728, 1957.

MacLearie E. C. and Gross, F. *Experimental Programs in Intensive Cycle Scheduling of Speech and Hearing Classes.* Columbus, Ohio: Ohio Department of Education, 1966.

Mowrer, D. O. Accountability and Speech Therapy in the Public Schools. *Asha, 14(3),* 111–115, 1972.

Mowrer, D. O. *An Experimental Analysis of Variables Controlling Lisping Responses of Children.* Doctoral Dissertation, Arizona State University, 1964.

Mowrer, D. O. *Methods of Modifying Speech Behavior.* Columbus, Ohio: Merrill, 1977.

Neal, W. R. Speech Pathology Services in Secondary Schools. *Language, Speech and Hearing Services in Schools, 7(1),* 6–16, 1976.

Norris, D. The Cleveland Study. In *Experimental Programs for Intensive Cycle Scheduling of Speech and Hearing Therapy Classes.* Columbus, Ohio: Ohio Department of Education, 1966.

O'Toole, T. J. and Zaslow, El. Public School Speech and Hearing Programs: Things are Changing. *Asha, 11,* 499–501, 1969.

Pfeifer, R. C. *An Experimental Analysis of Individual and Group Speech Therapy with Educable Institutionalized Mentally Retarded Children.* Ed.D. Dissertation, Boston University, 1958.

P.L. 93-380 *Education Amendmendments of 1974 of the Rehabilitation Act of 1973.*
P.L. 94-142 *Education For All Handicapped Children Act, Nov., 1975.*
P.L. 95-661 Title II of Elementary and Secondary Education Act of 1978, Nov., 1978.
Regulations of the Commissioner of Education Part 200 Handicapped Children. Albany, New York: The State Education Department, 1980.
Sokoloff, M. A. *A comparison of Gains in Communication Skills Resulting from Group Play Therapy and Individual Speech Therapy Among A Group of Non-Severely Dysarthic Speech Handicapped Cerebral Palsied Children.* Ph.D. Dissertation, New York, 1959.
Sommers, R. K. et al. Effects of Maternal Attitudes upon Improvements in Articulation When Mothers are Trained to Assist in Speech Correction. *Journal of Speech and Hearing Disorders,* 29, 126–133, 1964.
Sommers, R. K. et al. Factors in the Effectiveness of Group and Individuals Articulation Therapy. *Journal of Speech and Hearing Research,* 9, 144–152, 1966.
Sommers, R. K. et al. Factors Related to the Effectiveness of Articulation Therapy for Kindergarten, First and Second Grade Children, *Journal of Speech and Hearing Research,* 10, 428–437, 1967.
Sommers, R. K. et al. Factors in the Effectiveness of Articulation Therapy with Educable Retarded Children. *Journal of Speech and Hearing Research,* 13, 304–316, 1970.
VanHattum, R. J. Evaluating Elementary School Speech Therapy. *Exceptional Children,* 25, 411–415, 1959.
VanHattum, R. J. Program Scheduling. In R. J. VanHattum, *Clinical Speech in the Schools,* Springfield: Thomas, 1969.
Weaver, J. B. and Wollersheim J. P. *A Pilot Study Comparing the Block System and the Intermittent System of Scheduling Speech Correction Cases in the Public Schools.* Champaign, Illinois: Champaign Community Unit Schools, 1963.
Weidner, W. Brecksville Study. In *Experimental Programs for Intensive Cycle Scheduling in Speech and Hearing Therapy Classes.* Columbus, Ohio: Ohio Department of Education, 1966.
Weston, A. J. and Harber, S. K. The Effects of Scheduling on Programs in Paired Stimuli Articulation Therapy. *Language Speech and Hearing Services in Schools,* 6(2), 96–101, 1975.
Wilson, F. Efficacy of Speech Therapy with Educable Mentally Retarded Children. *Journal of Speech and Hearing Research,* 9, 423–433, 1966.
Work, R. et al. *Designing Facilities for Language Speech and Hearing Programs in Florida Public Schools.* Tallahassee, Florida: Florida State Department of Education for Exceptional Children Section, 1973.

Chapter 10

THE THERAPY PROGRAM

RHONDA S. WORK

In a world of almost constant communication, the importance of language is increasingly being recognized. Language has always played an important role, not only in learning, but in all aspects of school programs. With an increase in the quantity and quality of programs for the communication handicapped, an emphasis on language has emerged. The once prevalent case load of articulation problems has gradually diminished as the emphasis has shifted to language disorders. As case loads have decreased, the number of students with severe communication disorders being seen for therapy has increased. Federal and state legislation have created an expanded role for the school speech-language pathologist. Professionally, we are entering a new decade as speech-language pathologists providing remediation for a wide variety of disorders of language, fluency, voice, and articulation.

The discussion in this chapter is intended to explore the scope of the therapy program. It is not intended to be a discussion of specific therapy procedures. Instead, it will center on selected aspects of the program that, when taken as a whole, can increase success. Each aspect or component is a part of the whole—an integral part that cannot stand alone but must become interlocked with all the others for the delivery of appropriate and productive services.

GENERAL CONSIDERATIONS

The need to develop a therapy program for the provision of comprehensive services to the speech-language handicapped has been enhanced by mandates to serve exceptional students and from demands for accountability in program development, management, and evaluation. The term "therapy program" may be defined in two ways: (1) as the overall program, which encompasses services to all communication handicapped students or (2) as the individual program, which is designed for a single student. Whether we are referring to a total program or an individual program, there are some general considerations that form the foundation for the program. These considerations include the evolution of a program philosophy, an understanding of the educational impact of speech-language disorders on learning, the need for an interdisciplinary approach to the identification and remediation processes, and the development of a conceptual framework.

Program Philosophy

An indispensible requirement of any therapy program is the establishment of a basic philosophy for the development and implementation of the communication disorders program. Although speech-language pathologists may have varied approaches to the remediation process and may differ in the techniques employed, a basic philosophy would be one that reflects the central role of communication in the educational, social, and emotional life of the child. The development of a philosophy should be based on goals and objectives that are designed to meet the varying communication needs and skills of the individual. It should insure that the needs of each child remain central to the provision of services. The State of Florida has adopted in its document describing services to speech-language impaired students the following philosophy: "Adequate communication skills are essential to academic, social and economic success; therefore, every student manifesting a communication disorder shall have the right to appropriate services from the language and speech program. These services shall be designed to improve communication skills to a level commensurate with physical and mental ability" (1979, p. 25). Once a philosophy is adopted it is paramount that the speech-language pathologist make known this philosophy along with program goals and objectives to school administrators, teachers, parents, and other professional personnel within the community.

Educational Impact

The impact of communication, in particular language, on the learning process has been well documented. The expanding body of literature in language, information processing, and reading has provided knowledge of the fundamentals of learning and communication. Lieberman et al. (1977) have noted the effect of research in speech perception and reading problems; Sanders (1977) has demonstrated the influence of language on both auditory and visual perception; and Rees (1974) has indicated that word decoding interacts with the reading comprehension process, in part as a result of the interpretation of spoken utterances as strings of phonemes or as the process of linguistic decoding (phonological analysis).

That language development can serve as a measure of children's potential for academic success was reported by Hutchinson et al. (1976) in a study related to the development of The Florida Language Screening System (FLASC). The FLASC was designed to meet the need for a standardized language screening instrument for kindergarten and first grade students. Comparisons between the FLASC and the Metropolitan Readiness Test (MRT) in the areas of reading, writing, mathematics, and speech were conducted. The MRT, a test designed specifically to assess a child's potential in school, predicted overall progress and progress in the four specific areas only slightly better than the FLASC, a test designed to measure language difficulties. Thus, the concept of the interrelationship of communication and learning is necessary to an understanding of the impact of communication disorders on the educational process.

Interdisciplinary Approach

The development of a basic philosophy for the speech-language program and the understanding of the educational impact of a communication disorder serve well as a basis for the implementation of a therapy program. With the advent of P.L. 94-142, the speech-language pathologist has become less of a separatist and more of a participant in providing services in the schools. Ainsworth (1965) discussed these two roles and defined the separatist as an "independent professional who is responsible for diagnosing and treating the speech disorders of children. This point of view assumes that the responsibilities of the specialists are fulfilled when he successfully carries out the clinical activity for which he has been trained." He defined the participant role as one that "conceives of additional responsibilities which can be summarized by saying that the speech specialist is obligated to make a direct contribution to, and thus be an integral part of, the on-going educational program" (p. 495). Thus, the speech-language pathologist has the responsibility to become an active partner with other school personnel in the total education of the student.

As services to exceptional students have expanded, the need for professionals to work together has become apparent. The concept of the interdisciplinary team has become a reality. It is within the framework of these teams comprised of individuals such as the school administrator, teachers, speech-language pathologist, audiologist, guidance counselor, psychologist, and social worker that planning for optimal learning may occur. Interdisciplinary teams offer the opportunity for each professional to communicate the perceived needs of the student and to plan the management of the student's program. These teams also offer the opportunity for the individual members to learn about the contributions of the various disciplines. As a member of the team, the speech-language pathologist has an extraordinary opportunity to impart significant information regarding communication disorders, the impact of language on learning, and the appropriateness of the therapy program. McBride and Levy (1979) imply that the success of the team will be the result of formal and informal interaction among group members while determining the interrelationship of the student's language, thought, academic skills, motor skills, and social-emotional behavior. By pooling the resources of many specialists the potential is there for meeting the needs of the individual student more quickly, thoroughly, and successfully.

Conceptual Framework

The nature of the therapy program will be dependent on the identified needs of the child, the conceptual framework within which the speech-language pathologist works, and most important, the motivation of the individual. The development of a conceptual model based on rationales for evaluation and instruction is essential to the development of a total communication disorders program. This basic premise must be recognized by the speech-language pathologist as a foundation for the initiation of services. As stated earlier, SLPs may vary in their approach to therapy, but the need for a conceptual model as well as a basic philosophy is a requirement for successful programming. Simon (1979) describes the model as "a dynamic model—one that is continuously being refined by new clinical insights and research findings. It should never be a static, blindly accepted model proposed by a test, a program or another professional" (p. 111). For the model to be effective, it will need to reflect all aspects of the communication process, i.e. reception, cognition, and expression. It will need to take into account competence in the phonologic, morphologic, semantic, syntactic, and pragmatic aspects of the communication process. Finally, not to be ignored are the aspects of articulation, fluency, and voice. Without a comprehensive model coupled with a basic philosophy, the speech-language pathologist will struggle in a quagmire of uncertainty and will find the therapy program to be inefficient, ineffective, and uninspiring for both herself and the student.

POPULATION TO BE SERVED

The traditional model used to describe the population of clients to be served in the schools is found in the P.L. 94-142 definition of speech impaired: "... means a communication disorder, such as stuttering, impaired articulation, a language impairment, or a voice impairment..." (1977, pp. 4278–4279). More recently, populations are being described by student category as well as by type of communication disorder. As a result, therapy programs are expanding beyond the room where the speech-language pathologist conducts small group instruction and are moving into the classroom and even the home. The development and implementation of the therapy program become a major chess game that requires innovative moves and expert manipulation. The ability to maintain a traditional program while at the same time incorporating elements of newer philosophies and approaches requires skill on the part of the speech-language pathologist and understanding on the part of school personnel.

The Traditional Population

Communication disorders have most frequently been divided into two basic categories: speech and language. Speech disorders have commonly included articulation, fluency, and voice, while language disorders have included phonology, morphology, syntax, semantics, pragmatics, and prosody. Implementing therapy programs based on these classifications has led to the establishment of the well-known model of three to four students every half hour for twice a week therapy. Clients with similar problems or from the same classroom are frequently placed in the same group. Group and individual therapy are planned according to the type and severity of the problem with voice and stuttering clients often seen individually and articulation and language students seen in groups.

In the past, children with articulation disorders received primary attention with consideration also given to fluency, voice, and some language disorders. More recently there has been a tremendous increase in recognition of and concern for the language handicapped. Parallel to this recognition has been an intensification of diagnostic and programmatic activities for the language impaired. This shift in emphasis has ignited an evolution in scheduling. As a more diverse population of students with communication disorders has entered the schools, the traditional model has been altered to include elements representative of more frequent service to more severe populations and service to differentiated populations.

The Preschool Population

The preschool years have been viewed as "years of great significance in the life of a child for a great many reasons. No aspect of development during these years is more important for his future life than his language development. It colors the attitudes, the potentials for learning, and the acquisition of foundational equipment not only for these years but in a measure for the rest of the individual's life" (Strickland, 1951, p. 68). That the first five years of the child's life are considered to encompass the optimal period for language growth is evident. Early development is considered to be important to later progress; thus, by identifying deficits in children at as young an age as possible, programs can be designed to prevent or reduce the impact of a potential learning problem. More specifically, recent studies have identified disorders of language as major components of later reading disabilities in children (Hall and Tomblin, 1978; Garvey and Gordon, 1973; Strominger and Bashir, 1977). Each of these studies has supported the assumption that the preschool language impaired child will most likely demonstrate problems in reading and writing. The establishment of therapy programs during critical development periods of the preschool child becomes not only an ideal, but a mandate—a commitment to children. It would appear, then, that early identification, intervention, and remediation may prevent later academic failure or an accumulation of problems into a multiple disability.

In many areas the role of the speech-language pathologist has expanded to include services to the preschool population. The therapy program may include direct intervention or indirect programming depending on the needs of the population and the resources available to the school system or the speech-language pathologist. The range of services within the therapy program might include (1) consultation to the classroom teacher of the preschool handicapped regarding normal and abnormal speech and language development, (2) presentation of lessons to the classroom for general speech stimulation and language development, (3) scheduling of therapy sessions for selected children identified as having communication disorders, (4) full-time preschool programs designed specifically for the speech-language impaired and/or (5) provision of service to parents, in the home or in a preschool center, regarding the development of appropriate communication behavior and skills.

The Regular Education Population

As speech-language pathologists have become more involved with the moderately to severely communication handicapped student, alternatives for services to the more mildly handicapped have been implemented. Less frequent and shorter therapy sessions may be scheduled. The extension of training from the therapy room to the classroom through the use of aides, other paraprofessionals, and volunteers is becoming more popular. Some aides are used with taped programs or other programs such as described in Chapter 1. In addition, there is a great deal that can be done in the regular classroom and with its curriculum to provide experiences for strengthening language and speech skills. The classroom teacher has daily opportunities to incorporate oral language activities into subject matter. The interrelationships among the language areas of listening, speaking, reading, and writing are varied and highly intricate. The teacher who is sensitive to these interrelationships can create an atmosphere for learning that includes many opportunities for listening and speaking as well as for vocabulary building and grammatic usage.

The educational system is becoming more aware of the premise that language is the primary means through which the curriculum is presented. The speech-language pathologist has the opportunity to provide consultant services to the regular classroom by observing the curriculum and classroom activities in an effort to assist in matching teacher and learner style. The speech-language pathologist may do some demonstration teaching, may provide technical assistance in the use of a language-based curriculum, and may offer suggestions for materials and other support services. The opportunities for expanded services to the classroom are there and merely require ingenuity, understanding, and receptivity on the part of all involved professionals.

The Severely and Profoundly Handicapped Population

Within more recent years, school districts have become responsible for the provision of services to the severely and profoundly handicapped individual. It is acknowledged that this individual has the right to be able to relate, to the extent possible, to the environment. This ability to relate is dependent upon the development of cognition, which is considered by many to be the precursor of language and communication. In this context, communication is defined in its broadest sense as the sending and receiving of a message between two persons. It is the transmission of ideas and thoughts through verbal and nonverbal means, for example, talking, winking, pointing, crying, waving, or smiling. Language, in a more limited sense, is a system within the bounds of communication that includes the transmission of gestural, oral, and written language. As a communication specialist, the speech-language pathologist has become more involved with programs for the profoundly handicapped.

Services to this population may be offered on a continuum of services from consultative based to a direct therapy model. The child's overall functioning level and potential for change must be taken into consideration when designing a therapy program with the professional judgment of the multidisciplinary team serving as the final determiner of the amount and type of service to be offered.

The scope of services offered by the speech-language pathologist might extend from evaluation of each client's cognitive, receptive, and expressive language skills to individual or group therapy based on intermittent or intensive cycling. Other responsibilities might include the development of instructional objectives to be incorporated in the educational plan implemented by the classroom teacher, recommendation of methods and materials to be used by the teachers and aides in achieving the objectives, and the reevaluation of each client's progress with the adjustment of objectives, as appropriate, on a regular basis. Certainly the speech-language pathologist has the obligation to provide or assist in the provision of teacher training and parent education. Finally, ongoing consultation regarding the language development process in the classroom is a role appropriate to the speech-language pathologist.

The Bilingual Population

The individual with a non-English native language, upon entering a classroom where English is spoken exclusively, faces the unseen burden of having to understand and cope with new concepts as well as a new language. This individual functions cognitively in his native language and must continually translate his second language (English) into his first (native) language so as to understand. The second language has not been learned sufficiently well to permit the use of two automatic, independent language systems.

To consider these children speech-language disordered would be improper. Their difficulty with English is not due to a language disorder but to a language difference. Differences may be found in the linguistic structure, the phonological system, and the inflectional use of voice. Differences also exist in the cultural background at verbal and nonverbal levels. During the influx of Vietnamese refugees to the United States in the 1970s, personnel in school systems suddenly became aware of the lack of knowledge or experience many of them had with far Eastern culture. The common activity of many speech-language pathologists of administering hearing tests became a perplexing situation until it was learned that the touching of the head by an unfamiliar or unknown individual is culturally prohibited in Vietnam. It is apparent that any instructional program for non–English-speaking students must take into consideration the linguistic and cultural differences of these individuals.

Speech-language pathologists are in a position to provide consultative services and in-service training to teachers working with those students who are acquiring basic communication skills. Before considering a student for enrollment in the program, the speech-language pathologist must determine if the basic language deficit is in the native language. The evaluation of language skills and the development of an appropriate therapy plan may prove difficult, but the assistance of bilingual paraprofessionals could be most useful. As Glass (1979) has suggested, the speech-language pathologist should not enroll a student if it is determined that the second language is still in transition. "It is misleading and inappropriate to regard as 'pathological' a child whose second language is still in transition; it is also misleading to overlook the bilingual child who may be struggling to learn a second language when his knowledge of his native language is faulty or deviant" (Glass, 1979, p. 512). In other words, it is helpful for the speech-language pathologist to become familiar with the culture and the native language of the bilingual population, to seek assistance in assessing the language of the child if little is known of the native language, and to insure provision of services based on the identified needs of the child.

The Dialectally Different Population

Freeman (1977) has stated that "dialectal differences cannot be construed as speech or language disorders. They are deviations from Standard American English which are based on rules of the dialect, not on the speaker's ability to understand or speak." Thus, the speaker of a dialect cannot be considered as communication handicapped based on the dialect alone, rather he must demonstrate a deviation or disorder within the dialect form to be so classified. The speech-language pathologist may assist the teacher in understanding the differences between dialect and disorder and may offer suggestions for recognizing these differences. The speech-language pathologist will need to be familiar with major dialects in the community to provide such information and to be able to select the appropriate individuals for therapy. By becoming familiar with the rules of the dialect, the speech-language pathologist can evaluate the language of the population and insure that only those students with disorders within the dialect system are considered for therapy. A serious deviation in the language functioning within the dialect will most likely be reflected in the use of the standard language system.

The Hearing Impaired Population

In 1971 O'Neill reflected, "It appears to me to be quite obvious that speech pathology and audiology should indicate in the strongest way a major commitment to the areas of language and the hearing-impaired" (p. 51). In this discussion the hearing-impaired individual is defined as one whose hearing loss is developmentally and educationally handicapping, no matter what the degree of loss or the age of onset. The concern of the speech-language pathologist is developing proficiency of communication and purpose of communication. The hearing-impaired client needs training not only in speech-language, auditory training, and speech reading but also in understanding of self and relating to the total environment. Communication development must relate to the mechanics of communication — voice quality, rate, rhythm, fluency, articulation, and grammatical use; the content of communication—vocabulary, sentence structure and clarity of thinking; and applied skills in communication—in group discussion, conversation and impromptu speaking (Marge, 1964). The speech-language pathologist should provide appropriate services to the hearing impaired on a direct therapy basis and serve as a consultant to all individuals in the hearing impaired student's environment. Perhaps the most important role for the speech-language pathologist in the educational community aside from therapy is the provision of support for the classroom teacher. Many classroom teachers have had little, if any, experience with a hearing-impaired student so that the simple explanation of preferential seating opens new understanding for the teacher. As Northcott (1972) stated, "The challenge and the charge to the speech and hearing specialist is to assume a catalytic role in providing direct services for the hearing impaired child, the classroom teachers and resource specialists who support the child during the school day, and his parents" (p. 18).

Other Special Populations

Speech-language impairments are commonly associated with other handicapping conditions including cleft palate, cerebral palsy, mental retardation, emotionally disturbed, specific learning disabilities, and visually impaired. Even the gifted population includes individuals with communication problems. In each instance, special techniques for remediation may need to be incorporated with standard approaches to effect change in the communication process. As with any population, the role of the speech-language pathologist may include both direct and indirect services to the client, the teacher, and the parent. The determination of an appropriate communication program may be the primary responsibility of the speech-language pathologist, but cooperative team planning and management will be required to avoid fragmentation of services provided by all disciplines on behalf of the client. The integration and coordination of all services will have a potential impact on the child's ability to learn and to interact in his or her environment.

THE THERAPY PROCESS

Speech-language pathology as a profession in the schools must be based on at least two concepts, one faithful to the requirements of a sound process for therapy and the other that reflects an understanding of the ongoing educational program. The therapy program may be considered, in part, an element of the total instructional program, but, by its very nature, its uniqueness and individuality must be preserved. Interdisciplinary planning is essential to meeting the needs of the child, but the therapy process becomes the responsibility of the speech-language pathologist.

When developing the therapy process, the communication needs of the client serve as the pivotal point around which curricula and methodologies are selected. The curriculum is an organized design using time, material, and tasks. It is composed of all the experiences and activities in which children participate. The development of a curriculum for the communication handicapped should include experiential components that follow a natural sequence for optimum learning. The curriculum should be designed to provide for comprehensive assistance by the speech-language pathologist to the many and divergent populations requiring assistance in speech and language.

Methodologies are part of the curriculum and are defined as those selected approaches to therapy which provide a systematic plan for remediation based on the identified disorder. Methodologies should be based on professionally recognized approaches to therapy and should include a rationale for the use of the specific approach developed in accordance with the specific needs of the child as determined by the evaluation process.

Screening, Evaluation, and Therapy

The development of an appropriate and effective therapy program must, by necessity, be based on efficient identification and a thorough evaluation of the client's communication skills. Sommers and Hatton discuss case selection in Chapter 8. The process of diagnosis does not stop with the enrollment of the client in the therapy program. Assessment becomes an ongoing process that continually evaluates the child's progress, determines program success, and provides new goals and direction.

Screening is a process by which a rapid assessment is made of a given population to obtain those potential candidates who may fit a particular profile. The screening process is a rapid assessment that provides the professional staff with a cursory profile of the communication abilities of each student tested and that identifies the greatest possible number of students with significant deviations from the communication norms. Screening results are not to be used to place students in therapy. Rather, these results assist the speech-language pathologist in determining which students need additional diagnosis.

Evaluation of language, articulation, fluency, voice, hearing sensitivity and perception, and the peripheral speech mechanism is necessary to the determination of communication competence. In some instances, more emphasis may be placed on one area rather than the other depending on previous knowledge of the child's communication skills. A case history including medical, developmental, family, and social information is necessary for understanding the child's present behavior. Additional information such as physical examination results, academic history, psychological evaluation and educational assessment should be included in the gathering of data. The child's profile should include factors in the student's developmental history, home situation, and school environment that might relate to the communication disorder. A suggested form for recording appropriate history is included in Chapter 7. Once all the data are collected, integrated, and analyzed, the speech-language pathologist is prepared to develop and implement an appropriate therapy program.

Provision should be made for the use of specialized tests, materials, and equipment appropriate to the diagnostic process. When selecting evaluation instruments, consideration should be given to the sociocultural and linguistic home environment to avoid identifying a student as handicapped solely on the basis of dialect or native language performance.

Assessment should be designed to provide maximum information about the client's communication skills, and results should suggest directions for planning and implementing a therapy program. If results are reported by describing the significant behaviors observed, a sound therapy program can be designed. Whenever there is any doubt as to an area of communication competence, the speech-language specialist needs to initiate further diagnostic procedures or seek additional assistance or information from available resources prior to planning the therapy program.

The speech-language pathologist working in a school setting usually does not function as a member of a medical team. She must, however, establish a system of referral to medical agencies and medical personnel both within and outside a school system. It is imperative that medical opinion be sought prior to the inclusion of some children into the therapy program. The rather surprisingly high number of young children demonstrating vocal nodules (Anderson, 1965; Wilson, 1961) and other pathologies, for example, makes it mandatory that all children requiring voice therapy be examined by a physician before they are entered into therapy. The implications are obvious: misdirected therapy may aggravate some problems, and the speech-language pathologist could be found guilty of malpractice. Similarly, children having recently experienced surgery for cleft palate or those showing an active oral pathology of almost any type should not be enrolled into therapy without gaining medical permission. Three other types of conditions would appear to be important enough to warrant noninclusion until medical permission has been gained. One of these is active ear pathology, the second consists of cardiovascular conditions, and the third comprises active seizures or controlled seizures due to medication. In all instances, the problems and their implications are ongoing ones, and it behooves the speech-language pathologist to take the precaution of securing proper medical consultation in conjunction with therapy. Generally, any medical referral and clearance that are required should occur prior to the initiation of therapy.

Sequential Therapy

Another important consideration for the development of the therapy program is the building of sequential steps as a result of evaluating diagnostic information and records of individual student progress. Communication skills develop sequentially, and any therapy program that is to be successful must be based on decisions using the knowledge of sequential development. Dayan et al. (1977) support the concept of sequential learning by stating, "Communication develops in a pattern. This pattern is called a sequence. Most, but not all, children develop a sequence for developing language. Some will go much slower than others. Some will jump ahead quickly" (pp. 9–10).

The speech-language pathologist has the knowledge and training to determine the appropriate learning sequence when designing a therapy program for the communication handicapped. It is the responsibility of the speech-language pathologist to determine this sequence for each student in the therapy program and to continually monitor the appropriateness of the sequential steps. As progress is or is not made, a reevaluation of the program should be conducted to determine, in part, if the proper sequence is being used. This reevaluation should be on a regularly scheduled time basis which becomes another component of the sequential process.

Individualized Therapy

Consideration of sequential development is accompanied by the understanding and implementation of individualized programming. No two children are the same, and no two children learn in exactly the same manner. Although similarities may exist among children, individual differences will dictate the need for individualized programming. Decision making for specific remediation should evolve from the child's total communication needs. Guidelines for making decisions regarding individual programming have been suggested by Rieke et al. (1977) and include questions such as "What does the child need in order to communicate successfully in his environment?" "What skills is the child currently demonstrating?" and "How do you facilitate the child's use of the newly learned skill in his natural environment?" (p. 6). Decisions made as a result of this kind of inquiry will assist in the individualization of the therapy program.

The Disorders and Therapy

Earlier in this chapter, a description of the populations to be served included discussion about categorization by type of disorder. This represents not only a traditional model but also an extremely viable model. A therapy program organized around the disorders of language, articulation, fluency, and voice represents a logical approach to the remediation process. Of course this organization must take into account the bases of each disorder and the resultant strategies appropriate to the remediation of the disorder.

It also must be recognized that these disorders do not form discrete categories but can overlap and may even coexist at any given point in time. Thus, program planning may need to cut across categories to account for the total communication needs of the individual. Any discussion of the development of a therapy program by category must assume the possibility of integrating therapy methods when more than one disorder exists. The skill of the speech-language pathologist will be essential to the development of a program that must include strategies for remediation of multiple disorders.

Intervention strategies in the language area should be selected on the basis of the child's age, developmental and readiness levels, utility and usefulness of present language performance in communication, and a reasonable prognosis for improvement. Consideration should be given to the type and complexity of the language required in the classroom, and goals should be established that reflect language usage in the child's communication environment. Since language usage influences all aspects of communication as well as the individual's ability to interact as a social being, remediation of language disorders should occur in an environment that uses all resources, including multi-sensory programming, parent-teacher-client interaction, and team approaches in content areas.

Articulation disorders require the development of intervention strategies based on number, severity, and type of misarticulations, age, sex, and listener reaction. The use of newly found speech skills in contextual situations and spontaneous conversation is the ultimate goal of the therapy program. Perhaps the most important aspect of this program is carry-over programming to develop speech skills to maximum usefulness in the shortest period of time. Some speech sound production may be the natural result of transitory misarticulations usually associated with maturational and learning periods. The speech-language pathologist needs to determine the appropriateness of therapy in these cases. It may be more appropriate to provide assistance to teachers and parents in the understanding of these maturational misarticulations rather than to provide therapy for the client. The speech-language pathologist may wish to develop strategies for use by parents and teachers that will reduce the impact of these misarticulations and help provide the child with experiences to promote speech development.

Therapy for fluency disorders should include consideration of the client's age, motivation, expectations for improvement, and self-perception of the problem as well as the severity of the problem. Effective clinical intervention may include procedures for a change in nonfluent behaviors and in attitudes. Counseling of students, parents, and teachers is an important component of the total program, and as noted in Chapter 2, the speech-language pathologist must recognize the need for appropriate counseling when the nature of the problem so indicates.

Approaches to voice therapy may take many directions depending on the type of disorder, organic, nonorganic, or whether related to pitch, quality, or intensity. Evaluation by a physician qualified to evaluate laryngeal structure and function is of utmost importance to determine presence or absence of pathology, and parents should be counseled as to the importance of this referral. Consideration needs to be given to the client's perception of the problem. Basic approaches to the remediation process should include teaching an understanding of the voice and its use, developing correct use of pitch, loudness, quality, and resonance. In some cases, referral for counseling may be appropriate before any improvement in voice quality can be realized.

PARAMETERS OF THE THERAPY PROGRAM

Sommers (1969) discussed the importance of the speech-language pathologist guiding the "therapy process." He stated, in part, that "this, then, implies that therapy, in a real sense, must extend beyond the four walls of the speech room" (p. 280). The process of planning a complete program of intervention must include interpretation of diagnostic data, case selection and scheduling, determination of therapeutic approaches, data recording, referral and consultation with other professionals and agencies, and parental involvement. The management of the therapy program requires techniques for effecting behavior change and the development of a program with appropriate content that will allow the client to develop communication competence to the limit of his or her potential. The capability of conducting the therapy program must include the use of appropriate strategies and techniques, the recording and analysis of communication behaviors, the implementation of generalization and transfer of newly learned skills, and periodic reevaluation of skills and of the therapeutic process. In planning for therapy, the speech-language pathologist must maintain flexibility so as to provide appropriate services for each client.

The Therapy Session

The speech-language pathologist must use ingenuity, must emphasize the importance of the services to be offered, and must exert leadership to provide these services despite the constraints of many variables such as those discussed in Chapters 8 and 9. In planning the therapy session, the speech-language pathologist must avoid the maintenance of a schedule that prevents responsiveness to special needs. Sessions need to be scheduled to accommodate the clinical requirements of the remediation process. The age of the client and the severity of the disorder certainly should have an effect on the frequency and duration of sessions. If the case load consists of a diversity of disorders, the sessions may vary according to the nature of the problem. Several sessions of intensive but relatively short periods of therapy per week may be successful in developing attending skills with the very young child while longer but fewer sessions per week may provide the necessary impetus for use of carry-over techniques in the older client.

One of the major decisions a speech-language pathologist must make when developing a therapy program is how many individual and how many group sessions should be scheduled. Part of this decision will be influenced by the many variables suggested earlier and by the case load size. A major factor may be the type of case load to be served and the severity of the problems within that case load. Previous studies of group versus individual therapy have been based on articulatory impaired children (Sommers 1964, 1966). Results suggested that group and individual therapy were equally effective. However, these results cannot be translated to therapy for more severe problems or even different problems. Until studies have been conducted in the area of language, voice, and fluency and based on several other parameters, we must make no assumptions as to the effectiveness of group or individual therapy in these areas.

When selecting children for group therapy, the speech-language pathologist needs to take into account the type of disorder each child exhibits and the point at which therapy should begin. The individualized therapy plan will provide the specialist with an understanding of the needs of the student and how that student will fit into a group situation. It must be understood that all children learn at different rates and have different learning styles, thus no amount of initial "matching" of disorders or needs will assure equal progress among all children. Frequently the speech-language pathologist finds that after several sessions, no two students are at the same point in therapy. The therapy sessions have to be molded to meet the needs of each student while planning for all the students in the group. This requires the ability to balance individual work with group activity throughout the therapy session.

Individual therapy provides the opportunity for intensive remediation, as the client is seen on a one-to-one basis. Frequently, students with more severe problems or with less common disorders are scheduled for individual therapy mainly because they do not fit into any group. Whether this is the reason or that the student would appear to benefit more readily from individual therapy, enrollment on an individual basis will provide more direct therapy. As the student progresses, the ongoing evaluation process may suggest that he is ready for group work. The speech-language pathologist has several options available, such as scheduling the child on a limited basis into an already established group, placing the child immediately into a group on a full-time basis, or establishing a completely new group by reshuffling part of the weekly schedule. It is the astute speech-language pathologist that can manage the case load efficiently and still provide appropriate therapy schedules for the students within the constraints of the everyday "school world."

Many school districts have incorporated the concept of the single school based speech-language pathologist. When assigned full-time to one school, the professional has an opportunity to develop therapy sessions on the same basis as a resource teacher. Sessions for severely impaired clients might occur five days a week for the major portion of the morning, and traditional sessions of one-half hour in length two to three times a week may be scheduled the remainder of the day for moderately handicapped persons. In some instances, the therapy program becomes a full-day special class with both communication and academic components incorporated in the curriculum. Cafaro (1973) expressed her bias for this approach by asserting that "... it is time for the clinician in the public school to assume the role of clinical teacher in a clinical classroom in order to meet the needs of the severely language handicapped more sufficiently" (p. 179). The implementation of this kind of program would transfer the therapy process from the itinerant setting to a classroom setting without diminishing provisions for the remediation of communication disorders from a classical point of view. In fact, the process should be enhanced due to the increase in contact time with each student.

Regarding the therapy process, Van Hattum (1964) maintains that each therapy session consists of five parts. The first of these deals with preplanning. This initial step includes a review of the child's past performances based on former techniques, goals to be attained next, and the activities used to incorporate the technique along with some idea concerning the success realized. The second step he labels preparation. As expected, this includes readying materials and equipment for the impending task. The third step consists of the therapy session, i.e. the face-to-face meeting between the children and the speech-language pathologist. Evaluation comprises the fourth step. During this time, the speech-language pathologist evaluates the relative success or failure of the planned activities and also the relative effectiveness of the materials and equipment that were used. The final step he terms "clean-up," which refers to the returning of appropriate materials, supplies, and equipment to their proper places and setting the room in order. It is his opinion that many speech-language pathologists (particularly beginning ones) focused on step three (the therapy session) to the exclusion of the four other aspects of therapy.

The therapy session, then, must be designed to provide an appropriate delivery system of remediation for all clients selected for therapy. It must be developed within the parameters of the school program and according to variables such as the client's age and motivation and the type and severity of the communication disorder. It must include a logical step-by-step procedure for an effective therapy process. It must not be arranged for convenience or ease of scheduling but rather for maximizing the potential of all students enrolled in the program.

The Individual Therapy Plan

Public Law 94-142 has mandated the development and use of an individualized education program for each handicapped child. This program may serve as the therapy plan or as a framework for the further development of an implementation plan. Whichever approach is adopted by the speech-language pathologist, the intent should be to provide a management tool for the remediation of the communication disorder.

Inherent in this plan is the assurance of a free, appropriate education based on long-range goals, short-term objectives, and evaluation procedures to determine the effectiveness of the program. Perhaps not as easily identifiable is the translation of these components into everyday lesson plans. If one looks, however, at the process as a hierarchy for planning, the transition from "program" to "lessons" is more readily perceived.

Goals encompass many specific objectives. The statement of goals for a client's program gives focus to learning activities, makes preparation more relevant, and facilitates communication with parents and other professionals about the student's needs. Short-term objectives reflect the intermediate steps between the present level of functioning and the anticipated goals. In discussing the provision of education programs for communication handicapped children, Falck (1978) noted that "educational objectives in the area of speech and language must specify type of intervention (individual, groups, or classroom techniques) as well as the target of intervention (the child, the parent, regular classroom teacher, and/or other personnel)" (p. 75). Stated another way, the speech-language pathologist must decide which goals are to be reached by the end of therapy and how these goals are to be reached. The "how" of reaching the goals becomes the selection of objectives that specify a terminal behavior, define the conditions under which the behavior is to occur, and describe the criteria for acceptable performance of the behavior. The inclusion of procedures, content, and methods that are relevant to the objectives further defines the process. As Mager (1962) has said, "When clearly defined goals are lacking, it is impossible to evaluate a course or program efficiently, and there is no sound basis for selecting appropriate materials, content, or instructional methods... A builder does not select his materials or specify a schedule for construction until he has his blueprints (objectives) before him" (p. 3).

The inclusion of the word "individualized" in describing requirements for educational programming under the provisions of P.L. 94-142 appears to have been highly intentional. Each child is to be provided with a plan tailored to her needs so that maximum progress can be anticipated. This philosophy is obviously based on the assumption that "individual differences are so strongly evident that it is inappropriate to expect that the same problems... exist for every individual in the same way within the group; or that intervention procedures should be standardized" (Muma, 1978, p.4). By observing and assessing the client's behavior, a starting point for therapy can be identified and the remediation program developed. Whether the communication deficit is in the area of language, articulation, fluency, or voice, the need to systematize therapy is crucial. Building sequential tasks, operationalizing these tasks, and analyzing the outcomes will provide a list of future tasks. Systematic observations and documentations will provide guidance for the therapy process. The use of checklists, clinical notes, daily logs, or behavioral charting devices has proven to be most successful for documenting progress, or the lack of progress.

Basic to the success of the individualized program is the selection of therapy techniques and methods. Written objectives may be pertinent, but without appropriate techniques, success of the program may be fleeting. The speech-language pathologist can insure success by establishing a rationale for the selection of techniques. Is the technique necessary? Will it accomplish what the SLP desires to be accomplished? Will it contribute to the total therapy plan? (Sommers, 1969). If these questions are applied to each stage in the development of the individual plan, a sequence of therapy will emerge leading to program goals.

An integral component of all individual planning is that which measures the effectiveness of objectives and goals along with the client's progress. Evaluation criteria should be directly related to the instructional objectives so that progress toward the objectives can be analyzed. Any changes in the program can be determined by the successful completion of objectives. Several forms of evaluation are available to the speech-language pathologist including observation, charting, criterion referenced assessment, or standardized tests. The choice of evaluation techniques will depend in part on the type of objective to be measured and the perceived progress of the client.

Therapy Techniques and Methods

As stated in the previous section, the selection of therapy techniques and methods is basic to the success of the individual child's program. The selection process is heavily dependent upon the experiences of the speech-language pathologist, an overview of the total therapy program, and the current status of the student in the therapy program. A rationale for the use of specific techniques and methods will evolve, and as the speech-language pathologist gains experience and constantly questions the need or appropriateness of a technique or a method, the outline for a therapy program for a typical type of problem will emerge. As a function of clinical training, experience, and some intuitive reasoning, the sequence of therapy steps will come into focus — the blueprint is drawn and a concept has emerged. Each of the techniques now relates to every other; the logic of the therapy regimen becomes clear, and the speech-language pathologist finds that he is better able to judge the worth of each technique and procedure in terms of the total therapy required for the problem at hand. When the concept has been developed, improvements in techniques and methods can be made.

The need for new techniques is obvious, for even the speech-language pathologist may tire of doing the same thing the same way. The lack of enthusiasm for the use of a technique or activity on the part of the speech-language pathologist is likely reflected in the children—who may find it easy to become bored on their own. Even an often used technique, however, may be vital in a total therapy program for a problem. Inherently, it may prove very effective and comprise a cornerstone in the overall program. How can the valuable ingredients of this technique be presented in a different and interesting manner? How many alternatives can be developed? Depending upon the uniqueness of the original technique the answer may be none, or one, or many. Fortunately, other techniques are usually available to offer suggestions about new ways of doing things.

The single best source for this information is a professional colleague. The probabilities of gaining a fresh idea concerning another way that this important technique or procedure can be presented are probably dependent upon either having another SLP observe the original technique being used or having a lucid description of it presented to him along with an account of why it is used, what is accomplishes, and a notion of the total therapy program for this type of problem. When speech-language pathologists are employed by one school agency, opportunities for interaction obviously increase, and both informal and formal training sessions can be devoted to the development of new techniques and procedures or in devising new ways to teach old techniques of importance. Under the conditions of being employed by different school districts, the speech-language pathologist must actively seek this type of assistance from nearby professional workers employed elsewhere. Usually the camaraderie of speech-language pathologists is such that ideas are exchanged socially. The supervisor of speech and language services may also be an important source for new techniques and procedures. This is particularly true if the supervisor is an experienced speech-language pathologist and has opportunities to observe the individual doing therapy. Ideas can be gleaned from professional publications such as speech-language pathology texts and from published and unpublished manuscripts, pamphlets, and term papers. Frequently, a survey of material of this type will uncover new ideas.

Other types of professional workers in school settings may stimulate new ideas. The experience of observing a regular or a special class teacher may suggest a way in which a commonly used teaching method may be amenable to change to make it effective with a particular type of communication disordered child. For example, the phonovisual method may be used to teach reading in a particular school system. The speech-language pathologist observing this teaching may feel that it could serve well, with some degree of modification, in teaching a brain-injured child speech and language. Similarly, the speech-language pathologist may be stimulated to develop additional techniques by observing a reading specialist work with selected children. Techniques of improving word attack skills or in reinforcing associations between letters and phonemes may suggest numerous ways of expanding technique for the enterprising individual. Perhaps techniques of teaching respiration to cerebral palsied children can be developed by observing the music teacher or methods of gaining better carryover of improved speech sounds can be developed by observing a physical education class. This broadening of horizons can frequently result in the development of unique and possibly very effective ways of doing therapy.

The Place of Materials and Equipment

Earlier Mager was quoted as saying, "A builder does not select his materials... until he has his blueprints..." (p. 3). A wise speech-language pathologist will select carefully the materials to be used based on the objectives chosen for the therapy program. Sometimes it is tempting to design objectives around the use of a new and exciting material, but quite obviously this may be a most inappropriate path to follow. This author was involved in a study designed to evaluate the effectiveness of the speech therapy program through an analysis of instructional materials use (Work et al., 1976). Several questions were postulated: How effective are materials? Are materials chosen according to the type of therapy planned? Are materials related to program objectives and goals? Project staff developed a procedure for evaluating materials used to provide speech-language pathology services to students with articulation problems. The study indicated that a system to evaluate the effectiveness of materials used in the clinical process could be implemented and further indicated that materials were chosen for use to meet the identified therapy objectives, rather than as the central aspect of the therapy program.

With an increase in the availability of commercially developed instructional materials, the speech-language pathologist has a major responsibility to determine the appropriateness of each new material for use in the program. Consideration must be given to the following: What is the purpose of the therapy objective? Will this material enhance the therapy process? Will it assist in the accomplishment of the objective, or will it become a game that detracts from the purpose of the therapy session? Is it durable? Is it attractive? Is it priced appropriately? Is it within budget allocations? There are many questions to be asked, all of which should lead to a final decision on use of the material. To assist in material evaluation, the speech-language pathologist may wish to seek and share experiences with co-workers. Many materials are displayed at state and national conventions, and the American Speech-Language-Hearing Association's monthly publication, *Asha*, includes a regular feature on book and material reviews.

The importance of materials and equipment to the therapy program cannot be denied. As suggested earlier, however, the materials should not become the central feature of the therapy session. Materials should be supplemental to the objectives and should provide a means by which the end may be accomplished. This applies especially to the use of games. For many years, students talked about going to speech to "play games." This image has changed over the years as the speech-language pathologist has become more involved with the severely handicapped and has shifted program emphasis to language and communication. There is a rightful place for gamelike activities but only as an integral part of the total therapy process. Many of the commercially produced speech-language materials today are designed as curriculum components rather than as "spinner games" or "dice games" and appropriately so. Therapy has become more of a curriculum-based activity similar to some classroom activities. This is obviously the result of a better understanding of the role of language in learning, which has led to an increase in the language therapy conducted by the speech-language pathologist.

Speech-language notebooks should be mentioned. For many years notebooks used by children in therapy have provided a great deal of support to the therapy program. They are usually made by the children themselves, who add practice material on a regular basis at the direction of the speech-language pathologist. The books can provide a vital information link between the speech therapy session, the teacher, and the parents. Also, hours of additional practice can be ensured with the use of an attractive, well-designed speech-language notebook. Children will take pride in their progress and accomplishment and will be eager to share their successes with their parents, sisters, and brothers. It is important to stress that these books can only be as successful as the material within them permits. The speech-language pathologist must be willing to take the time to find appropriate practice material for each student but must not become a slave to the process. Too often unnecessary time is spent during precious therapy time to hunt for material and to cut and paste it into the notebooks. Judicious use of the notebooks, as with any material, will prove a boon to the therapy program.

While materials are very essential, some cautions are in order. The first caution pertains to the competitive factor of material. One should be very careful whenever using highly competitive materials, since they may be distracting to therapy and may place the emphasis on competition itself. Competition may not be desirable for many children in the therapy program. If games are used as materials, they should be couched in terms of activities rather than talked about as games per se. Games must remain speech-language centered if the speech-language pathologist expects to accomplish speech-language centered goals.

Another caution is to avoid using the same materials over and over for the same children or for all children. The children and the SLP lose interest when the same materials are used repeatedly.

This is one reason why it is so important to develop a good variety of materials. Using the same materials session after session during the day regardless of the child's problem, purpose, goals, or stage of therapy is totally inappropriate. A wise speech-language pathologist will use a variety of materials every day. The last caution is to guard against using materials that are too time-consuming. A given activity or material probably should not take more than three-fourths of any therapy session. The remaining time can be used effectively to review and give assignments.

Any decision making regarding the use of materials will be dictated, in part, by monies available. School districts vary in their approach to budgeting. Some districts have a central budget system whereby all materials, equipment, and supplies are purchased for the program. Depending on the size of the program, each speech-language pathologist is assigned a designated amount of money to spend or is assigned specific materials to use throughout the year. In some instances, such as the use of large pieces of equipment or expensive materials, several speech-language pathologists are asked to share these items. In other school districts, the purchase of materials, equipment, and supplies may be the responsibility of each school, and the dollars made available will dictate the type and amount of material to be purchased by the individual speech-language pathologist. In other districts, the materials may be ordered districtwide and then prorated to the schools in proportion to the amount of time the speech-language pathologist is assigned to each school.

Upon employment in a school district, the speech-language pathologist needs to learn the budgeting system to determine the options available for purchasing basic therapy materials. It is not uncommon to find that many speech-language pathologists supplement the district purchased items with personally purchased items. Although not as common as perhaps a decade ago, speech-language pathologists do make their own materials. Perhaps this activity has become less frequent as the quality of commercially produced products has improved and as more products have become available.

Any attempt at listing specific materials, equipment, and supplies important to the therapy program would run the risk of omitting

Materials	Equipment	Supplies
Language Kits	Clock; stopwatch	
Programmed Therapy Kits	Automated teaching	Tongue depressors
Articulation Picture Cards	machines	Mimeograph masters &
Cubical Counting Blocks	Portable, high fidelity tape	paper
Workbooks	recorder	Scissors
Pre-recorded magnetic tapes	Portable pure tone screening	Paste, rulers
Pre-recorded cards & tapes	and threshold audiometer;	Cellophane & masking tape
Film strips	impedance audiometer	Newsprint
Flash cards	Mirror	Construction paper
Flannel board cutouts	Auditory training units &	Blank tape cassettes
Attendance register	headsets	Chalk, marking pencils,
Lottos & games	Pen flashlight	crayons
Pegboard picture cards	Pegboards	Pencils & erasers
Posters	Large, durable carrying case	Stapler & staples
Picture & story books	for materials	Paper clips, thumb tacks
	Chalkboards	Blank magnetic tape cards
	Pencil sharpener	Typing paper
	Minute Minders	File folders
	Flannel board	Index cards
	Wastebasket	Rubber bands
	Access to:	Sentence strips
	Film, filmstrip and slide	Bond paper
	projector	Letter envelopes
	Paper cutter	
	Overhead projector	
	Record player	
	Typewriter	
	Mimeograph machine	
	Telephone	

Figure 10-1. Suggested materials, equipment, and supplies.

some items. Perhaps a prudent approach would be to list items by general categories with the understanding that omission of any item is unintentional. Figure 10–1 serves as a guide, and each individual must complete his or her list based on the demands of the communication disorders program and the available resources.

A discussion of materials should not be limited to client-use materials. Equally as important is the need for the speech-language pathologist to maintain currency within the profession. This can be accomplished in a large part by establishing and maintaining a professional library and by attending local, state and national meetings where continuing education opportunities abound. Fisher

(1969) discussed the importance of a professional library and suggested that the mere possession of such a library was only half the story; the other half, of course, would be the regular *use* of such a library, including both the ongoing purchase of professional books and journals and an ongoing reading program to assure the improvement of professional skills.

It is apparent that materials can be an important aspect of any therapy program. They can provide motivation for the client. They can reduce the amount of time involved in lesson planning. However, they must be chosen carefully and used judiciously to assure the most effective therapy results. The astute speech-language pathologist will combine professional knowledge, clinical skills, and the use of appropriate materials in the development of the communication disorders program.

Facilities

Providing adequate facilities so that each client with a communication disorder will have the opportunity to develop and grow in his use of speech and language is an essential aspect of the therapy program. Why is the therapy room so important? Speech-language pathologists who have worked in a variety of facilities for several years report that there is a definite relationship between the quality of physical facilities and the results of therapy. Poor facilities tend to minimize motivation of both the child and the professional, whereas good facilities have a tendency to improve motivation. Poor facilities may create undesirable attitudes, be distracting to the children, and in some cases create fear within the children when they must work in small, dirty, cluttered, dark, and/or noisy cubbyholes. This is not to say that an effective speech-language pathologist cannot observe some very significant improvement in some of the children even in the poorest of facilities. Little can be done to change the size and the shape of the facilities, but a great deal can be done to improve the appearance, equipment, and furnishings. A learning environment that is roomy, clean, free of extraneous materials and noise, and is cheerfully decorated will provide an atmosphere for optimal learning.

As programs for the communication handicapped broaden, so will the need for varied facilities. Consider the following program formats that have an impact on facility design: self-contained classrooms for the severely language impaired; individual therapy for the profoundly handicapped child; provision of services in the everyday environment of the child; provision of services in special areas such as kiosks where students can practice their communication skills alone; provision of services to the secondary schools on a one period a day basis; and small group therapy for the mildly and moderately impaired. It is obvious that the instructional space for particular children with communication disorders will differ as the needs of the children differ. There is need for privacy, for small group activity centers, for adequate acoustical protection, for glare-proof and shadow-proof lighting, for ventilation and appropriate temperature control, and for adequate space for therapy and office needs.

For many years, the speech-language pathologist was relegated to the boiler room, the broom closet, the health clinic, or a corner of the library. Frequently the space was shared with the guidance counselor, reading specialist, physical education instructor, or the music teacher. Although these conditions still exist in some school districts, it is apparent that space allocation is improving steadily. Perhaps much of the improvement is due to the increased amount of time spent in each school for the therapy program. It was difficult to command adequate space when services were offered on a once a week basis. With more and more schools receiving full-time or nearly full-time services, the availability of adequate space becomes a foregone conclusion. A second factor that has had an impact upon improved facilities is that schools built within the last ten to fifteen years have been built with specific facilities provisions for programs such as communication disorders, guidance, reading, and other special services. Speech-language pathologists have had the opportunity to provide information regarding the minimal requirements for space allocation. The idea that the speech-language pathologist can work in any area, however inadequate it may be, is being rejected by educators and speech-language pathologists with more frequency. Thus, there is a much improved atmosphere for securing adequate facilities for speech-language therapy.

It should be noted, however, that the increase in availability of space has not always meant an improvement in conditions. It is extremely important that vigilance not be relaxed. The speech-language pathologist should take the initiative to secure the best available working area. This can be done by talking with the special education director, school administrators, and the board of education. These people need to be informed by the SLP and/or supervisor if physical facilities are unsatisfactory, as some of them may not be aware of the unsatisfactory working conditions. By attacking this problem tactfully and energetically, by talking with these individuals, and by preparing written reports and suggestions for improving the facilities, working conditions should improve. When new school buildings are being planned it is important to discuss physical facilities with the architect as well as with the board of education. It is the responsibility of every professional to assure that adequate facilities to meet the needs of the handicapped are available to every program.

The committee on Speech and Hearing Services in the Schools of the American Speech-Language-Hearing Association detailed its recommendations for housing as shown in Figure 10-2.

Parents

No single event has made as large an impact on parental involvement in speech-language programs as has P.L. 94-142. Prior to requirements for parental consent and parental participation in the development of individual education plans, parents of students receiving speech-language therapy knew little about the program or their child's participation in the program. That has changed dramatically. Now there is more opportunity for information exchange and parent counseling regarding speech-language development. Parents are becoming an important partner in their child's therapy program, providing reinforcement for newly learned skills. Since language and speech are an integral part of the child's total environment, the development of the parent component becomes an important aspect of the therapy program.

Webster (1977), in the preface to her text on parent counseling, commented that "Each parent of a handicapped child is different, as is each member of that family, and each situation with them" (p.xiii). It should follow, then, that the goals of parent involvement

Item	Minimal	Acceptable	Ideal
		ROOM	
Location	Near elementary classrooms and relatively quiet	Near lower elementary classrooms and relatively quiet	Near lower elementary classrooms and relatively quiet. Near administration unit with accessibility to waiting area, secretarial services, and other special service personnel
Size	150 sq ft	200 sq ft multipurpose room	250 sq ft to be used exclusively for speech and hearing services
Number	One	One	One room and adjoining office
Lighting			
Artificial	50 foot candles	50 foot candles	60–75 foot candles, indirect, plus floor lamp
Natural	One window	One window with shade	Two windows with blinds and draperies
Heating	Adequate central heating or space heater	Adequate central heating	Central heating with thermostat which can be controlled by clinician
Ventilation	One window which can be opened	One window which can be opened	One window which can be opened or air conditioning
Acoustical Treatment	None	Acoustical treatment of ceiling	Acoustical treatment of ceiling, door and walls, draperies, carpeted floor
Electrical power supply	One 110 V double plug	Two 110 V double plus conveniently located	Three 110 V double plugs conveniently located. Dimming mechanism to facilitate use of audiovisual equipment
Intercom	None	None	One listen/talk unit, connected to administrative offices
Rest room facilities	Available	Available	Adjoining rest room(s) facilities —for exclusive use of speech and hearing room only
Chalkboard	One 3' × 3' mounted or portable	One 3' × 5' mounted or portable	One 3' × 5' mounted on wall at appropriate height for children
Bulletin Board	None	One 4' × 4' mounted on wall	One 4' × 6' mounted on wall

Figure 10-2. Recommendation for facilities (ASHA, 1967).

Mirror(s)	Small hand mirrors	Small hand mirrors plus one 2' × 4' mounted on wall at appropriate height for children	Small hand mirrors plus one 3' × 5' which can be covered mounted on wall at appropriate height for children
Observation facilities	None	None	One-way-vision window 3' × 5' with listening facilities

FURNITURE

Desk	None	One small office desk	Two four-drawer office desks (one for room and one for office)
Chairs			
Adult	One chair	Three chairs, one office chair, two folding chairs	Two office chairs, two lounge chairs
Children	Six chairs that can accommodate both lower and upper elementary children	Six chairs that can accommodate both lower and upper elementary children	Five chairs appropriate for lower elementary children and five chairs appropriate for older children
Table	One approximately 32" × 4810%%, 24–30" high	One approximately 32" × 48", 24–30" high	One table appropriate size and height to accommodate younger and one appropriate size and and height for older children

STORAGE FACILITIES

Storage space	Two shelves	Small locked cabinet	Large locked cabinet, preferably in a small storage closet adjoining therapy room
File cabinet	None	Two drawer file cabinet with lock	Four drawer file cabinet with lock
Bookcase	None	Wall mounted or stand. Approximately 4' linear space	Wall mounted or stand. Approximately 8' linear space

Figure 10-2. *Continued*

will be almost as varied as the number of parents participating in the program. Some parents will need to be involved because they need to learn new ways to interact with their child. Some parents will need to learn how to foster their child's social and emotional development. Other parents may need the emotional support derived from the professional or other parents of communication handicapped children. Whatever the reason, the parents' needs will vary, and the speech-language pathologist must be alert to this.

The success of parental involvement is contingent upon a number of factors. The attitude of the professional must be a positive one which connotes that parents have a contribution to make. The speech-language pathologist must recognize that there is more than one way to involve parents and that the parents must be assisted in selecting the best ways to be involved with their child's program. Parents must be made to feel that they are an important part of the therapy program and that avenues for positive communication are available to them. The SLP must be able to communicate a feeling of acceptance and understanding while recognizing parental hostility, fear, indifference, or apathy. Parents often stand in awe of the school and the educational process or are ashamed of their child's handicap. By demonstrating understanding and acceptance, the speech-language pathologist breaks down these barriers and opens the door for parental involvement.

The extent to which parents should become involved is a decision to be made based on the individual needs of the child, the ability of the parents to participate, and the time available to the speech-language pathologist to monitor parents' activities with their child. Certainly minimum participation would be at the planning stage when the parents would be invited to assist in the development of the child's program. As the speech-language pathologist becomes better acquainted with the parents and observes the interaction of parent and child, certain judgments can be made regarding the type and amount of assistance the parent might provide in the therapy process. A cautionary note: premature parental involvement in the remediation process could lead to failure. There are certain aspects of any therapy program that must be conducted by the speech-language pathologist. Other aspects may become part of a home program, but only with carefully selected and monitored activities. However, to ignore the role of the parent because of concern about appropriateness and time constraints could very easily negate a potential factor that could lead to more rapid progress in the program.

Is it worthwhile for a speech-language pathologist to train parents to assist in the therapy program? When viewed in terms of articulation problems, research findings to date clearly say yes. This appears to be true for preschool articulatory defective children (Tufts and Holliday, 1959) and for school-age ones as well (Sommers et al., 1959; Sommers, 1962; Sommers et al., 1964). The evidence on school-age children was based upon three related experiments in which intensive training was provided to parents of children having articulatory problems during a period in which their children received daily speech therapy. In all three studies, the children whose mothers were trained to assist in correction made significantly greater improvements. The first study in this series demonstrated that this held more for certain types of speech errors than for others; the second study demonstrated that this was the case regardless of the intelligence of the children and generally irrespective of whether or not they received individual or group therapy; and findings from the third study revealed that this was true regardless of the attitudes of the mothers trained concerning child-rearing practices. Carpenter and Augustine (1973) conducted a training program for parents and concluded that "The use of trained parent-clinicians can ultimately provide a useful resource to aid the speech pathologist in modifying communicative behavior in some instances" (p. 54). In their study, four mothers of children with communication disorders were trained in specific techniques to effect change in certain aspects of language or prelinguistic behavior. All but one of the mothers were successful in using the program on a daily basis. Since children with language disorders seem to require frequent reinforcement and some degree of overlearning so as to improve, this study further supports the usefulness of parent training.

Although parents may prove of real value in the improvement of all types of speech-language disorders, training may take a different form depending on the disorder. It essentially has the same purposes, however, i.e. setting the stage for the extinction of poor language and speech habits, finding desirable ways of rewarding good speech performances, and generally seeking valuable ways of fostering good speaking situations. Because of the difficulties often inherent in improving language and speech, parents need understanding concerning the goals of therapy so that frustration and disappointments do not work adversely upon them or the child. However, the speech-language pathologist can select the most promising areas of endeavor and seek the parents' assistance. As in any phase of the therapy program, professional judgment will be the final determiner in the decision-making process.

Variables of Success

Any discussion of the therapy program requires an inspection of certain variables related to success. Frequently an understanding of these variables is based more on empiricism and experience rather than well-supported evidence or documented research. Intuition and common sense might suggest which factors and to what degree these factors may affect therapy outcome. The speech-language pathologist must consider carefully any factor that may enhance or impede progress and adjust the therapy program to accommodate the influence of the variable. In a manner of speaking, the SLP must become a detective always on the alert, always looking for clues, always putting the clues together to build a case for success. Variables that appear to influence therapy include motivation, carry-over, dismissal, and support services. By examining these particular variables and relating them to each student in the program, the speech-language pathologist should be able to maximize the likelihood of success.

Motivation

Although little is known about the effects of motivation upon the improvement of communication skills, it is assumed that both a general motivational factor and some specific motivational ones may be in operation. Occasionally poorly motivated children are discontinued in speech therapy by some speech-language pathologists who feel that their time is better spent with children who desire to improve and will make sincere efforts to do so. Perhaps increased motivation for improvement can be achieved by varying the length and frequency of sessions for these children. It seems probable that some poorly motivated children might respond best to frequent sessions (three or four weekly) of short duration (twenty minutes), particularly if more efforts were made to specify therapy goals from session to session that were capable of being realized by the children.

Perhaps motivation has been affected by inappropriate therapy techniques or lack of progress. Students who consistently face failure soon will become poor attendees at the therapy session, and lack of attendance will only reinforce the cycle of failure. The speech-language pathologist needs to examine the therapy plan and determine whether the objectives have been written in small enough increments to assure success. As objectives become broader and more general in nature, the amount of time required to complete the objective will increase. If the student does not see progress over a relatively short period of time, the chances of losing that most important influence—motivation—increase. It would appear, then, that therapy objectives should be written in discrete steps that will insure progress on a regular basis.

Another consideration of what may be the cause of poor motivation concerns lack of continuity in therapy. This continuity may be the result of the mobility of the family or of inadequate planning by the speech-language pathologist. We live in an age of constant flux whereby many families move from city to city, or within a town, thus interrupting the course of schooling. A child who enrolls in three schools within one year most likely will find it difficult to maintain a satisfactory level of commitment to school and to speech-language therapy. That the transfer of records between schools may take several months due to the difficulty of identifying where the student may have been previous to the new enrollment only adds to the problem of maintaining stability in a program. The speech-language pathologist may initiate an assessment and remediation program only to find that efforts have been duplicated when the educational records are received from the last known school. In some instances, a totally different therapy program may be planned by each of the involved professionals. At times, it is difficult to avoid these circumstances, and the speech-language pathologist must grasp the opportunity at hand and proceed with the best intentions on behalf of the student.

The need to develop an appropriate and effective therapy program based on sequential development and individualized programming was discussed earlier in this chapter. Inadequate planning by the speech-language pathologist not only leads to potential failure but also increases the possibility of poor motivation. As the student becomes less and less interested, both he and the professional become more frustrated. This is when the speech-language pathologist must evaluate the program design to determine if the therapy plan needs adjustment or improvement. Satisfactory progress and increased motivation should be the result of careful planning to meet more appropriately the needs of the student.

Carry-over

Among the specific problems faced by many speech-language pathologists is how to achieve client carry-over or the habituation of newly learned skills in spontaneous communication. A study by Sommers (1960) revealed that 134 of 176 speech-language pathologists responding to a questionnaire ranked carry-over of new sounds into spontaneous speech as the most difficult area in speech therapy. In a study designed to evaluate service effectiveness in a public school program conducted by this author (1973), data were analyzed regarding the time spent in therapy as related to six stages of articulation therapy. These stages were (1) cannot produce target phoneme or discriminate it from error phoneme, (2) can discriminate target phoneme, but cannot produce it, (3) can produce target phoneme in isolation, (4) can use target phoneme in any syllable position, (5) can use target phoneme in controlled speaking situations, and (6) can use target phoneme in unstructured speech. The distribution of time spent in therapy revealed an increase in therapy time as a function of therapy stage. Approximately one-half of the total therapy time was spent in stages 5 and 6 of therapy before reaching the terminal point and dismissal. In other words, 50 percent of therapy was devoted to two stages that represent the carry-over process.

The lack of carry-over on the part of some students was discussed by Sommers (1969), who cited six possibilities for this problem. The first of these, insufficient therapy, relates to the premature dismissal of students. Some students may not establish their newly learned language and speech patterns sufficiently well enough to maintain accuracy of production without support from the speech-language pathologist. The SLP needs continually to evaluate the student's progress and by so doing will probably learn not to make premature judgments about readiness for dismissal.

Additional causes related to the problem of carry-over cited by Sommers included superficial therapy, the nature of the problem, an inflexible program, poorly motivated children, and the "no spread of effect." If a criterion for successful performance is based on an inaccurate assessment or a lack of understanding of the child's disorder, the resultant therapy will be superficial and perhaps lead to remediation or "correction" that will prove to be unstable. Poor carry-over may be related to the nature of the problem. More severe and complex communication disorders present many problems to be solved, and the speech-language pathologist may determine that approximation of the targeted goal is acceptable, thus negating complete carry-over. The type of the disorder and the degree of its severity will dictate ultimately the success of the remediation process. Once again the need to evaluate each individual therapy program on a regular basis is evident as a means to effecting the optimum in carry-over.

Flexible scheduling and motivation, discussed earlier in slightly different contexts, can reflect the success of carry-over and need little elaboration here. Frequency of scheduling and intensity of therapy have a direct relationship to the habituation of newly learned skills. The speech language pathologist must determine just how much therapy is needed at each stage to insure continuing success, and as success is achieved, the student's motivation will be a positive factor leading to the next step in the process.

Finally, it appears likely that a major contributing factor to a lack of carry-over is the "no spread of effect" phenomenon. The speech-language pathologist in the schools who fails to seek the assistance of parents, teachers, and other persons to "set the stage" for carry-over may have a disappointing record. It might be said that therapy in isolation is therapy with limitation, and for some children this may mean a failure to carry over the use of correct patterns.

The carry-over problem has been found to be a critical one. Speech-language pathologists working in schools have resources available to them that may tend to mitigate this problem to a degree.

Dismissal

Dismissal is the ultimate goal of any speech-language therapy program. It is the culmination of all the planning and activity that have gone into each child's program. It is the representation of success and satisfaction. But dismissal doesn't just happen. It is the result of planning based on a set of sequential performance objectives that lead to a terminal goal(s). These goals become the dismissal criteria upon which the completion of the program is predicated. Dismissal criteria may reflect the complete remediation of the problem, or they may suggest cessation of the program based on anticipated maximum performance. Whichever of these postures they represent, dismissal criteria should be realistic and appropriate to the child's needs. In some instances, direct clinical intervention may be suspended to allow other factors, such as language experience or maturation, to influence the ultimate outcome.

Some general considerations for dismissal may be related to the type of disorder. For an example, dismissal criteria should clearly differentiate between students with normal speech skills (no errors) and those with satisfactory speech skills that may be in error but are not affecting or expected to affect communication. The mildly distorted /r/ phoneme may be acceptable to the student and all those concerned with the student's communication skills, while a severe lateralized /s/ and /z/ phoneme would be unacceptable until correction had been attained. Dismissal in each of these cases would be dependent upon separate criteria.

Dismissal criteria in language will be based on the nature of the disorder and the expected outcome of therapy. The determination of the student's readiness for dismissal should include results of formal reevaluation and informal tests, overall language functioning, observation of classroom performance, and reports of language performance in other situations including the home. Since language is pervasive to the total environment, a dismissal decision without these considerations would be inappropriate and premature.

For those students with fluency problems, dismissal should involve aspects pertaining to the student's perception of progress, actual reduction or modification of nonfluent behaviors, and maximum expected gains. If self-perception becomes a positive factor, often this becomes the single motivation for achieving other goals leading toward dismissal. On the other hand, the child and the speech-language pathologist must recognize when maximum benefit has been derived from therapy and dismissal should be considered even if only temporarily.

Dismissal criteria for voice cases may not be as definitive as in other areas of speech-language pathology. Voice improvement varies according to the standards of the community, the student, and the speech-language pathologist, the nature of organic factors, and the phonatory needs of the child. Voice improvement may not always be the only criterion for determining the effectiveness of therapy; improvement of damaged tissue may be necessary before any discernible improvement in voice quality is noted. A panel of "listeners" may assist the speech-language pathologist in making a clinical judgment as to the quality of the voice and its acceptability. The student's own report that his voice "feels" better also may be helpful in evaluating the appropriateness of dismissal.

There are occasions when a student leaves the school system prior to graduation and the completion of the therapy program. In these instances, the speech-language pathologist has the responsibility to refer the student to another agency for the express purpose of continuing the remediation program. The referral should include diagnostic reports, a copy of the individual student plan, an evaluation of student progress, and other pertinent records and reports. The parents and the student should be encouraged to seek additional assistance, but if they choose not to do so, the speech-language pathologist still has the professional responsibility to make an appropriate referral.

Dismissal, then, is the process whereby the student is removed from the therapy program as a result of meeting the requirements established in the dismissal criteria. When the speech-language pathologist has developed dismissal criteria based on performance objectives and when these objectives have been accomplished, the termination of therapy becomes a relatively easy decision and represents the final achievement of the therapy process.

Supportive Services

Available to the speech-language pathologist for assistance in the remediation program are many resources that can provide support to any phase of the therapy program. These supportive services may be represented by school personnel such as the classroom teacher, the teacher aide, the guidance counselor, the principal, the reading specialist, or the psychologist, to name a few. These services may be available from community agencies, clinics, hospitals, physicians, and service organizations. Many school programs cannot provide all of the services needed by the students on a direct basis. Therefore, it is imperative that the speech-language pathologist identify the available resources and initiate and procure those services necessary for the provision of a comprehensive program.

It was noted earlier that the interdisciplinary team approach offers the opportunity for planning an appropriate program based on an exchange of ideas and perceptions regarding the student's needs. The team approach should not cease operating at the planning level. Once the team has become active on behalf of a child, it should use every opportunity to share information regarding the progress of the student. As members of the team become better acquainted and more familiar with the various professional roles, they may rely on each other for assistance in a particular phase of the student's program.

The decisions to be made by the speech-language pathologist are "When should I involve someone in the therapy program?" and "Who should I ask to help me with the program?" Answers to both these questions will depend upon a number of interrelated factors. What is the student's disorder? How severe is it? Does the student respond well to a variety of instructors? Is the task one that can be taught by someone other than a speech-language pathologist? Will the activity serve as a reinforcement of learning? Is the other professional or paraprofessional truly interested in assisting in the therapy program? Can time be found in the individual's already busy day to assist in the therapy program? Does the administration support the involvement of additional personnel? How much time will be required by the speech-language pathologist to prepare for the training of the other individuals, and how much time will be needed to do the actual training?

Several projects have investigated the training and use of paraprofessionals as supportive personnel in a public school communication disorders program (Strong, 1972; Braunstein, 1972; Jelinek, 1976; Scalero and Eskenazi, 1976). Van Hattum reports on his experiences in Chapter 1. Although each project's design differed in the selection and training of personnel, the results were consistent. It was determined that supportive personnel with careful training and supervision could be used effectively in the public school speech-language program. As Braunstein concluded, "Carefully supervised, well planned, with clearly defined goals and responsibilities, the communication aide program can enhance public school speech therapy and provide opportunities to significantly expand, without diluting, the quality of services of the speech clinician serving the school" (p. 34–35).

The speech-language pathologist working in the schools has recourse to professional personnel who can assist rather effectively in a coordinated effort to provide comprehensive educational management of the child. The classroom teacher can become a major ally in the therapy program. It must be recognized that the teacher's day is extremely busy, and any request from the speech-language pathologist for assistance by the teacher should be realistic and relevant to classroom activities. The inclusion of the classroom teacher as an active co-worker in the therapy program should most often occur after the student has established the correct pattern of response but has not habituated its use. The teacher can encourage the child to use the newly learned skill in a variety of settings within the classroom, can implement specific activities suggested by the speech-language pathologist, and can report on the success of the student's attempts in these activities. The classroom teacher can also establish an atmosphere for language development and, with the guidance of the speech-language pathologist (if necessary), can create a language-based classroom for all the students' benefit.

Seaton (1975) conducted a study to evaluate the role of the school psychologist in the management of students with speech-language-hearing disorders. Through the use of a questionnaire and follow-up interviews with twenty-two certified school psychologists, she sought to determine their training in the evaluation and management of children with communication disorders, their use of instruments to evaluate these children, and their current involvement in the management of these children. She found that a limited number in the group had had any formal exposure to or training in speech-language pathology, but the large majority felt this training was necessary. It was noted also that there was a need for more definitive guidelines regarding appropriate tests and their uses. As a result, a significant number of the psychologists supported the multidisciplinary approach to evaluations as an effective and realistic avenue for the management of children with communication disorders. This was recommended even with the understanding of the time constraints for most personnel in school psychology and in speech-language pathology.

It would appear, then, that the speech-language pathologist should actively seek to develop interest among teachers, other professionals, and paraprofessionals in the remediation process and should evolve a systematic and concrete program for their inclusion in the total therapy program. A more integrated therapy program will give greater import to the work and will allow it to become a part of a greater effort to help children.

A second cluster of resource assistance can be found outside the school and includes agencies, clinics, hospitals, physicians, and service organizations. Every school speech-language pathologist needs to be familiar with and to use these sources as circumstances dictate. Most communities have health departments that provide physical examinations, medication, and information about and referral to other agencies. There may be dental clinics, mental health clinics, cleft palate teams, and early identification and evaluation teams, all of which can provide selected services. Where there are small communities without some of these agencies, the speech-language pathologist may need to look to multitownship cooperatives, district offices, or even state level agencies. Frequently the state office of education can provide information and may even have a directory of services available for use.

Local medical associations and their members are an excellent source of aid. If the speech-language pathologist has established lines of communication with the medical community, responses to requests may be more quickly and completely managed. Contact should be made with the various segments of the medical community, such as pediatricians and otolaryngologists, to provide avenues for open dialogue and to establish a viable referral system. Physicians are more than willing to participate in the diagnosis and remediation of communication disorders once they know with whom they are working in the speech-language pathology community. It is the responsibility of the speech-language pathologist to seek the assistance of the medical community to include in the program those aspects which require medical attention.

Referral to speech and hearing clinics may be appropriate for additional diagnostic or remediation services. Colleges and universities with speech and hearing clinics or medical departments can also provide diagnostic and therapy services. When fees are involved with any of these resources, financial aid can often be obtained from local service clubs. These organizations may assist with the provision of equipment such as the purchase of hearing aids or audiometers. Use of referral resources is a sign of professional competence, not weakness.

All of these agencies and organizations can be useful for many different purposes, including medical examinations and recommendations, diagnostic evaluations and therapy, prescription and prescriptive aids, partial or total payment of expenses, and parental involvement. To obtain maximum benefit from these resources, the speech-language pathologist must be responsible for initiating and following up referrals, coordinating services, and reporting all pertinent recommendations to the parents, teachers, and other involved school personnel. With the active use of supportive services, the speech-language pathologist will have a well-rounded program.

SUMMARY

It is apparent that the development of a comprehensive program of services to the speech-language-hearing handicapped is multifaceted and requires innovation, persistence, professional expertise, and dedication. The program must be based on a sound philosophy, the involvement of the interdisciplinary team, and the use of a conceptual framework. Understanding the impact of communication on language and learning is essential to both the program and the total educational needs of the child.

Every student should have the right to develop maximum competence in communication, and school programs have the continuing responsibility to meet the communication needs of their students. The school speech-language pathologist has the unique opportunity to build a dynamic clinical therapy program for the benefit of those students with communication disorders.

STUDY ACTIVITIES

1. Develop a program philosophy and suggest ways in which this philosophy can be shared with school personnel, parents, and other individuals, such as doctors.
2. What role should the speech-language pathologist play on the interdisciplinary team, and what methods would be most appropriate for educating the other team members about speech-language pathology?
3. What principles should guide the speech-language pathologist in discussions with school personnel concerning students enrolled in the therapy program?
4. Outline the similarities and differences in communicative proficiency among the various populations to be served. How would this affect planning for therapy?
5. Select an academic task from a school's curriculum and analyze the task in regard to language comprehension and usage.
6. What are some effective procedures for explaining the therapy program to different groups of people, e.g. teachers, administrators, PTA groups, service clubs in the community?
7. Discuss some specific activities that can be used by parents to assist in the therapy program.
8. What principles should guide the speech-language pathologist when referring students to other agencies for assistance in the remediation process?
9. How could the speech-language pathologist identify resources,

e.g. materials, programs, to be used in the therapy program for the student in a secondary school?

10. What other factors would appear to be essential in the development of an effective public school therapy program?

REFERENCES

1. Ainsworth, S. The Speech Clinician in Public Schools: "Participant" or "Separatist"? *Asha, 7,* 495–503, 1965.
2. Anderson, M. Voice Therapy Pilot Project. Hinsdale Public Schools. Illinois Speech and Hearing Association, *Newsletter, 5,* 4–6, 1965.
3. ASHA Task Force Report: Traditional Scheduling Procedures in Schools. *Language, Speech and Hearing Services in Schools, 4,* 100–109, 1973.
4. Braunstein, M. S. Communication Aide: A Pilot Project. *Language, Speech, and Hearing Services in Schools, 3,* 32–35, July, 1972.
5. Bureau of Education for Exceptional Students. *A Resource Manual for the Development and Evaluation of Special Programs for Exceptional Students: Speech and Language Impaired,* Vol. II-C. Tallahassee, Florida: Florida Department of Education, July, 1979.
6. Cafaro, M. D. Directions for Speech and Hearing Clinicians in the Public Schools. *Language, Speech and Hearing Services in Schools, 4,* 199–200, 1973.
7. Carpenter, R. L. and Augustine, L. E. A Pilot Training Program for Parent-Clinicians. *Journal of Speech and Hearing Disorders, 38,* 48–58, 1973.
8. Dayan, M, Harper, B., Molly, J. S., and Witt, B. T. Communication for the Severely and Profoundly Handicapped. Denver: Love Publishing Company, 1977.
9. Department of Health, Education and Welfare. Education of Handicapped Children. *Federal Register, 42,* August, 1977.
10. Engnoth, G. et al. Report on Housing. Committee on Speech and Hearing Services in Schools, American Speech-Language-Hearing Association, November, 1967.
11. Falck, V. T. Communication Skills—Translating Theory into Practice. *Teaching Exceptional Children,* 1978b.
12. Fellows, J. B. The Speech Pathologist in the High School Setting. *Language, Speech and Hearing Services in Schools, 7,* 61–63, 1976.
13. Fisher, L. E. In R. J. Van Hattum, (Ed.), *Clinical Speech in the Schools.* Springfield, Thomas, 1969.
14. Freeman, G. G. *Speech and Language Services and the Classroom Teacher.* Reston, Virginia: The Council for Exceptional Children, 1977.
15. Garvey, J. and Gordon, B. A Follow-up Study of Children with Disorders of Speech and Development. *British Journal of Disorders of Communication, 8,* 17–28, 1973.
16. Glass, L. Coping with the Bilingual Child. *Asha, 21,* 512–519, 1979.

17. Hall, P. K. and Tomblin, J. B. A Follow-up Study of Children with Articulation and Language Disorders. *Journal of Speech and Hearing Disorders, 43,* 227–241, 1978.
18. Hutchinson, E. C. Burgoon, H. M., Stinnett, W. D., Rutenberg, K. V., Work, R. S., and Ramsey, L. S. *The Florida Language Screening System: Report.* Tallahassee, Florida: Florida Department of Education, June, 1976.
19. Jelinek, J. H. A pilot Program for Training and Utilization of Paraprofessionals in Preschools. *Language, Speech and Hearing in Schools, 7,* 119–132, 1976.
20. Lieberman, I., Shankweiler, D., Camp., L., Heifetz, B., and Werfelman, J. *Steps Towards Literacy:* A Report on Reading Prepared for the Working Group on Learning Failure and Unused Learning Potential for the President's Commission on Mental Health. Washington, D.C., November, 1977.
21. Mager, R. F. *Preparing Instructional Objectives.* Belmont, California: Fearon Publishers, 1962.
22. Marge, M. Factor Analysis of Oral Communication Skills in Older Children. *Journal of Speech and Hearing Research, 31–46,* 1964.
23. McBride, J. and Levy, K. Language and Learning—an Integrative Approach. Paper submitted at the ASHA National Convention, Atlanta, Georgia, November, 1979.
24. McDonald, E. T. and Frick, J. Some Factors which Influence the Frequency and Duration of Treatment Sessions. *Journal of Speech and Hearing Disorders, 22,* 724–728, 1957.
25. Muma, J. R. *Language Handbook: Concepts, Assessment, Intervention.* Englewood Cliffs: Prentice-Hall, 1978.
26. Northcott, W. H. The Hearing Impaired Child: A Speech Clinician as an Interdisciplinary Team Member. *Language, Speech and Hearing Services in Schools, 3,* 7–19, 1972.
27. O'Neill, J. J. The Possible Role and Position of Speech Pathology and Audiology in Regard to Language Learning Disabilities, and Hearing-Impaired. *Asha, 13,* 51–52, 1971.
28. Rees, N. The Speech Pathologist and the Reading Process. *Asha, 16,* 255–258, 1974.
29. Rieke, J. A., Lynch, L. L., and Soltman, S. F. *Teaching Strategies for Language Development.* New York: Grune and Stratton, 1977.
30. Sanders, D. *Auditory Perception of Speech.* Englewood Cliffs, Prentice-Hall, 1977.
31. Scalero A. M. and Eskenazi, C. The Use of Supportive Personnel in a Public School Speech and Language Program. *Language, Speech and Hearing Services in Schools, 7,* 150–158, 1976.
32. Seaton, J. B. Communication Disorders: The School Psychologist's Role. *Language, Speech, and Hearing Services in Schools, 6,* 106–112, 1975.
33. Simon, C. S. *Communicative Competence: A Functional-Pragmatic Approach to Language Therapy.* Tucson, Arizona: Communication Skill Builders, 1979.
34. Sommers, R. K. In R. J. Van Hattum (Ed.), *Clinical Speech in the Schools.*

Springfield, Thomas, 1969.
35. Sommers, R. K. Factors in the Effectiveness of Mothers Trained to Aid in Speech Correction. *Journal of Speech and Hearing Disorders, 27,* 178–186, 1962.
36. Sommers, R. K. et al. Effects of Maternal Attitude upon Improvement in Articulation When Mothers Are Trained to Assist in Speech Correction. *Journal of Speech and Hearing Disorders, 29,* 126–133, 1964.
37. Sommers, R. K. et al. Training Parents of Children with Functional Misarticulation. *Journal of Speech and Hearing Research, 3,* 258–265, 1959.
38. Strickland, R. G. *The Language Arts in the Elementary School.* Boston: D. C. Heath and Company, 1951.
39. Strominger, A. Z. and Bashir, A. S. A Nine Year Follow-up of Language Delayed Children. Paper presented at the annual convention of the American Speech-Language-Hearing Association, Chicago, 1977.
40. Strong, B. Public School Speech Technicians in Minnesota. *Language, Speech, and Hearing Services in Schools, 3,* 53–56, 1972.
41. Tufts, L. C. and Holliday, A. R. Effectiveness of Trained Parents as Speech Therapists. *Journal of Speech and Hearing Disorders, 24,* 395–401, 1959.
42. Van Hattum, R. J. Personal Communication with R. K. Sommers, 1964.
43. Webster, E. J. *Counseling with Parents of Handicapped Children.* New York: Grune and Straton, 1977.
44. Wilson, K. D. Children with Vocal Nodules. *Journal of Speech and Hearing Disorders, 26,* 19–26, 1961.
45. Work, R. S., Hutchinson, E. C., Healey, W. C., Sommers, R. K., and Stevens, E. I. Accountability in a School Speech and Language Program, Part II: Instructional Materials Analysis. *Language, Speech and Hearing Services in Schools, 7,* 259–270, 1976.
46. Work, R. S., Hutchinson, E. C., Healey, W. C., Sommers, R. K., and Stevens, E. I. Evaluation of the Speech Therapy Program through Instructional Materials Analysis: Service Effectiveness. Unpublished study, 1973.

Chapter 11

LEARNING DISABILITIES AND AUDITORY PROCESSING

Lee I. Fisher

LEARNING DISABILITIES

Learning disabilities is a label used to categorize a nebulous group of significant disorders of learning. Many children and adults have been afflicted with these problems since the beginning of time, and the effect of these problems on their lives is very real. Little information regarding these learning disabilities was available prior to the 1960s. In fact, the American Association for Children with Learning Disabilities (ACLD) was not organized until April, 1963, when a symposium on perceptually handicapped children was held in Chicago, Illinois. More progress has been made in evaluating and serving students with learning disabilities during the last decade than had been accomplished during the last century. While we have made progress unraveling the intricacies of specific learning disabilities, there is still a great deal that is unknown about this group of significant learning disorders. Because of its impact on the profession, it is included in this text, which is primarily devoted more to matters pertaining to organization and management of school programs.

Much has been written on the problems of learning disabilities since the 1960s. The beginning of this chapter deals with the impact of recent state and federal legislation, a definition of learning disabilities, the incidence, the roles of the speech-language pathologist and the audiologist, and evaluation strategies. The majority of the chapter will address the relationships between specific learning disabilities and auditory processing. The following components of auditory processing will be discussed: definition, processing problems associated with the auditory pathways, incidence, involvement of the speech-language pathologist and the audiologist, review of auditory perceptual tests, development of a teacher's checklist, components of a diagnostic evaluation, need for child advocacy, and suggestions for remediation.

Legislation

Local, state, and federal legislation has created major changes in education and will continue to do so. Recent federal and state legislation now requires the provision of a wide variety of special education programs and services to meet the needs of all handicapped students.

One federal law, Public Law 94-142, has done more to upgrade the quality of services than any other event in the legislative history of special education in this country. This legislation has provided the impetus to initiate and expand special education programs and services. As a result, there has been a dramatic increase in the number of students being served. Many efforts have been made to describe the components of Public Law 94-142. Chapter 3 of this book addresses this topic in detail. One aspect of P.L. 94-142 deals with a free and appropriate education. Educational units throughout the country are currently dealing with the concept of determining the most appropriate placement and service program for each handicapped child. The requirement for parental involvement and permission for evaluation and placement is extremely important. This requirement has involved the parents in not only these processes but in the planning process during the development of a child's individualized education plan as well.

The mainstreaming concept is another concept that is very important to the ongoing needs of students with various handicapping conditions. This concept applies directly to nearly all students with speech-language-hearing problems. Public Law 94-142 will continue to have a significant impact on the provision of diagnostic and remediation programs for children with hearing, speech, language, and learning problems as educational units attempt to meet the needs of every handicapped student in the future.

Definition

There are many definitions of learning disabilities. This is not surprising in view of the complexity, the vagueness, yet the encompassing nature of the problem. Another reason for the variability in the definitions is that the problem has been approached from many angles, by professionals representing many different disciplines. For example, learning disabilities have been defined from physical, neurological, etiological, psychological, educational, linguistic, and conceptual bases.

The most recent definition of learning disabilities of the Department of Health, Education and Welfare appeared in the Federal Register on December 29, 1977. The definition reads as follows:

> Specific learning disability means a disorder in one or more of the basic psychological processes involved in understanding or in using language, spoken or written, which may manifest itself as an imperfect ability to listen, think, speak, read, write, spell, or to do mathematical calculations. The term includes such conditions as perceptual handicaps, brain injury, minimal brain dysfunction, dyslexia, and developmental aphasia. The term does not include children who have learning problems which are primarily the result of visual, hearing, or motor handicaps, of mental retardation, of emotional disturbance, or of environmental, cultural, or economic disadvantage. (*p.* 65083)

This definition is currently being used as the basis for identifying and serving learning disabled children in our country. While the definition does specifically include language problems and perceptual handicaps, the definition does not include children who have learning problems that are primarily the result of visual, hearing, or motor handicaps. The implication is that specific learning disabilities are not the result of auditory or visual *acuity* problems, but this concept is not clarified in the federal definition. Permanent auditory and/or visual acuity problems are not included as causes of learning disabilities in the federal definition but may coexist with learning disabilities. However, perceptual or processing problems associated with the auditory and/or visual channels may indeed be the most significant aspect(s) of a child's learning problems.

The term "specific" is important to use in conjunction with the words "learning disabilities," as it is possible to identify and isolate specific aspects of a learning disabled student that are more significant than other aspects of the problem. For example, dyslexia is a specific learning disability. Many people have shortened the label to "learning disability" from "learning disabilities." Rarely does one find a student with only an isolated disability. If so, the disability may be specific and severe, such as in the case of a child who is reading at the pre-primer level when enrolled in high school. Most children with learning problems have more than one specific learning disability. Therefore, the preferred term is "specific learning disabilities." A description of a student's specific disabilities is essential for a clear understanding of the nature, extent, and severity of the specific learning disabilities existing in the student's life at that point in time. Frequently, different children experience similar learning disabilities. However, each child's problems are unique and often in a state of change.

MAJOR LEARNING PROBLEMS

There are numerous causes and contributing factors of learning problems in children. The majority of these causes and contributing factors of significant learning disorders may be identified as follows:

- Auditory and/or visual acuity problems
- Auditory and/or visual processing problems
- Speech and/or language problems
- Subnormal intellect
- Specific learning disabilities
- Emotional disturbances
- Physical disabilities
- Developmental immaturity
- Prolonged illness due to infection, metabolic disturbance, or malnutrition
- Inadequate motivation
- Poor basic knowledge resulting from irregular school attendance, moving from school to school, or poor instruction

Many learning disorders are the result of or are associated with some form and/or degree of cerebral dysfunction, minimal brain

dysfunction (MBD) or organic brain damage. There are several major types of cerebral dysfunctions, according to Block (1979).
1. Global cerebral dysfunction, which is often referred to as minimal brain dysfunction. There are two subgroups in this classification: one subgroup is called hyperkinetic behavior syndrome, and the second subgroup consists of specific learning disabilities.
2. Speech and language disorders.
3. Mental retardation.
4. Encephalopathy or organic brain damage.
5. Convulsive disorders.
6. Emotional disturbances and/or behavior disorders.
7. Childhood psychoses.

The majority of all learning problems in children are the result of these causal and contributing factors. A given child may experience difficulty learning as a result of a single causal factor. However, complex learning problems often result from multiple handicapping conditions.

It is well established that cerebral dysfunction is the major causal factor of significant learning disorders in many children. Likewise, it is well established that significant learning disorders frequently result from other causes and contributing factors such as sensory deprivation, illness, cultural deprivation, and lack of stimulation. Speech-language disorders may or may not be caused by cerebral dysfunction.

The literature contains frequent references to the concept of cerebral dysfunction as the major causal factor of learning disabilities. According to Millichap (1977)

> Minimal brain dysfunction (MBD) was first described by Alfred A. Strauss in 1940 and more recently by a task force appointed in 1964 by the National Institute of Neurological Diseases of the United States Public Health Service and the National Society for Crippled Children and Adults. The definition includes children of or near average intelligence, with learning and/or certain abnormalities ranging from mild to severe, which are associated with subtle deviations of functions of the central nervous system. These are characterized by various combinations of deficits in perception, conceptualization, language, memory, and control of attention, impulse, or motor function (PP. 3–4).

Millichap indicates that alternative terms have been used to describe various syndromes of MBD with titles such as hyperactive syndrome, hyperkinetic syndrome, minimal brain damage, perceptually handicapped child, specific learning disabilities, and learning disorders. The choice of term is dependent on the most prominent presenting symptom(s) and the individual preference of the investigator or practitioner. None of these terms are entirely satisfactory because of the lack of uniformity of the manifestations and causes of the syndrome, according to Millichap.

Clemmens and Glaser (1967) suggested that specific learning disabilities are those persistent problems in academic achievement that are associated with demonstrable or presumed neurologic dysfunction in children whose intellectual capacity otherwise seems adequate.

In 1966, Clements indicated that the diagnostic and descriptive categories included in the term minimal brain dysfunction refer to children of near average or higher general intelligence with learning or certain behavioral abnormalities ranging from mild to severe, which are associated with suspected dysfunction of the central nervous system. These aberrations may arise from genetic variation, biochemical irregularities, perinatal brain insults, illnesses or injuries sustained during the years critical for the development of the central nervous system, or unknown causes. During the school years, a variety of persistent learning disabilities is the most predominant manifestation.

Weiner (1965) noted that the word "minimal" used in minimal brain dysfunction does not refer to a necessarily minor or unimportant impairment but, rather, to brain involvement that is not readily and grossly demonstrable.

Characteristics of Learning Disabilities

The major characteristics of learning disabilities most frequently associated with global cerebral dysfunctions are as follows:
1. Failure to achieve in relationship to intellectual ability that is at least within the normal range. There may be a wide discrepancy between verbal and performance scores on intellectual tests
2. Hyperactivity
3. Distractability

4. Short attention span
5. Auditory processing problems
6. Visual processing problems
7. Inconsistent performance within a day or from day to day
8. Poor gross and/or fine motor coordination
9. Speech-language problems
10. Academic deficiencies
11. Low frustration tolerance
12. Neurological abnormalities (so-called "soft" neurological signs)
13. Impulsivity
14. Emotional lability

Although this list is not all-inclusive, it does include most of the common characteristics of learning disabilities. No effort was made to place this list in priority order. A given child may have one or many of these symptoms. Frequently there are multiple symptoms, but all of these symptoms are not necessarily present in each child experiencing problems with learning disabilities. Likewise, the severity of each of the symptoms varies considerably from child to child, resulting in a unique combination of characteristics at a given point in time for each child. These characteristics may vary in intensity and consistency, resulting in significant learning problems.

Incidence of Learning Disabilities

There is a great disparity in the incidence of learning disabilities among authorities. These figures vary from less than 2 percent to in excess of one-fourth of all children. Boys experience learning disabilities more frequently than girls. Obviously, a major aspect of incidence relates to the severity of the problem(s) a given student is experiencing in learning. For example, in the specific learning problem of dyslexia, the problem at times is so severe that the student cannot read even after years of intensive regular and special help. On the other hand, there are probably very few children who do not experience some form of difficulty with some aspect of learning to read. In the area of auditory processing there are more than a dozen specific problems a child may experience, each of which may vary in intensity and in duration.

According to Millichap (1977), "Approximately four percent of children under twelve years of age are hyperactive and have signs of minimal brain dysfunction, or at least one in every classroom. Some authorities have estimated the incidence as high as ten percent in school children between five and twelve years of age, and one report claimed a total of three million children with MBD in the U.S.A." (p. 4). Obviously, a major aspect of incidence relates to the severity of the problems children experience.

Bader (1976) reported on a research study, "Minimal Brain Damage in Children," completed in 1969 under the direction of Myklebust. In this study 2,767 third and fourth graders were given intensive psychological, medical, and educational evaluations. The conclusion of the study indicated that 7.5 percent of the children experienced severe learning disabilities, and 15 percent of the children were underachievers with mild to moderate learning problems. A pilot incidence study was conducted by the Rocky Mountain Educational Laboratory in Greeley, Colorado, in 1969 for the U.S. Office of Education. In this study 2,400 second graders in an eight-state area were evaluated. Extensive educational, psychological, and medical evaluations were completed. The conclusion of the study was that 4.6 percent of these students experienced severe learning problems, and an additional 6 percent experienced mild to moderate learning problems. Estimates vary but seem to range from 1 percent to 7.5 percent of children with severe learning disabilities and 5 percent to 40 percent of children with learning problems that are creating underachievers, according to Bader.

The real incidence of learning disabilities falls between a range of 2 to 15 percent of school-age children. The 2 percent figure includes the most severe and diverse problems in need of special education programs and services. The 15 percent figure is a more inclusive figure including the less significant and less involved but still identifiable problems. At any rate there are a significant number of children affected by the problems associated with specific learning disabilities. These young people need help in overcoming their learning problems and in reaching their potential.

ROLES OF SPEECH-LANGUAGE PATHOLOGISTS AND AUDIOLOGISTS

Speech-language pathologists and audiologists have significant leadership roles in evaluating and serving students with learning disabilities and in expanding the body of knowledge about this significant group of learning disorders. There is an increasing awareness of the existence and importance of auditory processing problems and their significance in language and learning processes. Auditory processing and language are critical and integral aspects of all learning. Audiologists should be highly qualified to evaluate auditory processing skills and to serve as a resource for remediation theories in audition. Speech-language pathologists should be highly qualified in diagnosing and remediating language and auditory problems. In 1976 the American Speech and Hearing Association published a position statement on learning disabilities supporting the involvement of speech-language pathologists and audiologists in evaluating and serving learning disabled students, and fortunately this is occurring with increasing regularity.

In 1979 the Executive Board of the American Speech-Language-Hearing Association established a committee to review and revise the position statement on learning disabilities published in 1976. The committee felt it was necessary to reaffirm the role of the speech-language pathologist and the audiologist in learning disabilities. As a result, the following statement was prepared indicating that speech-language pathologists and audiologists must be included as members of multidisciplinary teams assessing and planning programs for children with language learning disorders. This committee (1979) published the following:

> The Role of the Speech-Language Pathologist and Audiologist in Learning Disabilities
>
> Children with learning disabilities are a heterogeneous group and include individuals with language disorders who manifest an inability to listen, think, speak, read, write, spell or do mathematical calculations. These individuals require the services of a variety of qualified specialists currently practicing within educational and clinical settings. A clear understanding of language behavior and language disorders reduces the likelihood of professionals adopting a single model for assessment and intervention and

acknowledges that language is not an isolated skill. Language is a necessary skill for success in academic, social, and emotional development. The language disordered individual demonstrates problems in language knowledge and use and frequently demonstrates disruption in higher order thinking, in learning the school curriculum and managing the language of instruction.

Public education assumes that a child enters school with an intact oral language system. The design and formulation of school curriculum is based upon the same assumption without regard for the central role of language in learning academic content areas. It is well known that children with language disorders are at high risk for academic failure of varying degrees and types.

Federal regulations for identifying children with learning disabilities (*Federal Register,* Vol. 42, No. 250, December 29, 1977) indicate that an individual may have a specific learning disability when there is a severe discrepancy between achievement and intellectual ability in one or more of the following areas: oral expression, listening comprehension, written expression, basic reading skill, reading comprehension, mathematics calculation, and mathematics reasoning.

Of major concern to speech-language pathologists and audiologists are those individuals whose primary disabilities are characterized by disorders of language acquisition, comprehension and production.

It is therefore essential that qualified professionals participate actively in the:

1) assessment of individuals suspected of having learning disabilities in order to determine the presence or absence of a language disorder;
2) assessment, program planning and program development for individuals who have language disorders and language based learning disabilities;
3) delivery of programs and services to language disordered individuals on a direct or indirect basis as appropriate.

Agencies having responsibility for providing programs and services to individuals with learning disabilities must ensure that qualified speech-language pathologists and audiologists are members of the multidisciplinary assessment and instructional team. (P. 1015)

Speech-language pathology and audiology training programs are now incorporating courses into their curricula pertaining to auditory processing and learning disabilities. These courses should be required of all students, since there is a direct relationship between auditory processing, language development, and language function; speech-language pathologists and audiologists encounter children with these problems in schools, clinics, hospitals, and in private practice. Speech-language pathologists and audiologists must also be capable of working with other professionals in an interdisciplinary effort to serve students' needs in the most effective manner.

Briefly, let us consider the relationship between specific learning disabilities and speech-language deviations and disorders.

At this point in time, students with significant specific learning disabilities are generally served by a learning disabilities teacher in a variety of program models ranging from resource programs to self-contained classes. Students with speech-language disorders are served primarily by speech-language pathologists who provide diagnostic evaluations and schedule the children for individual or small group therapy on a regular basis. The speech-language pathologist also often provides consultative assistance. Since language is the most important and critical aspect of almost all learning, there are very few children who experience difficulty with learning disabilities who do not also have some degree of difficulty with oral language skills. It is important to note, however, that many children who experience speech-language deviations and disorders do not have specific learning disabilities. Consequently, some children with language problems are served most effectively by speech-language pathologists, some are served most effectively by learning disabilities teachers, but the largest percentage of these students can be served most effectively through the joint efforts of these professionals working together to create improvement in the child's language skills. As professionals, we realize that language is central to all learning and is the joint responsibility of the parents, classroom teacher(s), speech-language pathologist, language learning specialists and/or a learning disabilities teacher in addition to others in the child's environment. Those persons who work in elementary and secondary schools recognize that we can no longer work effectively on an independent basis but can use our skills most productively by working cooperatively with other professionals in a unified effort to improve the language skills of each student.

There are many labels that are used to describe specific learning disabilities. Some of these terms are academic or educational disabilities, language disabilities, or language learning disabilities. These labels are often used interchangeably. During the identification of a specific learning disability, an evaluation team must determine if there is a severe discrepancy between achievement and intellectual ability in one or more of the following areas: (1) oral expression, (2) listening comprehension, (3) written expression, (4) basic reading skills, (5) reading comprehension, (6) mathematics comprehension, and (7) mathematics reasoning. Consequently, it is important to determine the existence and degree of academic or educational disabilities. However, the existence of a deficit in one or more academic or educational areas, such as reading, math, or spelling, is, in reality, the result of the learning problem, so we can conclude that academic or educational disability is not the most appropriate terminology. If one accepts a definition of language as including all the encoding and decoding skills involved in the areas of phonology, morphology, syntax, and semantics, the term "language disabilities" may seem to be a more appropriate label. However, upon closer examination of this label, it is readily apparent that many children who experience speech and language problems do not have specific learning disabilities. There are also children who experience difficulty with speech and language problems in addition to having one or more specific learning disabilities. From a semantic viewpoint, the term "language learning disabilities" may indeed be the most appropriate label. A close examination of the areas of discrepancy listed above suggests that language is indeed involved in all these areas. Therefore, the term "language" is indeed appropriate to use in conjunction with learning disabilities, as the learning pertains to the abilities to achieve in talking, listening, writing, reading, and mathematics. Consequently, speech-language pathologists and audiologists may consider the term "language learning disabilities" as an appropriate label for children with these problems.

EVALUATION STRATEGIES

There is a critical need for early identification of children with specific learning disabilities. Frequently problems are not identified until they have been reinforced and have become more serious in the middle and upper elementary grades. These problems must be identified as early as possible to provide early service programs for these children. Identification programs should begin during the preschool years and should be intensified as a student progresses through elementary and secondary school. In fact, Public Law 94-142 now requires early identification and treatment programs in all states.

In the past ten years we have developed numerous evaluative tools for determining the presence and severity of specific learning disabilities. Learning problems must be identified and diagnosed in each student. This can best be done by a multidisciplinary team using a differential diagnostic approach. The evaluation design should include the following:

1. Family history
2. Medical, birth, and developmental histories
3. Auditory acuity and processing evaluation
4. Visual acuity and processing evaluation
5. Speech-language evaluation
6. Psychological evaluation
7. Physical and neurological examination
8. Educational evaluation

Learning disabilities can best be identified and diagnosed through a comprehensive interdisciplinary approach. Each aspect of this evaluation process lends important information to the current functioning of the total child. Whenever a segmented or individualistic approach is taken in the evaluation of a student, one does not obtain a clear or a complete picture. There is also danger in omitting some aspects of this evaluation, again resulting in an incomplete impression. For example, for a number of years this writer served as a speech clinician doing speech, language, and hearing evaluations with an interdisciplinary team in the public schools. At the time it seemed as though "everything" was being considered. The writer then had an opportunity to serve as a speech-language and hearing consultant to a child evaluation clinic for a period of several years. It was a rewarding learning experience to have a pediatric neurologist as a member of the team, routinely providing information on physical and neurological evaluations, which proved to be highly significant. Likewise, the social worker's contributions as a part of this team provided significant input on family history as well as birth and developmental history. An educational consultant's evaluation of academic areas was often imperative in making a complete assessment.

The professionals on the team should include a psychologist, speech-language pathologist, audiologist, educational specialist, social worker, and a pediatric neurologist, if possible. Such a team can best use their interdisciplinary skills in the evaluation process and in the process of planning appropriate remediation. In small school districts all of these team members may not be available, so speech-language pathologists should make an effort to work closely with the other professionals who are available.

AUDITORY PROCESSING PROBLEMS

Some of the most perplexing learning problems in children are related to or are the result of auditory processing difficulties. At first this may seem to be a rather trite statement. However, consider that the majority of what humans learn is acquired through the auditory and/or the visual senses. The statement becomes more meaningful as you think about the manner in which humans communicate. During the first few years of life nearly all language is processed and learned through the auditory channel. As a child continues to grow and as the meaning of words becomes more complex, the auditory pathway becomes more significant in the language learning process. Fortunately the majority of children experience little or no difficulty with this complex miracle of learning. However, some children are less fortunate and experience frustration and difficulty learning through the auditory channel. These children need help in overcoming these processing problems and the associated frustrations they experience in their daily lives.

Auditory problems certainly are as old as time. Little thought was given to these problems and their involvement in the learning process until the turn of this century. In fact, little was known about the cause or the significance of auditory learning problems until the 1960s and 1970s, and still little is known about the complexity of auditory processing. Speech-language pathologists and audiologists have a vital role in evaluating and serving these students and in the quest for knowledge so these problems can be dealt with more effectively. Similarly the profession is increasing efforts to delve into the heart of communication—the way humans process language. Many audiologists who have been primarily involved in the measurement of acuity in the past are now becoming more involved in evaluating all aspects of the total auditory learning mode. There is still much to learn in this exciting area. As a profession we need to forge ahead and increase our knowledge and ability to serve the communication handicapped, including those children and adults with auditory processing problems. It is hoped that in the future audiologists will provide more leadership in this search for knowledge and will inform professionals in related disciplines regarding the significance of auditory processing deficits.

Specific Auditory Processing Problems

In this chapter the term "auditory processing" will be used as the preferred term instead of "auditory perception." Processing is a broader term than perception, per se, and is related to all of the specific aspects in the chain of events that encompass the processing of language and other auditory events. The literature contains many definitions of auditory processing. Eisenson (1972) refers to perception as a process of categorization and stresses that perception for language deals with series of sequences of stimuli that have temporal order. Barr (1976) defines perception as receiving, processing, and classifying sensory information for coding into familiar symbols. Berry (1969) defines auditory perception of speech as the temporal management of information. Butler (1980) defines auditory perception as temporal management of auditory input or the immediate short-term processing of information received aurally. The latter definition is similar to the definition Witkin used in 1969 to define auditory perception as immediate short-term processing of information received aurally.

Auditory processing includes all of the abilities and skills involved in processing information received aurally. An auditory processing deficit is a dysfunction or a disruption of the ability to perceive and process auditory signals within the central nervous system.

Auditory processing involves several separate but often interrelated abilities and skills. Numerous models of the components of auditory processing can be found in the literature. The major components of auditory processing include the following:

Sensitivity
Attention
Attention span
Recognition
Identification
Association
Localization
Discrimination
Figure-ground
Integration of information
Short-term, long-term, sequential memory
Closure

These components are not listed in degree of importance, nor is this necessarily a complete list of all potential aspects of auditory processing. The list does represent, however, what are considered to be the major components of auditory processing. These components involve abilities and skills in the process of decoding — comprehension — storage — retrieval — and the encoding of language. Following are brief descriptions of components of auditory processing.

Sensitivity: Sensitivity refers to a person's ability to perceive and respond to a wide range of sound(s). The terms sensitivity and acuity are often used interchangeably and denote the sharpness, clearness, and distinctness with which one is able to hear sound. Auditory sensitivity is commonly measured in decibels over a diverse range of frequencies and intensities. When evaluating a student it is important to know if the student has experienced a history of hearing loss, the time of onset, severity, frequency, and duration of loss. Likewise, it is important to know the current status of the student's hearing sensitivity from an educational standpoint.

As a result of being responsible for the supervision of screening and testing approximately one-half million children during the past ten years, this writer is convinced that there are very few children who do not experience some degree of hearing loss, especially during their first few years of life. During these early years children are most vulnerable to ear infection and temporary fluctuating hearing loss. This hearing loss may have a significant educational impact, especially since it occurs during the critical language-learning period. Therefore, it is important to attempt to determine whether a child has experienced any prior hearing loss, as this information may provide important clues to a child's current difficulty. Some children have numerous ear infections before they enter school. These infections are usually accompanied by mild to moderate hearing loss for a period of time. Children who experience recurrent middle ear problems and associated fluctuating hearing loss may be delayed in their language development and/or academic development up to a year or more by the beginning of second grade.

A team of pediatric researchers at The University of Tennessee (Zinkus, 1979) believes they have identified for the first time a preventable cause of learning disabilities. During this study it was found that children who suffered repeated ear infections or who had chronic inflammation of the middle ear during the first three years of life—the critical years of language development—were prone to disturbances in auditory processing that could later interfere with their learning to read, spell, and perform mental arithmetic. Such children also tend to have difficulties following a sequence of verbal instructions and answering verbal questions that require attention to an entire sentence. Zinkus, a member of the research team, reported that early recognition and treatment of middle ear disease could prevent later learning problems. Infants can be rapidly and inexpensively evaluated. Children with middle ear problems that could affect their auditory perception may be treated even before the age of one year. It was found that children with a history of a severe or chronic middle ear inflammation showed significant delays in speech and language development, especially in acquiring an initial vocabulary of four to ten words and in formulating sentences. On intelligence tests the children did poorly on measures that involved auditory skills, although tests dependent on visual skills were normal according to the study.

Katz (1978) described the effects of conductive hearing loss on auditory function. Katz indicated, "There is a good deal of support for the conclusion that there can be brain dysfunction as a result of conductive loss. Although the association of mechanical ear problems with cerebral processing disorders seems strange in light of the prevailing thought, there are too many indicators of this relationship for audiologists, otologists, and speech-language pathologists to ignore."

Katz and Illmer (1972) reported a high incidence of conductive hearing loss among learning disabled children who were tested in two studies. Learning disabled children (20% of a total school population) were tested in hearing and auditory perception as well as other areas. These children ranged from the kindergarten to high school level. In both studies, 33 percent of the learning disabled children were found to have hearing losses. The greatest percentage were children with conductive problems of slight to mild degrees. The losses were not always bilateral and were frequently fluctuating. The children with conductive losses had more severe auditory perceptual problems than the learning disabled children with normal hearing or those with sensory-neural problems.

Although one might associate difficulty in speech-in-noise skills primarily with brain stem dysfunction, phonemic synthesis, and auditory speech, these appear to tell us more about brain function. Further evidence relating possible brain dysfunction has been noted in both children and adults with conductive losses.

Children with learning disabilities, many of whom have conductive impairments, display abnormalities on the Staggered Spondaic Word (SSW) Test (Katz, 1968) of central auditory function.

The results of Katz and Burge (1971) and Katz and Illmer (1972) have been supported by the results of Lewis (1976). He reported that children who consistently failed audiometric, tympanometric, and otoscopic examinations over a four-year period had considerably poorer auditory perceptual performance than children who consistently passed these tests. Test differences were noted in discrimination ability in quiet and discrimination in noise, on the Wepman Auditory Discrimination Test (1958) phonemic synthesis, and language function. Some conclusions follow:

Conductive hearing losses are like earplugs in that they restrict the sounds of the environment from stimulating the cochlea, thereby depriving the auditory system of normal activity.
The effects of deprivation may be far reaching and no doubt involve the retrocochlear system and the brain.
The effects of deprivation depend on

   a. the age of onset.
   b. the duration of the loss.
   c. the degree of loss.
   d. whether the loss is unilateral or bilateral.
   e. whether the problem is constant or variable.
   f. the frequency tested.
   g. the test procedure.

The greater the hearing loss and the longer the period of deprivation, the more extreme the retrocochlear signs.
Disruption in auditory perception and language (presumably cerebral functions) are associated with fluctuating hearing loss, especially unilateral problems and with early age of onset.
Even after the mechanical blockage has been removed, abnormal auditory function may persist.
Some aspects of hearing might be depressed while others are enhanced depending on the time, test frequency, and the test procedure.
Stimulating a deprived ear or one with conductive hearing loss seems to improve hearing function. (Pp. 884–885)

By definition, sensorineural hearing loss is not one of the causes of learning disabilities but often causes significant learning problems. Therefore, it is important that this factor not be disregarded in the evaluation process. However, students with specific learning disabilities may have some degree of sensorineural or mixed hearing loss in addition to their learning disabilities. Such students experience multiple handicaps—both of which may have a significant effect on the student's ability to learn.

Attention and Attention Span: Attention and attention span are not the same. They are aspects of attending behaviors that are critical to the learning process. Under *attention* the main question to be raised is Can the child attend to auditory stimuli or is the child so distractable and/or hyperactive that attention is nonexistent? The next question to be answered is Can the child attend to a variety of stimuli and under what conditions? This is often a subjective observation and may vary from minute to minute or from day to day. Some children with severe learning problems cannot attend to auditory stimuli for even a few fleeting seconds. Other children seem to be highly selective in their attending behaviors. Occasionally poor attending behaviors may be attributed to poor listening habits and lack of motivation to listen, but many learning disabled children cannot attend because of this specific auditory processing problem. Likewise, *attention span* is critical to learning. Professionals frequently refer to a child as having a "short attention span" but do not describe how short the attention span is or describe the listening conditions. Attention span does vary for most children, from a few seconds to several hours, depending on the subject, interest in the subject, the presence or absence of background noise, physical alertness of the child, intellectual ability. For example, a student may be able to attend on a one-to-one basis for more than an hour in a quiet room but may not be able to attend in a classroom for more than a few minutes because of distractions in the environment. When evaluating a child, observe whether the child can attend and, if so, does the attention span last for a few seconds, less than two minutes, two to five minutes, five to fifteen minutes, or in excess of fifteen minutes? The listening conditions should be recorded as well as the specific length of the attention span. Consider how frustrating it must be for a second grade child with an attention span of less than two minutes to sit in a classroom and be bombarded with auditory information all day long. Some children literally drift in and out of school throughout the entire day even though they are physically present. One train of thought suggests that if you could get and hold a child's attention and develop excellent listening skills in the child, all other auditory problems would be resolved. This belief is not held by this writer, as it is felt that attention and attention span are two directly related factors in the auditory processing chain of events. Fortunately, with time, skill, and patience, effective clinicians and teachers can often develop and improve attending behaviors in highly distractable children with poor listening skills.

Recognition — Identification — Association: There are several different skills involved in the recognition, identification, and association of auditory sounds. It is important to know if a child can *recognize* and *identify* given sound(s) based on previous experience and/or meaning. Likewise, it is important to know if a child can categorize sound(s) into meaningful and nonmeaningful units and to *associate* sounds and symbols. A person derives considerable meaning from the recognition and identification of nonlinguistic environmental sounds. However, the majority of comprehension results from the linguistic association between sound and meaning. This may occur at the morpheme, phoneme, and/or word level and may or may not be integrated with visual processing skills. Butler (1980) described auditory analysis as the ability to separate a series of sounds that have been presented as a meaningful whole and to identify the component parts; to perceive not only the auditory sequence but the placement of sounds within the sequence as well. Another skill, auditory synthesis, was described by Butler as the ability to integrate a series of sounds that have been presented separately into a meaningful whole. During the evaluation process a child's ability to recognize and identify sounds should be determined. Can the child readily recognize phonemic sounds accurately and associate them with symbols or experiential events? In reality, the ability to recognize and identify sounds often occurs in an automatic fashion and at a subconscious level. Consider for a moment the importance of this factor in the process of two people communicating. Words and thoughts must be recognized and identified conceptually if communication is to occur.

Kroth (1971) has described auditory association as the ability to relate meaning to particular environmental sounds and/or spoken words. A child may be able to recognize a sound but may not know its meaning or significance. Furthermore, the child may be able to hear speech but may be unable to relate a combination of specific sounds to a meaningful unit. When a person has difficulty associating sound and meaning, the response may frequently be inappropriate if there is a response.

Localization: Mencher (1974) defines *auditory localization* as spatial orientation. Generally this factor is considered of major importance in the presence of a significant hearing acuity problem. This skill is also an important element in auditory processing problems. Rapid changes in the direction of sound generate anxiety, creating chaos in the learning situation. This factor also plays a role in figure-ground discrimination and may have added significance in view of some recent thinking about the importance of the right ear in processing and the left hemisphere in storing language in some children.

Discrimination and Figure-ground: Discrimination of sound(s) in quiet and in the presence of competing sound(s) represents one of the most interesting and important components of auditory processing. In the past speech-language pathologists and audiologists have placed emphasis on discrimination of speech sound(s) in quiet listening conditions. This skill is important for learning but is not felt by this writer to be as important as discrimination of connected discourse in the presence of competing speech and/or noise.

Until the early 1970s little consideration was given to the significance of understanding in the presence of competing messages. In fact, today most audiologists continue to evaluate discrimination in quiet and not in the presence of various levels and types of background noise. There are basically three factors in noise interference. The first is the type or complexity of noise. The second is the intensity in relation to the signal. The third factor is the location of the noise in relation to the signal. Most children and adults experience little or no difficulty discriminating in a quiet environment and generally score near 100 percent on this task. However, as the intensity of background noise increases up to and exceeds the intensity of the speech signal, the competing noise interference has a dramatic effect. Rupp (1977) has indicated that speech noise is more contaminating to listener efficiency than noise that does not contain competing speech. Listening in quiet is easy for most persons; however, today's environment provides few truly quiet listening opportunities. Generally we listen to speech with a multitude of competing sounds and messages. Therefore, it is important to know if a student can sort out the *figure* (speech) from the *background* (competing speech and/or noise) and can selectively attend and concentrate on the speech and minimize the effects of the background even if the competing message is speech itself. There appears to be a critical level of noise interference. When the intensity of the competing signal comes to within approximately ten decibels of the intensity of the speech signal, it begins to have a significant effect on a person's discrimination ability.

Figure 11-1 presents two articulation curves for a single list of words. In one case the words were presented in isolation. In the other case the words appeared as parts of a sentence. Note that the same words are always more intelligible in sentences than in isolation. Words become more intelligible as the signal to noise ratio changes as the signal exceeds the intensity of the noise or competing message. At zero signal to noise ratio only 40 percent of words are intelligible in isolation, and only 74 percent of words are intelligible in sentences. At a plus 18 decibels signal to noise ratio note that 80 percent of the words are intelligible, and 98 percent of the same words are intelligible in sentences. The implication is that if speech is spoken at a conversational level of 50 decibels in the classroom, the noise should not exceed 32 decibels or it will begin to interfere with intelligibility. This implication is significant, since noise levels often reach or exceed 50 or 60 decibels in school classrooms and speech is often softer than 50 decibels.

When the intensity of the competing signal, especially if the competing signal is speech, reaches the level of the speech signal, discrimination drops markedly. In many cases when the intensity of the noise exceeds that of the speech signal by approximately 5 to 10 decibels, the original speech signal is obliterated, and discrimination drops to a range of 0 to 20 percent of intelligibility. Listening in the presence of background noise is indeed a signifi-

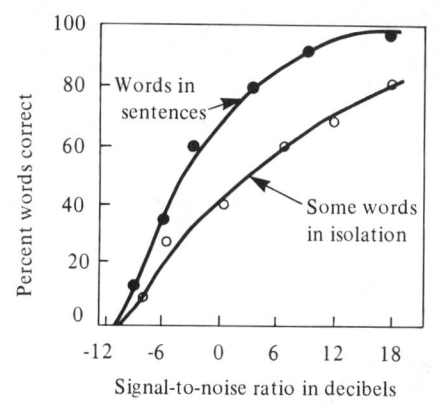

Figure 11-1. Two articulation curves for a single list of words. From Miller, Heise, and Lichten, 1951.

cant factor in auditory processing and should definitely be included in the evaluation process. This is especially important in modern education as open spaces and large classroom facilities are common in the public schools. Students are confronted with listening to the teacher, other students, and a host of environmental noises in these settings. These difficult listening situations create real problems for students with this type of auditory processing deficit.

Rupp et al. (1977) indicated that the presence of noise as a background factor in the majority of listening environments in our society cannot be disregarded. These authors drew several interesting conclusions in a recent research study of speech discrimination norms in different noise environments. General findings were as follows: White noise is less disabling than speech-spectrum noise; speechlike noise is more disabling than white noise or trafficlike noise; spatially separated noise is less disabling than speech mixed with noise from the same soundfield speaker; the greater the intensity of the noise, the more disabling are its effects; and individual performance variability increases as noise level increases. Rupp advocates that routine measurement of discrimination efficiency in some kind of noise environment become standard practice in current basic audiologic assessments.

In 1978 Downs and Crum reported on a study of processing demands during auditory learning under degraded listening conditions. Downs and Crum reported the following:

> Previous research has demonstrated that prolonged listening in the presence of background noise can produce delays in speech and language development, as well as deficits in speech perception and educational achievement. Specifically, learning difficulties have been attributed to reduced speech intelligibility in adverse listening conditions. However, the current results indicate that other factors also are involved. Although all speech signals were highly intelligible, processing demands during auditory learning were significantly greater under competition than under quiet conditions. This difference was reflected in the ease with which the learning task was performed....
>
> ... This result is an indication that noise present in home or educational environments may produce deleterious effects on learning performance of children. Increased effort would be required to attend selectively to an auditory signal. If this effort is not expended, there will be a concomitant decrease in learning performance... Similarly, if effort is allocated, but is not adequate to fulfill attentional demands of a learning task, performance

also will falter. These two possibilities are quite reasonable with respect to noise conditions in many educational environments where signal-to-noise ratios lower than the +6 dB level used in this study have been reported (Paul, 1972; Sanders, 1965). Long reverberation times present in many classrooms (Crum, 1974; Finitzo-Hieber, 1975; Thomas, 1960; Tolk, 1972) may further increase processing demands. With the recent prevalence of open-span classrooms in our schools, further detrimental effects are likely to occur from the interaction of reverberation and noise. Because the presence of ambient noise has been shown to increase processing demands during auditory learning, greater emphasis must be focused on acoustical design of educational environments.

The present experiment also demonstrated that detrimental effects of noise were evident regardless of signal presentation level ... (and that) ... a background noise as low as 14 decibels sensation level affected processing demands. A possible explanation is that processing demands during auditory learning depend on the relationship of signal to noise, rather than absolute noise level. Thus, it can be proposed that no listener (normal-hearing or hearing-impaired) is immune from deleterious effects of noise on auditory learning.

... Because the present study indicated increased processing demands for normal-hearing subjects listening in a background of competing speech, one may speculate that processing demands may be greater in noisy situations for a person with an auditory perceptual disorder. (Pp. 711–712)

Auditory memory: The ability to remember what a person has heard is likely the most significant factor in the auditory processing chain of events. There are basically three types of memory functions, namely, short-term memory, long-term memory, and sequential memory skills. There are many references to the concept of short-term memory in the literature, but there is widespread discrepancy as to the meaning of "short." Some refer to short-term memory as immediate recall lasting only a few seconds. The other end of the continuum is that short-term memory includes up to a twenty-four-hour period, a week, or even a month in duration. This writer feels that short-term memory can be subdivided into immediate recall lasting only a few seconds up to daily short-term memory skills involving auditory retention for a given day. In certain situations some children experience difficulty with immediate recall of events. In other cases immediate recall is satisfactory, but children have difficulty remembering events that occurred within a given day. Long-term memory is the ability to recall events in excess of a twenty-four-hour period. Within the concept of long-term memory there may be a subdivision of recall of events up to approximately a week in time for events in the immediate past, and those involved in the long-term past would be events recalled in excess of a week in duration. Evaluation of students with memory deficits often reveals that children experience much greater difficulty and frustration with short-term memory skills than with long-term memory deficits.

One can arbitrarily separate short-term, long-term, and sequential memory skills. In reality, however, there is constant interaction among these factors in the learning process. There is disagreement as to *how* information is stored in the cortex. There is also disagreement as to what is specifically involved in short-term, long-term, and sequential memory skills. For example, one could contend in the case of immediate recall that the information may not enter long-term storage and may not be learned, per se. One could also contend that short-term deficits involve difficulties in confusion and recalling information in a logical sequential manner and that long-term memory involves such aspects as vocabulary, semantics, language rules, and the phonetic aspects of language. However, this is only speculation, and in reality it is difficult to sort out the true implications of the parameters of short-term and long-term memory skills.

A third aspect of memory is auditory sequential memory. Simply stated, this is the ability to sequence a series of events just as one has heard and perceived them. There is often a difference in a child's ability to recall sequentially words, digits, and connected discourse, but this may be due, in part, to the type of stimulus material used. Sequential memory is essential to the development of good learning skills. Consider the child who cannot recall more than two or three events in order but who is exposed constantly to classroom instructions containing a series of several complex and detailed instructions. Obviously the child may be easily frustrated, may misunderstand, and may recall little from these instructions. Auditory sequential memory skills appear to break down in a somewhat consistent manner. First a child will confuse the sequence of words within the sequence, then the child may substitute words or phrases, then the child may omit words or phrases. This is followed by a combination of these factors. In severe cases, the law of recency comes into effect, and the child can remember only the last word or two of an entire sequence of sentences or instructions. Fortunately in many cases, with time, effort, and skill, auditory memory can be increased and can be developed.

Auditory Closure: This skill may be defined as the ability to synthesize phonemes into a meaningful word. Mencher (1974) has defined closure as the ability to complete the missing parts of the message. He indicates that

> Good auditory closure is necessary for the development of the appropriate phonetic skills required in sound blending and is thus closely tied to the child's ability to read, spell, speak, and write. Though we may not hear every sound or every word, auditory closure enables us to correctly analyze the signal and fill in when a portion of the message is not heard or perceived. When closure is not feasible, large gaps remain in words, concepts do not form, nor do ideas become integrated. Because of the inability to grasp situations readily, there is no clear picture of the sound environment. Sequencing of events becomes extremely difficult. Imagery is either distorted or impossible to achieve, and relationships between concepts are usually irrational and nonexistent. Original or unfamiliar speech becomes less fluent and more hesitant, and it becomes more difficult to use society's language as a medium for thought. Indeed, thought becomes confused, and it does not take long for the child to become conditioned to the fact that it is best not to offer any of his own ideas. Soon he learns that it is even better not to listen. (P. 979)

Richardson (1977) defines auditory closure as

> ... a means of decoding the sets of impulses that represent the entity in the environment. At best, the relationship between the impulses and the stimuli is only partial. Some stimuli are lost in the transmission through the environment, and some are lost in the transduction in the cochlea, and some are lost enroute to the high centers of the brain. Such disturbances as faulty or distorted sound production, stimulus obliteration by loud noise and shifts of listener attention may cause gaps in the sequences of impulses that are available for decoding, yet meaning can be achieved through the process of closure. This process is possible because of the manner in which objects are perceived: immediately, without analysis and as a whole. The neurological basis for the perception of a whole is not yet entirely understood. (p. 285)

This listing of auditory processes includes the major problems involved in the totality of processing language through the auditory system. Obviously these factors are interrelated, overlapping, and associated with complex neurology and functioning of the cerebral cortex, which is still very much a mystery—and a miracle!

Incidence of Auditory Processing Problems

A Cry for Help

The incidence of auditory processing problems varies considerably, depending upon the definition, severity level, and one's viewpoint. Incidence figures for auditory processing problems range from fewer than 2 percent to upwards of 20 percent. The percentage varies considerably with the degree of significance of a given problem or combination of processing problems. This writer believes that approximately 5 percent of the elementary student population has significant difficulty with one or more aspects of auditory processing. If one were to evaluate a large number of learning disabled students in classes for learning disabilities at all grade levels, one would likely find at least half of this population with significant difficulty with one or more aspects of auditory processing. Likewise, auditory processing deficits may contribute to and/or coexist with other types of handicapping conditions such as retardation, deafness, and visual impairment.

Classroom teachers, special class teachers, and various professional disciplines are referring more students from the mainstream of education for evaluation and possible assistance with auditory processing than in the past. As more of these professionals become even more cognizant of the impact of auditory processing difficulties and what can be done to help students overcome these problems, help will be sought for these students with increasing regularity. Consequently, speech-language pathologists need to be prepared to serve an increasing number of students with auditory processing problems.

In addition to seeking general input on student referral forms, such as a hearing evaluation, vision evaluation, speech and language evaluation, and psychological evaluation, many school systems and educational agencies are also asking for a description of the present concerns. When one reviews these written comments, it is apparent that teachers and support personnel are often aware of a student's processing difficulties. For example, the following are some comments written on referrals. A psychologist referring a child noted, "severe depression of verbal functioning suggests possible language and/or auditory processing problems." A classroom teacher noted, "This child is very distractable and inattentive. Because of this, completing assignments seems to be a difficult task for him. This is interfering with his progress in all areas of curriculum. He is more capable than his progress shows." Another teacher wrote, "John appears to hear okay in quiet but has great difficulty concentrating in a noisy environment. Please give him a thorough auditory evaluation." A mother requested that her daughter be checked for auditory discrimination as she often misunderstood what the parents said. A speech-language pathologist referred a child and noted that the language deficit suggested the possibility of significant auditory processing problems. Another child was referred by a psychologist with the indication that the psychological assessment indicated possible auditory processing problems. A classroom teacher noted the child's short attention span, distractability, and inability to remember short, simple instructions and requested an auditory perceptual evaluation. The list of comments could continue on and on. Three years ago there was only an occasional request for a processing evaluation. Currently referrals are increasing daily. The speech-language and audiology profession provides a significant service evaluating these perceived needs and serving students with identified auditory processing problems in an effort to help them reach their communication potential.

Vital Objectives: Approximately five years ago when this writer began to assume responsibility for the evaluation of auditory processing problems, several goals and objectives were developed. These goals and objectives included reviewing the majority of auditory perceptual tests available at that time, selecting or developing a recommended auditory processing diagnostic test battery, developing and standardizing a checklist of auditory problems to use as input from referents, preparing lists of available auditory processing materials, and providing in-service for classroom teachers, special teachers, and other professional staff. Initially the task appeared to be an easy one: Simply buy all the tests on the market, examine and evaluate them, and select the one or ones that were best suited to meet the perceived needs. Purchasing the tests was the only easy aspect. Approximately twenty different instruments were reviewed, each designed for evaluating one or more aspects of auditory processing. To evaluate these instruments, the writer developed a common form with the following items:

Title:
Author:
Ages and/or grades:
Function(s) tested:
Method of stimulation:
Skills involved:
Norms:
Time to test:
Description of the test:

The analysis of these instruments was very revealing. For example, it was learned that there are very few true auditory tests on the market, since most of them involve not only auditory skills but also visual, cognitive, motor, and verbal skills. Consequently, with many instruments one evaluates more than auditory processing, and what the focus is on is questionable. It was also learned that many of the discrimination tests on the market involve discrimination in quiet and do not evaluate discrimination function in the presence of competing sound(s). Most of the commercial tests on auditory processing evaluate only one or two aspects of processing and only a few, such as the battery recommended by Willeford (1977), and the Goldman, Fristoe, Woodcock Diagnostic Auditory Test Battery (1974), evaluate a wide range of auditory skills. Many of the tests take considerable time to administer, some involving as much as three or four hours. The norms available on many of the tests are very limited, especially with a wide range of children. This review was discouraging! At first it seemed like an easy task to develop an auditory processing battery rather than use commercial tests that were currently available. This also proved to be a difficult task.

FISHER'S AUDITORY PROBLEMS CHECKLIST

Development

As increasing requests for auditory processing evaluations were made, it became evident that it would be beneficial to collect information about the perceived problem or problems from the referring source. Whenever an auditory processing evaluation is being considered, there is a need to obtain pertinent information about the student's processing skills. A review of the literature revealed that a simple checklist of auditory problems could not be located. Recently, Grispino (1979) reported on the development of a twenty-nine item Language and Auditory Perceptual Checklist. However, normative data is not available for this checklist.

The following criteria were planned when the concept of a checklist was originated: The checklist should include problems related to all major components of auditory processing; contain simple, straightforward language; be quickly and easily administered and scored; be normed on students in kindergarten through sixth grade; discriminate between students with "normal" processing skills and those who may have significant problems; and, be used to obtain information from classroom teachers, speech-language pathologists, and other professionals, as well as parents. The checklist should be useful as a screening instrument.

After the initial planning stages, a number of auditory processing models were reviewed. The purpose of this review was to study and select the most important components from the various processing models for inclusion in the checklist. It was determined that the following components should be included: acuity, attention, attention span, discrimination, short-term memory, long-term memory, sequential memory, comprehension, speech and language problems, auditory-visual integration, motivation, and performance. A list of twenty-five simple descriptive items was selected for the checklist. The items for each of the components are as follows:

Acuity:
1. Has a history of hearing loss.
2. Has a history of ear infection(s).

Attention:
- 3. Does not pay attention (listen) to instruction 50 percent or more of the time.
- 4. Does not listen carefully to directions—often necessary to repeat instructions.
- 5. Says "Huh?" and "What?" at least five or more times per day.

Attention Span:
- 6. Cannot attend to auditory stimuli for more than a few seconds.
- 7. Has a short attention span.
- 8. Daydreams—attention drifts—not with it at times.

Figure-Ground:
- 9. Is easily distracted by background sound(s).

Discrimination:
- 10. Has difficulty with phonics.
- 11. Experiences problems with sound discrimination.

Short-term Memory:
- 12. Forgets what is said in a few minutes.
- 13. Does not remember simple routine things from day to day.

Long-term Memory:
- 14. Displays problems recalling what was heard last week, month, year.

Sequential Memory:
- 15. Has trouble recalling a sequence that has been heard.
- 16. Experiences difficulty following auditory directions.

Comprehension:
- 17. Frequently misunderstands what is said.
- 18. Does not comprehend many words—verbal concepts for age/grade level.
- 19. Learns poorly through the auditory channel.

Speech and Language Problems:
- 20. Has a language problem (morphology, syntax, vocabulary, phonology).
- 21. Has an articulation (phonology) problem.

Auditory-Visual Integration:
  22. Cannot always relate what is heard to what is seen.

Motivation:
  23. Lacks motivation to learn.

Performance:
  24. Displays slow or delayed response to verbal stimuli.
  25. Demonstrates below average performance in one or more academic area(s).

As can be seen, each item was described in a phrase or a short, simple sentence. It was apparent that there was overlap in some of the items, and some of the items could appear under two or more headings. The twenty-five items were written, and input was obtained from various professionals. After a trial administration period the items were rewritten, regrouped, and the entire scale was redesigned. The final checklist contains twenty-five items pertaining to what is believed to be a combination of all the major components of auditory processing. Each item was assigned a value of 4 percent. Identifying information contains only the student's name, district and building, date, grade, and the name and position of the observer. The observer is simply instructed to place a checkmark before each item that is considered to be a suspected problem. After checking the items, one simply counts the items not checked and multiplies by four to obtain the total percentage. A student with no observed processing problems would obtain a perfect score of 100 percent. As developed, the checklist takes less than two minutes per child to complete. The checklist is shown in Figure 11-2.

A plan was devised to develop normative data on forty students (twenty boys and twenty girls) at each grade level from kindergarten through sixth grade. The 280 students in this study were selected at random from four different rural and urban school districts varying in population. In addition to this normative data the checklist has been normed on forty students who were referred for a hearing acuity test but upon examination were found to have normal hearing acuity. Participating classroom teachers were given a brief presentation on the purpose of the checklist and were given simple instructions for completing the checklist. The data were

FISHER'S AUDITORY PROBLEMS CHECKLIST

Student's Name _____ District/Building _____

Date _____ Grade _____ Observer _____ Position _____

Please place a check mark before each item that is considered to be a concern by the observer:

_____ 1. Has a history of hearing loss.
_____ 2. Has a history of ear infection(s).
_____ 3. Does not pay attention (listen) to instruction 50% of the time.
_____ 4. Does not listen carefully to directions—often necessary to repeat instructions.
_____ 5. Says "Huh?" and "What?" at least five or more times per day.
_____ 6. Cannot attend to auditory stimuli for more than a few seconds.
_____ 7. Has a short attention span.
(If this item is checked, also check _____ 0–2 minutes _____ 5–15 minutes
the most appropriate time frame) _____ 2–5 minutes _____ 15–30 minutes
_____ 8. Daydreams—attention drifts—not with it at times.
_____ 9. Is easily distracted by background sound(s).
_____ 10. Has difficulty with phonics.
_____ 11. Experiences problems with sound discrimination.
_____ 12. Forgets what is said in a few minutes.
_____ 13. Does not remember simple routine things from day to day.
_____ 14. Displays problems recalling what was heard last week, month, year.
_____ 15. Has difficulty recalling a sequence that has been heard.
_____ 16. Experiences difficulty following auditory directions.
_____ 17. Frequently misunderstands what is said.
_____ 18. Does not comprehend many words—verbal concepts for age/grade level.
_____ 19. Learns poorly through the auditory channel.
_____ 20. Has a language problem (morphology, syntax, vocabulary, phonology).
_____ 21. Has an articulation (phonology) problem.
_____ 22. Cannot always relate what is heard to what is seen.
_____ 23. Lacks motivation to learn.
_____ 24. Displays slow or delayed response to verbal stimuli.
_____ 25. Demonstrates below average performance in one or more academic area(s).

Scoring: Four percent credit for each numbered item *not* checked.

Number of items *not* checked _____ × 4 = _____.

Figure 11-2. Fisher's Auditory Problems Checklist.*

gathered and analyzed by computer. Preliminary results of diagnostic testing following use of the checklist suggest that the checklist is a valid instrument for obtaining information about auditory processing and has potential use as a screening instrument.

Checklist Findings

Some of the findings of the study were as follows. On an item

---

*Available from Life Products, Box 332, Bemidji, Minnesota 56601.

analysis of the twenty-five individual items, the items most frequently checked as problems by the total group as well as the group referred for hearing tests are as follows:

Total Group	Teacher Referrals	
Random Selection, Grades K–6 $N = 280$	Teacher Suspected Hearing problem(s) Grades K–6 $N = 40$	
20%	78%	Difficulty following auditory directions.
22%	70%	Short attention span.
24%	73%	Easily distracted by background sound(s).
30%	76%	Daydreams—attention drifts—not with it at times
34%	83%	Does not listen carefully to directions; it is often necessary to repeat instructions.

It is interesting to note that the five items most frequently checked by both groups are in the areas of attention, attention span, listening in the presence of background noise, and difficulty with short-term and sequential memory skills. Note that the significant increase in the percentage of times these items was checked in the figures above by the group referred for a hearing test by their teacher.

In an analysis of the total group the majority of students did relatively well and obtained a median score of 92.4 percent and a mean score of 86.8 percent. In fact, 42 percent of the total population of students had no apparent auditory problems and obtained a score of 100 percent. It is also significant to note that a number of students scored one or two standard deviations below the norms (*see* Figure 11-3).

Group	Mean % Correct
Kindergarten	92.0%
First	89.9%
Second	87.0%
Third	85.6%
Fourth	85.9%
Fifth	87.4%
Sixth	80.0%
Total Group ($N = 280$)	86.8%
Cutoff Score Suggesting Need for Further Evaluation	72.0%
One *SD* Below Group Mean	68.6%
Two *SD* Below Group Mean	50.4%

Figure 11-3. Normative data for Fisher's Auditory Problems Checklist.

In a comparison of male versus female performance, boys did poorer than girls. In fact, there were twenty more girls than boys who scored 100 percent on the checklist in the total study. However, scores that were one standard deviation or greater below the mean were similar for males and females.

In a grade analysis of the data one of the most interesting findings was discovered. One would generally expect auditory skills to improve with age, at least to a point. It is interesting to note that kindergarten students scored the highest, as a group, and sixth graders scored the lowest on the checklist. As age (grade levels) increased, scores on the checklist decreased. It was noted that students with increasingly low scores experienced difficulty with several different processing skills, and the deficit is not an isolated problem.

In addition to the normative data on students in regular classrooms, data were also collected on a group of forty kindergarten through sixth grade students who were referred for a hearing test but who had normal hearing acuity. For years we have been evaluating teacher referrals by doing an audiometric pure tone hearing test. Eighty to eighty-five percent of the students pass these hearing acuity evaluations. For years this writer has seen the looks of disbelief as classroom teachers have been told, "This child's hearing is okay!" As time continued the writer often suspected that the teacher knew the student had some difficulty with auditory processing. It now appears that classroom teachers have been selecting appropriate students for "hearing" evaluations, many of whom may have processing problems.

Classroom teachers were asked to complete Fisher's Auditory Problems Checklist on forty students they referred for suspected hearing problems. The hearing sensitivity of each student when evaluated with a pure tone audiometer was within 0 to 10 decibels at all frequencies in both ears. One of the most exciting aspects of the study was found in this group. The range of scores on Fisher's Checklist varied from a low of 12 percent to the highest score of only 80 percent. The mean for this group was only 50.5 percent compared to a mean of 92 percent for kindergarten students, 80 percent for sixth grade students, and a mean of 86.8 percent for the total group of 280 kindergarten to sixth grade students selected at random. The results strongly suggest that consideration should be given to evaluating teacher referrals in the area of auditory processing whenever a child is singled out by the classroom teacher as being a suspect with a "hearing" problem.

As a final step, a cutoff score for the checklist was established to suggest the need for an in-depth diagnostic evaluation. A chi square analysis of the data on all 320 students resulted in selecting a cutoff score of 72 percent and below as the best choice for determining the need for diagnostic testing. A cutoff score of 72 percent on the checklist would identify 11.6 percent of the total kindergarten to sixth grade population with potential auditory processing problems in more than one area of processing. This cutoff score would have selected thirty-seven of the forty students (92%) who were referred for a hearing test but who had normal hearing acuity as suspected auditory processing problem cases. Since these data have been established, the checklist has been used on a regular basis whenever an auditory processing evaluation is done. Over 92 percent of the students falling below the cutoff score of 72 percent have been determined to have one or more auditory processing problems when a diagnostic battery was used. The results of this study indicate that classroom teachers, through the use of this checklist, can effectively select students with auditory perceptual problems who are in need of an in-depth diagnostic evaluation. The checklist may be used as a screening device as well as for obtaining information from those who live and work with a child whenever an auditory processing diagnostic test is being considered.

Evaluation of Auditory Processing Problems

Auditory, language, and speech evaluations are integral aspects in the process of evaluating a child's learning problems. Fortunately we no longer expect a professional to work in isolation when evaluating children and to make judgments on the nature and severity of all of the student's communication and learning problems. In nearly every clinical and educational setting, evaluation and diagnosis are the responsibilities of an interdisciplinary team of professionals.

Each interdisciplinary team member plays a vital role in

the evaluation and diagnostic process. Each interdisciplinary professional uses her/his expertise in evaluating the total child. Speech-language pathologists and audiologists should be core members on the diagnostic team for all clinical and educational settings. Audiologists should strive to be the most knowledgeable team members in the evaluation and diagnosis of acuity and auditory processing problems. Speech-language pathologists should strive to be the most knowledgeable team members in evaluating the child's language and speech skills. The combined skills—auditory, language, and speech—are primary considerations in the evaluation process. The child's communication skills are paramount and should always be considered. However, speech-language pathologists and audiologists should not assume the total responsibility for the evaluation process except in extremely isolated situations. In doing so it is easy for the professionals to overstep their boundaries of professional knowledge and responsibility. The same thought holds true for the remediation process. Volumes have been written on the evaluation and diagnosis of auditory acuity, language disorders, and speech problems. Considerably less has been written about the evaluation of auditory processing deficits. It is interesting that in a recent ERIC (Educational Resources Information Center) search, over 100 articles were written about one aspect of visual processing and less than ten articles were discovered in the same area of auditory processing. Efforts in research in the area of auditory processing of language need to be intensified.

The element of time is important to consider. Speech-language pathologists and audiologists should take sufficient time for adequate diagnosis of problems but on the other hand should not take an excessive amount of time for this purpose. In most cases, a speech-language pathologist should be able to complete an evaluation of a child's speech and language skills in a two-hour time frame. Likewise, an audiologist should be able to complete an evaluation of a child's acuity and processing within approximately a two-hour time frame. It is recognized that there are situations where considerably more time may be necessary in the evaluation process. There are also times when professionals may take considerably less time for an evaluation. The two-hour period is only an arbitrary guideline. It sometimes appears that our profession has a tendency to overevaluate rather than underevaluate, especially in working with children on an ongoing basis. Periodic reevaluations should be completed for any child receiving assistance in an effort to determine the ongoing nature of the problem and needs of the child in keeping with the requirements of Public Law 94–142.

What tests should be included in an evaluation of auditory processing problems? This is a question with which professionals are currently struggling. Some clinics and educational programs have considered this question and have developed an evaluation design. In many clinics and educational settings at the current time audiologists and speech-language pathologists are being deluged with requests for auditory processing evaluations, and professionals are asking the question, "What test(s) should we administer?" As previously mentioned, there are a number of commercially produced auditory processing tests available at this time. Many of these tests evaluate only one aspect of processing, but others are designed for a more comprehensive evaluation.

Willeford (1974, 1975, 1976, 1977, 1978) has done extensive work in evaluating auditory processing problems of learning disabled children. He has made significant research contributions in the areas of dichotic and diotic listening tasks. Dichotic tasks involve the simultaneous presentation of different signals to both ears. Diotic tasks, on the other hand, require the listener to decipher a signal that has been combined with a different signal in one or both ears. Willeford has used an experimental battery of tests for learning disabled children. These tests involve procedures that challenge two aspects each of cortical and brain stem integrity as confirmed on adult patients with carefully defined lesions. The battery involves tests of (1) dichotically competing messages (sentences); (2) filtered CNC words; (3) a binaural-fusion technique involving the dichotic presentation of complementary portions of sharply filtered spondaic words; and (4) an alternating speech task. Norms were established for youngsters who were judged to have adequate intelligence and average health and who were performing successfully in school. More than 90 percent of the children referred with suspected central auditory problems have failed one or more of the tests in the battery. Binaural fusion is the task most often failed, and alternating speech is the task least often failed. Both tests, interestingly, are measures of auditory functions at the brain stem level. However, the data clearly suggest that these tests challenge different subcortical processes. Willeford has added a Test of Compressed Speech (Beasley, 1972) and the Synthetic−Sentence−Identification Test with Ipsilateral Competing Message (SSI−ICM) described by Jerger and Jerger (1975). The total battery provides three measures each of cortical and subcortical processes. Willeford is continuing to expand his normative data for learning disabled children. Results suggest that a complete test battery should include dichotic and diotic listening tasks.

There are at least four different approaches to evaluating auditory processing disorders. The first approach is to evaluate the specific components of auditory processing problems such as attention span, discrimination in quiet and in competing messages, and auditory memory. The second approach is to evaluate the processing problems with speech-language measures, including phonology, morphology, syntax, and semantics. The third approach to evaluation is to use a variety of academic tests to determine academic deficiencies in areas such as reading and mathematics. The fourth approach is to evaluate processing deficits with a battery of site of "lesion" tests in an effort to study where the breakdown may occur in the central nervous system. Perhaps site of dysfunction would be a more appropriate term, as children with auditory processing problems may not have a "lesion" per se. An evaluation battery based on site of dysfunction may be the most scientific approach. This is unknown, since "site of lesion" testing with patients with known lesions is still in the developmental stages but becoming more promising as site of lesion batteries become more sophisticated. This approach is also difficult because of the concept that many auditory processing disorders are associated with a dysfunction in the central nervous system, which may be intermittent, rather than a "lesion," which may cause consistent and perhaps more serious and dramatic damage.

All these approaches have merit. There is a need to evaluate the specific components of auditory processing problems described in this chapter, but the battery may also include tests from these other approaches. The selection of the individual tests or group of tests becomes the responsibility of the person(s) evaluating the child who has been referred for an auditory processing evaluation.

Components of a Diagnostic Evaluation: An auditory processing battery should consist of several components. Based on the research with the checklist of auditory processing problems, and the knowledge and experience of auditory problems, a battery consisting of the following components was developed:

1. Hearing sensitivity
2. Fisher's Auditory Problems Checklist
3. Discrimination of words and sentences in quiet and in noise
4. Short-term, long-term, and sequential memory skills
5. Attention and attention span
6. Other selected auditory and language tests

The current status of the child's hearing sensitivity is considered along with the history of previous acuity problems. In the event of the existence of a hearing loss, the implications of the loss are important and are always given due consideration.

Fisher's Auditory Problems Checklist is administered by the classroom teacher(s) and is also given to others working with the child in some cases. After the checklist is returned, the child's score is compared to the normative data, and the types of problems noted by the teacher or referent are analyzed. During the past three years of extensive use of the checklist, it has been learned that in excess of 90 percent of the children who scored below the cutoff score of 72 percent on this checklist did indeed have one or more processing problems when a comprehensive diagnostic evaluation was administered.

When administering the discrimination tests it is necessary to have a sound-treated acoustical environment and a speech audiometer. Words and sentences are administered at conversational level of 50 decibels with a zero signal-to-noise ratio. If the child scores below 75 percent on these tasks, the tasks are repeated with a +10 decibel signal-to-noise ratio. If the child scores below 85 percent on the tasks, words and sentences are administered in quiet. The test materials should be recorded, if possible. Scores of 75 percent and below in zero signal-to-noise ratio indicate some degree of difficulty in understanding. A score of 50 percent or below in a zero signal-to-noise ratio is felt to be very significant.

As previously mentioned, children frequently have excellent discrimination in quiet but have significant difficulty discriminating in noise, often scoring as low as or below 50 to 60 percent in a zero signal-to-noise ratio. One of the real problems at this time is that we do not have adequate normative data on discrimination in various types and intensity levels of noise and other competing message stimuli. The student's scores will vary, depending upon the type of stimulus material used, the type of competing message, the signal-to-noise ratio, and whether or not the material is live or recorded.

Kalikow et al. (1978) have been involved in research on the Speech Perception in Noise Test. This test may have potential value for use in such a battery. Some type of dichotic and/or diotic competing message test(s) should be used for assessing various discrimination functions.

Perhaps one of the most important questions at this time is the significance of this problem. For example, when a child fails to understand 35 percent of the words in the presence of zero signal-to-noise ratio, does this necessarily mean that the child is capable of understanding only 65 percent of what is heard in the environment under similar listening conditions? It is likely that there is such a direct relationship, but considerably more research needs to be done on this question. We need more normative data of connected discourse at different signal-to-noise ratios.

One of the major problems in the area of auditory processing is that of auditory memory skills. A combination of words and/or digits, commands, and sentences should be used in evaluating short-term and sequential memory skills. There are various measures available for this purpose. The digit span of the Wechsler Intelligence Scale for Children (1974) is a good subtest to administer. Wepman (1973) has developed a word and digit test, which may also be used. Selected tests from the Detroit Tests of Learning Aptitude (1967) or Goldman-Fristoe-Woodcock Auditory Skills Test Battery (1974) may also be used. There are a variety of other tests that may also be used for assessing auditory memory skills. In evaluating memory skills the test observations are perhaps as important as the test scores. During the memory subtest it is often easy to observe where the breakdown occurs in a child's memory pattern. For example, some children will be able to recall and sequence five commands correctly with no problem. Another child of the same age may remember the commands but may confuse them and omit some of them. Another child may remember only the first or last command. Observing the child's nonverbal expressions during this time often reveals that the child is aware of the problem, and the level of frustration is apparent. Tests used for this portion of the test battery should be primarily auditory in nature. When using a picture test, for example, one is also evaluating visual perceptual skills. It is easy to understand how a child may become easily frustrated when he or she cannot remember more than one or two commands in a given sequence yet is confronted with a continuous barrage of instructions in the classroom. It is also important to compare auditory memory skills with visual memory skills as administered by the psychologist or educational consultant to see if both areas are affected or to learn if one sensory channel is stronger than the other.

Attending behaviors are currently evaluated by subjective observation and recording of actual behaviors. Attention span can and should be measured in time in response to various auditory stimuli. Throughout the child's evaluation the examiner should make notations on the child's attending behaviors and length of attention span. Can the child attend to different types of auditory stimuli? If so, is the attention span less than thirty seconds, up to two minutes, two to five minutes, five to ten minutes, ten to twenty minutes, a half hour, or in excess of an hour? Also note whether there is variability in the child's attending skills, depending upon the type of material used, the manner in which it is presented, and whether there is any variability in the child's attention and attention span from the beginning to the end of the session. Note whether the child is distractable, fidgity, hyperactive, or hypoactive. At times it is apparent that a child's attention and attention span are excellent but there are other processing problems. Some children can attend well in a one to one quiet environment but are highly distractable in a classroom environment, and some children cannot attend to auditory stimuli for more than a few seconds even in a one to one quiet environment.

Selective Special Auditory Processing Tests

The lack of normative data for many of the tests that are currently available leaves much to be desired. Many of the tests have been normed on adults and not on children; when norms are available, they are often on small groups of children or are developed on a restricted age range. In some of the normative data, there is a chance that a single test item will make a marked difference in the child's test score and results. There will continue to be many variables in the tests and normative data designed in the future. Tests should be valid and reliable. One of the most urgent needs at this time is for better normative data. In many cases selective special tests are administered to seek additional information on one or more aspects of processing. These tests are selected from the tests that are currently available.

The following list does not include many language tests for phonology, morphology, syntax, and semantics, or educational achievement tests, many of which are also certainly appropriate evaluative instruments for aspects of auditory processing.

Alternating Speech Test, Willeford, J., 1976, Jack Willeford, 1013 Valley View Rd., Fort Collins, Colorado 80524.

Assessment of Children's Language Comprehension, Foster, R., Giddan, J., and Stark, S., 1973, Consulting Psychologists Press.

Auditory Discrimination Test, Wepman, J., 1973, Language Research Associates, Inc.

Auditory Memory Span Test, Wepman, J., and Morency, A., 1973, Language Research Associates, Inc.

Auditory Pointing Test, Fudala, J., Kunze, L., and Ross, D., 1974, Academic Therapy Publications.

Auditory Sequential Memory Test, Wepman, J., and Morency, A., 1973, Language Research Associates, Inc.

Binaural Fusion Test, Willeford, J., 1976, Jack Willeford, 1013 Valley View Rd., Fort Collins, Colorado, 80524.

Binaural-Separation Test, Willeford, J., 1976, Jack Willeford, 1013 Valley View Rd., Fort Collins, Colorado, 80524.

Boston University Speech Sound Discrimination Test, Pronovost, W., 1953, Go-Mo Products.

Composite Auditory Perceptual Test, Witkin, B., Butler, K., Hedrick, D., and Manning, C., 1973, Alameda County School Department, Hayward, California.

Compressed Speech Test, Beasley, D., 1972, D. Beasley, Memphis State University.

Detroit Tests of Learning Aptitude, Baker, H., and Leland, B., 1967, Bobbs-Merrill Company, Inc.

Differentiation of Auditory Perception Skills, Reagan, C., and Cunningham, S., 1976, Communication Skill Builders.

Filtered Speech Test-Frequency Distorted Speech, Willeford, J., 1976, Jack Willeford, 1013 Valley View Rd., Fort Collins, Colorado, 80524.

Flowers Auditory Test of Selective Attention, Experimental Edition, Flowers, A., 1975, Perceptual Learning Systems.

Flowers-Costello Test of Central Auditory Abilities, Flowers, A., Costello, M., and Small, V., 1970, Perceptual Learning Systems.

Goldman-Fristoe-Woodcock Auditory Memory Tests, Goldman, R., Fristoe, M., and Woodcock, R., 1974, American Guidance Service, Inc.

Goldman-Fristoe-Woodcock Auditory Selective Attention Test, Goldman, R., Fristoe, M., and Woodcock, R., 1976, American Guidance Service, Inc.

Goldman-Fristoe-Woodcock Sound-Symbol Tests, Goldman, R., Fristoe, M., and Woodcock, R., 1974, American Guidance Service, Inc.

Goldman-Fristoe-Woodcock Test of Auditory Discrimination, Goldman, R., Fristoe, M., and Woodcock, R., 1970, American Guidance Service, Inc.

Illinois Test of Psycholinguistic Abilities, Revised Edition, Kirk, S., McCarthy, J., and Kirk, W., 1968, University of Illinois Press.

Ipsilateral-Contralateral Competing Message Test (Male and Female Competing Sentences), Willeford, J., and Billger, J., 1980, Jack

Willeford, 1013 Valley View Rd., Fort Collins, Colorado, 80524.

Kindergarten Auditory Screening Test, Katz, J., 1971, Follett Publishing Company.

Lindamood Auditory Conceptualization Test, Lindamood, C., and Lindamood, P., 1971, Teaching Resources Corp.

Lyness Auditory Perception Test, Levels A and B, Lyness, S., 1975, Wayne County Intermediate School District, Detroit, Michigan.

Screening Test for Auditory Perception, Kimmell, G., and Wahl, J., 1969, Academic Therapy Publications.

Short Term Auditory Retrieval and Storage Test, Experimental Edition, Flowers, A., 1972, Perceptual Learning Systems.

Slingerland Screening Tests for Identifying Children with Specific Learning Disability, Slingerland, B., 1970, Educators Publishing Service, Inc.

Specific Language Disability Test, Malconesius, N., 1967, Educators Publishing Service.

Speech Perception in Noise, Kalikow, D., Stevens, K., and Elliott, L., 1977. "Development of a Test of Speech Intelligibility in Noise Using Sentence Materials with Controlled Word Predictability," *Journal of the Acoustical Society of America, 61,* 1337–1351.

Staggered Spondaic Word Test, Katz, J., 1968, Hearing and Speech Department, Menorah Medical Center, Kansas City, Missouri. Also available from AUDITEC, St. Louis, Missouri.

Synthetic-Sentence-Identification Test with Ipsilateral Competing Message, Jerger, J., and Jerger, S., 1975, AUDITEC, St. Louis, Missouri.

Test of Auditory Comprehension, Developed by Audiologic Services of Los Angeles County Schools, 1979, Foreworks.

Test for Auditory Comprehension of Language, Carrow, E., 1973, Teaching Resources Corporation.

Test of Listening Accuracy in Children, Mecham, M., Jex, L., and Jones, J., 1973, Communication Research Associates, Inc.

Test of Nonverbal Auditory Discrimination, Buktenica, N., 1975, Follett Publishing Co.

Visual Aural Digit Span Test, Koppitz, E., 1977, Grune and Stratton.

Following the completion of the diagnostic evaluation it is important to summarize the results of the tests and the observations in a diagnostic report. The report should contain specific diagnostic test result data, normative comparisons, observations on behavior during testing, results of sensitivity testing, information obtained on Fisher's Auditory Problems Checklist, discrimination scores in noise and in quiet, results of dichotic and diotic tests, results on tests of short-term and sequential memory skills, information on attention and attention span, and results of selected tests that were administered. A special section should be devoted to diagnoses, and a final aspect of the report should include general and specific recommendations for programming based upon the child's needs.

THE REMEDIATION PROCESS

Much has been written on the remediation of learning problems and specific learning disabilities. Relatively few articles, chapters, and books have been written on remediation of auditory processing problems. One reason for this is that much of what has been written about visual and auditory processing is thoroughly embedded in all of the literature. Education is deeply rooted in the concept that learning can and does occur as a result of working with the handicapped. The degree of progress is dependent on the type and amount of stimulation and severity of a given child's problem(s). Professionals in the field of communication must be committed to providing direct and/or indirect services resulting in learned change and improvement. It is envisioned that direct remediation will include efforts directed to remediate the specific auditory processing deficits and considerable effort to improve the student's language skills as a result of language therapy. We do not know if we can assist a student in overcoming a problem until we have made an effort to do so. This writer firmly believes that audiologists and speech-language pathologists should be directly involved in the remediation process of students with significant auditory processing learning disabilities. There is a great deal that is not known about the extent to which a specific problem or set of problems can be resolved through the remediation process and what is the most effective means of resolving these problems. Likewise, the remediation approach varies from problem to problem. For example, experience has shown marked improvement in the development of auditory short-term and/or sequential memory skills in some children as a result of specific work in this area. However, we may not be able to achieve the same results in improving a child's ability to discriminate in the presence of background noise. In the latter case, the most effective treatment at this time appears to be creating changes in the child's environment, thus reducing the need to do critical listening in the presence of background noise.

There is little research to prove or disprove that specific forms of remediation are or are not effective. Research on the effectiveness of given materials is difficult to evaluate in view of the need to control a number of diverse human variables. Commercial materials are often developed and marketed without research studies to support their value.

Some of those who contend that remediation is ineffective point to studies in visual perception that support their views. Controlled research studies of remediation methods and materials are certainly needed in auditory processing. The point of view this writer would emphasize is that speech-language pathologists and audiologists should make an effort to try to remediate significant auditory processing problems. This can be done by direct work with the child, use of specific methods and/or materials, and by providing consultative help for the teacher(s) and parents in an effort to help the child overcome the specific auditory processing problem(s). We will not be successful with all children but can cause significant change in some children, which makes the effort worthwhile. If an auditory processing problem is the primary cause of a language learning problem and if we can indeed make progress toward resolving that problem, we have been successful in our endeavors.

The use of medication in treatment of learning disorders has been widely discussed in the literature. There are divergent views on the use of medication with learning disabled children. These views range from no use of medication to use of medication with the majority of learning disabled children. This matter should be explored with appropriate medical authorities whenever it is felt that medication may have an effect on the child's learning style. Medication has been used effectively to reduce hyperactivity, increase attention span, and to decrease distractability when educational approaches may have resulted in failure prior to the trial of medication. Speech-language pathologists and audiologists need to work closer with physicians in considering the need for and the benefits of medication for selected children. Whenever a child is given medication to assist in the learning process, we should continue to work closely with the child's physician, parents, and school personnel in monitoring the perceived effects of the medication.

There is no question that the majority of language and learning improvement occurs as a result of direct intervention with children with specific auditory processing and learning problems. Speech-language pathologists currently provide remediation for communication disorders of learning disabled students. This is very much as it should be. However, it is important to realize that speech-language pathologists do not have total responsibility for the management of many of these learning disabled students. This responsibility rests with the resource or special teacher(s) in many cases. Unfortunately, there are far too few audiologists in the schools to serve even the needs of the hearing impaired without considering the needs of children with significant auditory processing problems. Furthermore, to date, the majority of audiologists working in the schools have been too occupied with identification and follow-up of acuity problems to become involved with diagnoses and remediation of auditory processing problems.

There are a number of general remediation principles for working with students with auditory processing problems. These remediation principles were designed for those professionals who provide direct service to the child, such as a learning disabilities teacher, resource teacher, speech-language pathologist, audiologist, and others.

General Principles for Assisting Students with Auditory Processing Problems

1. Schedule the student for some help. Auditory processing problems will likely not be resolved by themselves. If you cannot help, arrange assistance from someone else.
2. You must obtain and maintain the child's attention if learning is to occur. It is far better to break a session into short, intensive learning periods rather than continue without the student's attention. When attention is lost, stop, take a brief break, and try to regain his/her attention.
3. The student should clearly know the specific task(s) on which you are working. Adult designed activity is meaningless unless it is meaningful to the student. Ask the student to repeat the task to you to make sure it is understood.
4. Do not intentionally overload the student's auditory memory system. If a student can repeat only three digits and confuses or forgets more than two commands, do not expect him or her to understand lengthy, detailed instructions and directions.
5. Reduce competing background noise to a minimum. Remember that speech noise as a competing signal is more debilitating than any other noise.
6. Zero in on the specific deficit(s). Work on the specific deficit(s) at least 50 percent of the time the student is with you. Target specific behaviors with appropriate materials. Unfortunately, most learning disabled students spend the majority of resource time trying to catch up or keep up and little or no time working on specific deficits.
7. Daily instruction is critical. If instruction cannot be scheduled on a daily basis, reinforcement should be provided by others in the student's environment. Two one-half hour sessions a week represent only about 1 percent of a student's waking hours.
8. Choose high interest materials. Little research has been done to prove remediation value of most materials. However, specific processing problems can be minimized or resolved with direct intervention. As professionals, we should make a sincere effort to try to help the child overcome his/her problems

through direct/indirect intervention.
9. A resource model, in and of itself, is generally highly effective. The material you use may not be as important as the effects of the one-to-one relationship. The success of the resource model is felt to be due to two factors: (a) you greatly improve figure-ground relationship, and in this way can better gain and hold the child's attention, reduce auditory and visual background distractions; and (b) the one-to-one relationship provides many opportunities for positive reinforcement.

There are a number of practical suggestions for working with students with auditory processing problems, which are more specific in nature and have been designed for the classroom teacher.

Practical Suggestions for Assisting Students with Auditory Processing Problems

1. Instructions and directions should be short, simple, and repeated because the student with auditory problems may not be able to process rapid, difficult material.
2. Question the student often to check on the level of understanding of the material being presented.
3. Provide short (5 to 15 minutes), intensive periods of instruction for the student with a short attention span.
4. If the student's visual perceptual skills are good, emphasize visual learning and encourage the student to watch the speaker as the person is talking. Provide visual clues whenever possible to reinforce the spoken word.
5. Set up a reward system for developing good listening habits. Provide frequent positive reinforcement for the student for auditory efforts.
6. Sometimes a gentle touch or other reminder may be used to call the student's attention to the auditory stimulus.
7. Frequently check the student's comprehension of words used in directions and instructions.
8. Plan weekly class, group, or individual activities involving receiving and following verbal directions of varying number and complexity.
9. A student with auditory memory deficiencies might be given

attention clues—for example, a nonverbal signal for a specific student to listen carefully.
10. Ask the student to follow a series of directions, working from simple to complex.
11. Try to gain the student's full attention before you speak to him or her.
12. The student with auditory processing problems may benefit as much from preferential seating, if not more, than a student with a hearing loss. Seating the student close to the source of instruction will reduce the figure-ground problem and may improve his or her attention and attention span.
13. For students who have difficulty studying in the presence of background noise, consider some of the following suggestions:
    a. Attempt to reduce the background noise in the classroom as much as possible. Remember that speech itself as a competing stimulus causes the greatest difficulty. In critical learning activities, only one person should be speaking at a time. Low-frequency broad-band noise creates the second most critical listening environment. Whenever possible, reduce or eliminate mechanical sounds.
    b. Initiate a short (15 to 20 minute) quiet time for independent study at least once or twice a day.
    c. Locate a quiet place in the building where students may go to study.
    d. Have ear plugs and/or headsets available for students to use as desired for study periods.
    e. Purchase or build an inexpensive study carrel or partitions made with acoustical materials.
    f. Reduce competing activities during the communication process as much as possible.

Materials

During the past decade materials development for working with handicapped students has exploded. A few years ago it was difficult to find materials for working with specific problems in dealing with the handicapped. Today hundreds of different types of commercial materials for working with students who have a multitude of learning problems are available. This is also true for materials dealing with auditory processing problems. Often materials in and of themselves are not effective. It is often the time and manner in which the materials are used that produce effective results. Considerable difference will be found in the commercial materials—some materials are of little basic value, while others are of great value and have proved to be effective. It is incumbent upon the professional, therefore, to select and/or recommend specific materials that are likely to be the most effective in assisting with the remediation process when working with specific children. These materials range in price from no cost to in excess of one thousand dollars for a complete set. In 1976 Rupp developed a list of commercially available programs appropriate for remediation of auditory processing difficulties and listed the address of publishers. There are other such lists in the literature, and most special education publishing companies currently stock some materials dealing with auditory processing.

Some materials that have been found to be generally effective in working with students having auditory processing problems are as follows:

Materials for Assisting Students with Auditory Problems

1. *Auditory Training Manual*, by S.E.C.D.C.
    Approximate Cost: $7.50 plus postage
    Order from: University of Iowa Campus Stores
    Iowa Memorial Union, Room 30
    Iowa City, IA 52242

2. *Auditory Processes* by Gillet
    Approximate Cost: $3.00
    Order from: Academic Therapy Publications
    1539 Fourth Street
    San Rafael, CA 94901

3. *Activities for Developing Auditory Perception* by Behrmann
    Approximate Cost: $2.00
    Order from: Academic Therapy Publications
    1539 Fourth Street
    San Rafael, CA 94901

4. *Auditory Perception Training Program* (Auditory Memory; Auditory Motor; Figure-Ground; Discrimination and Imagery)
    Approximate Cost: $275.00
    Order from: Developmental Learning Materials
                        7440 Natchez Avenue
                        Niles, IL 60648

5. *Perceive and Respond Auditory Discrimination Program* (Volume 1, Environmental Sounds; Volume 2, Auditory Discrimination; Volume 3, Auditory Sequential Memory)
    Approximate Cost: $210.00
    Order from: Modern Education Corporation
                        P. O. Box 721
                        Tulsa, OK 74101

6. *Activities for Auditory Learning Skills*
    Approximate Cost: $4.95
    Auditory Classification and Language Sequencing
    Approximate Cost: $7.95
    Auditory Memory for Directions
    Approximate Cost: $7.95
    Auditory Memory for Sounds
    Approximate Cost: $7.95
    Order from: Milliken Publishing Company
                        1100 Research Blvd.
                        St. Louis, MO 63132

7. *Auditory Discrimination in Depth* (Selective Listening, Identifying and Classifying Speech Sounds, Tracking Speech Sounds, Spelling, Reading)
    Approximate Cost: $77.00
    Order from: Teaching Resources Corporation
                        100 Boylston Street
                        Boston, MA 02116

8. *Sound, Order, Sense, Level I*
    Approximate Cost: $24.00
    Sound, Order, Sense, Level II
    Approximate Cost: $24.00
    Order from: Follett Publishing Company
                        1010 West Washington Blvd.
                        Chicago, IL 60607

9. *Auditory Memory Training Exercises and More Auditory Memory Exercises* by Carol Smith
   Approximate Cost: $ 3.25
   Order from: Alexander Graham Bell Association
   3417 Volta Place, NW
   Washington, DC 20007

10. *Basic Practice in Listening — Games and Activities* by Lloyd Harnishfeger
    Approximate Cost: $ 4.50
    Order from: Love Publishing Company
    6635 East Villanova Place
    Denver, CO 80222

11. *Auditory Skills Curriculum*, Developed by Audiologic Services and Southwest School for the Hearing Impaired, Office of Los Angeles County Superintendent of Schools
    Approximate Cost: $30.00
    Order from: Foreworks
    7112 Teesdale Avenue — Dept. C.
    North Hollywood, CA 91605

12. *Auditory Perceptual Enhancement Program*
    Volume 1 — Auditory Memory/Chunking
       Techniques $70.00
    Volume 2 — Auditory Discrimination $95.00
    Volume 3 — Following Directions $85.00
    Volume 4 — Improving Listening Skills — Critical
       Listening and Speed Listening $45.00
    Order from: Foreworks
    7112 Teesdale Avenue — Dept. C.
    North Hollywood, CA 91605

13. *Auditory Processing Curriculum*, Donnell, G., et al.
    Approximate Cost: $20.00
    Order from: Curriculum Materials for the Hearing Impaired
    Northwestern Illinois Association
    145 Fisk Avenue
    DeKalb, IL 60115

SUMMARY

During the past decade many significant advancements have been made in the areas of learning disabilities and auditory processing, but much remains to be learned about these intriguing problems. There is no question that learning disabilities constitute a major problem in education. While the specific cause(s) may be unknown in some cases, it is generally felt that specific learning disabilities result from "global" cerebral dysfunction(s). Speech-language problems are common in learning disabled children and may or may not be the child's primary disability. Likewise, many children with significant speech and language problems do not have learning disabilities. Children with learning disabilities often exhibit many common symptoms such as failure to achieve, distractability, hyperactivity, processing problems, speech-language problems, and academic difficulties. Many different incidence figures exist, but approximately 5 percent of school-age children experience significant learning disabilities in need of remediation, whereas up to 15 percent of the population may have isolated and less disabling, but still identifiable, disabilities. There is a need for early identification, and an interdisciplinary approach is recommended in evaluating a child's difficulties. Speech-language pathologists and audiologists should be involved in evaluating the speech-language and auditory processing skills of children with suspected learning disabilities. During the past decade there has been an explosion of new programs developed for learning disabled children. Much of the impetus for this development has resulted from state and federal legislation. Program models include a continuum of services, such as consultative services, itinerant services, resources programs, special class programs, and self-contained class programs.

Auditory processing problems are often an integral part of a child's specific learning disabilities. However, processing problems may coexist with other major learning problems, such as retardation, hearing impairment, language disorders, and other learning problems. All of the abilities and skills involved in processing information received aurally are included in auditory processing. The many components of auditory processing may exist in isolation, but a child often experiences difficulty with several of these components. Attention and attention span, listening in the presence of competing messages, and short-term memory are the most significant components of auditory processing. At least 5 percent of school-age children experience significant difficulty with one or more aspects of processing. As time continues, classroom teachers and a wide variety of professional support personnel are seeking help in evaluating and serving students with auditory processing deficits.

Fisher's Auditory Problems Checklist was developed as a result of a need to obtain information about a student's processing skills from teachers, parents, and others working with the child. This instrument is not a formalized test but a checklist containing twenty-five items describing observed concerns in the various major components of processing problems. Diagnostic data on children evaluated with scores below the cutoff of 72 percent on the checklist indicate that over 90 percent experienced documented difficulty in one or more areas of processing. It is recommended that this checklist be used whenever a teacher referral is made for a hearing assessment to collect information on possible auditory processing problems. The checklist may also be used as a screening instrument to identify children who may be in need of a diagnostic evaluation.

Speech-language pathologists and audiologists should be involved in evaluating children with suspected auditory processing problems.

There is no ideal battery of tests for evaluating children with auditory processing deficits. The most sensible approach is to evaluate the specific components of auditory processing as advocated in this chapter. The test battery, however, may include tests from several of the above diagnostic evaluation approaches. As professionals, we are confronted with selecting the most appropriate test(s) for the person with suspected processing difficulties. Diagnostic testing has confirmed a wide range of auditory processing problems in existence in today's population. These problems range in complexity and severity. The group includes children who need consultative help, are identified and being served as learning disabled, children whose disorders have been identified and are being served by speech-language pathologists, and children who are being served jointly by a number of professionals representing different disciplines. There are and will continue to be children in need of programming who are not currently receiving help.

The current state of the art suggests that we have a significant start in the quest for knowledge in the areas of learning disabilities and auditory processing, but much remains to be learned. There is much we do not know about auditory processing at this time. Auditory processing problems are difficult to evaluate because of the multiplicity of variables, but we must forge ahead in our search for additional knowledge, in research, in developing better normative data, and in developing more appropriate remediation programs for the future. These significant needs challenge speech-language pathologists and audiologists to discover new methods for dealing with these problems more effectively.

STUDY ACTIVITIES

1. Visit a learning disabilities class program in the public schools.
2. Familiarize yourself with at least ten different auditory processing tests.
3. Test your own discrimination with two different competing message tests at zero signal-to-noise ratio and +10 signal-to-noise ratio.
4. Do sound-level measurements of noise levels in three public school classrooms. Take the measurements in one wooden structure without acoustical treatment, one classroom in a new facility with carpet and acoustical treatment, and one open-spaces classroom.
5. Give Fisher's Auditory Problems Checklist to a group of school-age students and compare with mean data reported on the checklist.
6. Read the article by D. W. Downs and M. A. Crum *Processing Demands During Auditory Learning Under Degraded Listening Conditions. Journal of Speech and Hearing Research, 21(4)*, 702–715, 1978.

REFERENCES

Albert, M. L. Auditory Sequencing and Left Cerebral Dominance for Language. *Neuropsychologia, 10,* 245–248, 1972.
American Speech and Hearing Association. Report of a Committee on the role of the speech-language pathologist and audiologist in learning disabilities. *Asha, 22,* 1015, 1979.
Bader et al. *Learning Disabilities—A Handbook.* Des Moines, Iowa: Iowa Association for Children with Learning Disabilities, 1976.
Baker, H. J. and Leland, D. *Detroit Tests of Learning Aptitude,* rev. ed., Indianapolis: Bobbs-Merrill Co, 1967.
Barr, D. F. *Auditory Perceptual Disorders.* Springfield: Thomas, 1976.
Beasley, D., Forman, B., and Rintleman, W. Perception of Time-Compressed CNC Monosyllables by Normal Listeners. *Journal of Auditory Research, 12,* 71–75, 1973.
Beasley, D., Schwimmer, S., and Rintleman, W. Intelligibility of Time-Compressed CNC Monosyllables. *Journal of Speech and Hearing Research, 15,* 340–350, 1972.
Berry, M. F. *Language Disorders of Children.* New York: Appleton-Century-Crofts, 1969.
Block, W. I Am a Child with "MBD." What Does That Mean to You and Me? Paper presented at Human Diversity in Education Conference, Cedar Rapids, Iowa, 1979.
Butler, K. G. Auditory processing and dysfunction. *XVIth Int. Congress of Logopedics and Phoniatrics, Interlaken, 1974.* Basel, Switzerland: Karger, 1976.
Butler, K. G. Auditory Perceptual Training. *Acta Symbolica, 3,* 123–125, 1972.
Butler, K. G. Disorders of other aspects of auditory function. In R. J. Van Hattum (Ed.), *Communication Disorders—An Introduction.* New York: Macmillan, 1980.
Clements, S. D. Minimal Brain Dysfunction in Children. U.S. Public Health Service Publication No. 1415, 1966.
Clemmens, R. L. and Glaser, K. Specific learning disabilities I. Medical Aspects. *Clinical Pediatrics, 6,* 481–486, 1967.
Crum, M. *Effects of reverberation, noise and distance upon speech intelligibility in small, classroom size acoustic enclosure.* Doctoral dissertation, Northwestern University, 1974.
Darley, F. L. (Ed.). *Evaluation of Appraised Techniques in Speech and Language Pathology.* Reading: Addison-Wesley, 1979.
Department of Health, Education, and Welfare, Assistance to states for education of handicapped children, P.L. 94-142, Procedures for Evaluating Specific Learning Disabilities. *Federal Register, 42,* 250, 65082–65085, 12–29, 1977.
Department of Health, Education, and Welfare, Education of Handicapped Children, P.L. 94-142. *Federal Register, 42,* 163, 42473–42518, 8–23, 1977.
Downs, D. W. and Crum, M. A. Processing Demands during Auditory Learning under Degraded Listening Conditions. *Journal of Speech and Hearing Research, 21,* 702–713, 1978.

Dublinske et al. Serving Children with Learning Disabilities. *Language Speech and Hearing Services in Schools, 11,* 69–70, 1980.

Eisenson, J. *Aphasia in Children.* New York: Harper and Row, 1972.

Elliott, L. L. Performance of Children Aged 9 to 17 on a Test of Speech Intelligibility in Noise Using Sentence Material with Controlled Word Predictability. *Journal of the Acoustical Society of America, 66,* 651–653, 1979.

Finitzo-Hieber, T. *The influence of reverberation and noise on the speech intelligibility of normal and hard of hearing children in classroom size listening environments.* Doctoral Dissertation, Northwestern University, 1975.

Goldman, R., Fristoe, M., and Woodcock, R. W. Goldman-Fristoe-Woodcock Auditory Skills Test Battery. Circle Pines: American Guidance Service, 1974.

Grispino, L. M. Research oriented checklists to help prove educational performance. Paper presented at American Speech Language Association Convention, Atlanta, 1979.

Healey et al. Position statement of the American Speech and Hearing Association on Learning Disabilities. *Asha, 18,* 282–290, 1976.

Hirsh, I. J. *The Measurement of Hearing.* New York: McGraw-Hill, 1952.

Jerger, J. (Ed.), *Modern Developments in Audiology.* New York: Academic Press, 1973.

Jerger, S. and Jerger, J. Clinical validity of central auditory tests. *Scandanavian Audiology, 4,* 147–163, 1975b.

Jerger, S. and Jerger, J., Extra- and Intra-axial Brainstem Auditory Disorders. *Audiology, 14,* 92–117, 1975a.

Kalikow, D. N., Stevens, K. N., and Elliott, L. L., Development of a Test of Speech Intelligibility in Noise Using Sentence Materials with Controlled Word Predictability. *Journal of the Acoustical Society of America, 61,* 1337–1351, 1977.

Katz, J. and Burge, C. Auditory Perception Training for Children with Learning Disabilities. *Menorah Medical Journal, 2,* 18–29, 1971.

Katz, J. and Illmer, R. Auditory perception in children with learning disabilities. In J. Katz (Ed.), *Handbook of Clinical Audiology.* Baltimore: Williams and Wilkins, 1972, pp. 540–563.

Katz, J. (Ed.), *Handbook of Clinical Audiology.* Baltimore: Williams and Wilkins, 1972.

Katz, J. The Effects of Conductive Hearing Loss on Auditory Function, *Asha, 20,* 879–885, 1978.

Katz, J. The SSW Test: An interim report. *Journal of Speech and Hearing Disorders, 33,* 132–146, 1968.

Keith, R. (Ed.). *Central Auditory Dysfunction.* New York: Grune and Stratton, 1977.

Kirk, S. and McCarthy, J. *Learning Disabilities Selected ACLD Papers.* Boston: Houghton Mifflin Company, 1975.

Kroth, J. *A Programmed Primer in Learning Disabilities.* Springfield: Charles Thomas (1971).

Lewis, N. Otitis Media and Linguistic Incompetence. *Archives Otolaryngologica, 102,* 387–390, 1976.

Mencher, G. T. and Stick, S. L. Auditory Perceptual Disorders: "He won't outgrow them." *Clinical Pediatrics, 13,* 977–982, 1974.

Miller, G. A., Heise, G., and Lichten, W. The Intelligibility of Speech as a Function of the Context of the Test Materials. *Journal of Experimental Psychology, 41,* 329–335, 1951.

Millichap, J. G. *Learning Disabilities and Related Disorders.* Chicago: Year Book Medical Publishers, 1977.

Paul, R. L. Referred to in J. Katz (Ed.), *Handbook of Clinical Audiology.* Baltimore: Williams and Wilkins, 1972, p. 757.

Pinheiro, M. Tests of central auditory function in children with learning disabilities. In R. Keith (Ed.), *Central Auditory Dysfunction.* New York: Grune and Stratton, 1977.

Richardson, S. O. Learning disabilities: An introduction. In S. Kirk and J. McCarthy (Eds.), *Learning Disabilities Selected ACLD Papers.* Boston: Houghton Mifflin Company, 1975.

Rupp et al. Speech Discrimination Norms for CID W-22 Word Lists in Different Noise Environments. *Journal of Michigan Speech and Hearing Association, 13,* 59–67, 1977.

Rupp, R. R. Commercially available resources for clinicians, tests appropriate for assessing auditory perception and processing, programs appropriate for remediation of auditory processing difficulties, addresses of publishers, Ann Arbor: Audiology Area, University of Michigan Medical School (1976).

Sanders, D. Noise Conditions in Normal School Classrooms. *Exceptional Children, 31,* 344–353, 1965.

Thomas, H. Architectural acoustics as a fundamental factor in the design of schools for the deaf. In A. Ewing (Ed.), *The Modern Educational Treatment of Deafness.* Manchester, England: Manchester Univ. Press, 64, 1-64/5, 1960.

Tolk, J. Acoustics, intelligibility of speech and electroacoustic systems in classrooms. In J. Katz (Ed.), *Handbook of Clinical Audiology.* Baltimore: Williams and Wilkins, 1972, p. 766.

Wechsler, D. Wechsler Intelligence Scale for Children—Revised. New York: Psychological Corporation (1974).

Weiner, G. et al. Psychological Correlates of Low Birth Weight. *Pediatrics, 35,* 434, 1965.

Wepman, J. Auditory Discrimination Test. Chicago: Language Research, 1958.

Wepman, J. Auditory Memory Span Test. Los Angeles: Western Psychological Services, 1973.

Wepman, J. Auditory-Sequential Memory Test. Los Angeles: Western Psychological Services, 1973.

Willeford, J. and Billger, J. Auditory perceptual dysfunction in learning disabled children. In J. Katz (Ed.), *Handbook of Clinical Audiology,* Chap. 34, 2nd ed. Baltimore: Williams and Wilkins, 1978.

Willeford, J. Assessing central auditory behavior in children: A test battery approach. In R. Keith (Ed.), *Central Auditory Dysfunction.* New York: Grune and Stratton, Inc., 1977.

Willeford, J., Central auditory function. In K. Donnelly (Ed.), *Communication*

Disorders: Learning Disabilities, Chap. 14. Boston: Little, in press.

Willeford, J. Central Auditory Function in Children with Learning Disabilities. *Audiology and Hearing Education,* December/January, 1975–76.

Willeford, J. Central auditory function in children with learning disabilities. Paper presented at American Speech and Hearing Association Convention, Las Vegas, 1974.

Willeford, J. Differential Diagnosis of Central Auditory Dysfunction. *Audiology: an Audio Journal for Continuing Education,* Vol. II, No. 4. New York: Grune and Stratton, Inc., 1977.

Willeford, J. Evaluation of central auditory disorders in learning disabled children. *Learning Disabilities: an Audio Journal for Continuing Education,* Vol. II, No. 2. New York: Grune and Stratton, Inc., 1978.

Willeford, J. Sentence tests of central auditory function. In J. Katz (Ed.), *Handbook of Clinical Audiology,* Chap 22, 2nd ed. Baltimore: Williams and Wilkins, 1978.

Witkin, B. R. Auditory Perception—Implications for Language Development. *Journal of Research and Development in Education, 3,* 53–79, 1969.

Zinkus, P. W. *Learning Disabilities Linked to Ear Disease,* Newsletter of National Hearing Association, 2, 1, 1979.

We, and the people at Charles C Thomas, Publisher would like to assist you with ideas for therapy. To do so, we'd like to have you send us YOUR FAVORITE DIAGNOSTIC OR THERAPY TECHNIQUE.

We will compile these and make them available through a publication. Each item selected for publication will be credited to the person submitting it. The individual submitting the suggestion will be responsible for not violating copyright laws. Previously unpublished ideas are preferred.

The four best suggestions, as judged by the editors, will receive a copy of the text and $25.00. Other material used will not be reimbursed, but submitters will be credited.

Send your suggestion with your name and professional affiliation as you would like to have it appear by June 1, 1983, to Dr. Dolores Battle or Dr. Rolland J. Van Hattum, State University College at Buffalo, 1300 Elmwood Avenue, Buffalo, New York 14222.

Do you have a motivating game (therapy oriented) you have devised that works well?

Do you have a carryover technique that has proven very successful?

Do you have a method of eliciting a sound production that is unique and successful?

Do you have suggestions for materials and techniques for assisting junior and senior high students?

What method of aiding language development or providing remediation has been successful for you?

How can group therapy be improved?

What voice therapy approach works well for you?

Any suggestions that other SLPs might find helpful are welcomed. Help others and help yourself at the same time.

AUTHOR INDEX

A

Abeson, A. 110, 111, 315
Adair, M. 316
Ainsworth, S. 109, 144, 161, 174, 512, 558
Albert, M. 619
Albritton, T. 323
Alpiner, J. 356, 442
Aller, K. 218, 220, 244
Altman, R. 320
Anderson, J. 179, 202, 220, 230, 232, 233, 243, 316
Anderson, M. 524, 558
Andrews, J. 316
Atkinson, M. 110
Augustine, L. 546, 558
Ausenheimer, B. 459, 507
Ansoff, H. 316
Aram, D. 348
Audette, R. 316

B

Backus, O. 456, 507
Bader, J. 568, 619
Baker, H. 605, 619
Baker, R. 15, 36
Baldes, R. 235, 243, 244
Balow, B. 320
Barker, K. 244
Barr, D. 575, 619
Bashir, A. 516, 560
Baskerville, R. 15, 37
Battle, D. 448
Baynes, R. 370, 442
Beasley, D. 600, 605, 619
Beasley, J. 499, 507
Benne, K. 318
Berger, K. 364, 443
Bernstein, C. 316
Berry, M. 365, 442, 575, 619

Beste, P. 218, 220, 244
Bietzel, B. 458, 507
Billger, J. 605
Bingham, D. 456, 497, 507
Black, M. 109, 147, 174
Blanchard, M. 468, 474, 481, 482, 507
Blaschke, C. 316
Block, W. 565, 619
Bloom, H. 316
Bloomer, H. 316
Boone, D. 316
Braunstein, M. 15, 36, 554, 558
Brandenberg, R. 316
Brickman, W. 109
Brooks, R. 316
Brown, C. 308
Brown, J. 244
Bruder, E. 316
Bruner, J. 109
Buck, M. 461, 507
Buktenica, N. 606
Bullock, L. 316
Burge, K. 578
Burgoon, E. 559
Burr, J. 109
Burton, T. 316
Butler, K. 575, 605, 619

C

Caccamo, J. 316
Cafaro, M. 530, 558
Calvert, D. 316
Camp, L. 559
Campbell, B. 109
Carpenter, R. 546, 558
Carrow, E. 366, 442, 606
Carter, E. 461, 507
Cegelka, P. 321
Chandler, M. 320
Clase, J. 364, 442

Clements, S. 619
Clemmens, R. 566, 619
Coaker, F. 318
Coates, N. 94, 95, 109, 442
Cofey, C. 15, 36
Coffield, W. 109
Collins, P. 347
Colucci, S. 317
Connolly, A. 320
Conway, L. 15, 37
Conway, M. 316
Coombs, P. 317
Cooper, E. 317, 357, 443
Costello, M. 605
Cramer, W. 244
Crouch, Z. 244
Crum, M. 584, 585, 619
Crystal, D. 317
Culatta, R. 244, 317
Cunningham, G. 347
Cunningham, S. 605
Curlee, R. 317

D

Dale, P. 317
Darley, F. 109, 367, 379, 411, 412, 436, 437, 442, 444, 477, 507, 619
Davis, G. 317
Davis, T. 15, 37
Dayan, M. 525, 558
Deal, R. 370, 442
Dean, S. 109
Dell, C. 372, 442
Dempsey, D. 317
DesRoches, C. 366, 442, 507
Dickey, S. 443
Diebold, J. 317
Diedrich, W. 244, 317
Diehl, C. 357, 442
DiGiammarino, F. 317
Donnell, G. 615
Dopheide, W. 357, 443
Dorwood, B. 317
Downs, M. 584, 619
Drucker, P. 317
Dublinske, S. 106, 197, 244, 251, 317, 355, 442, 450, 451, 497, 507, 620
Duguay, M. 15, 37

Dunn, K. 112
Dunn, L. 442
Dunn, M. 456, 507
Dunn, R. 112
Dyer, 317

E

Edison, T. 26
Ehren, T. 381, 390
Eisenson, J. 109, 575, 620
Elliot, L. 318, 620
Emerick, L. 318, 370, 442
Engnoth, G. 558
Erickson, R. 369, 444
Ervin, J. 458, 507
Eskenazi, C. 15, 36, 554, 559

F

Faircloth, M. 367, 442
Faircloth, S. 367, 442
Falck, V. 531, 558
Fellows, J. 558
Finitzo-Hieber, T. 585, 620
Fink, A. 318
Fisher, L. 176, 539, 558, 561, 591, 594, 596, 601, 607, 617
Flanders, N. 318
Fleisher, D. 318
Flowers, A. 605, 606
Forbes, R. 318
Foster, R. 604
Freeman, G. 144, 149, 154, 161, 167, 174, 175, 358, 443, 520, 558
Freilinger, J. 217, 218, 234, 243, 244
Freire, P. 318
Frick, J. 499, 508, 559
Fristoe, M. 367, 443, 590, 602, 605, 620
Frohreich, L. 270, 321
Fudala, J. 367, 443, 604
Furst, N. 321

G

Gallager, J. 256, 318
Garbee, F. 109, 146, 174, 442
Garrard, K. 4, 36, 95, 109, 467, 477
Garvey, J. 516, 558

Author Index

Geers, A. 318
Giddan, J. 604
Glaser, K. 566, 619
Glass, L. 519, 558
Goings, R. 243
Goldman, R. 367, 443, 590, 602, 605, 620
Goldstein, R. 320
Gordon, B. 516, 558
Grady, M. 318
Granger, C. 318
Green, M. 113
Griffin, K. 318
Grimes, J. 251, 317
Grispino, L. 591, 620
Gross, F. 457, 463, 508

H

Hahn, E. 467, 479, 481, 508
Hale, J. 270, 321
Halfond, M. 318
Hall, P. 516, 558
Hannah, E. 316
Hansen, K. 109
Harber, S. 459, 509
Harnishfeger, J. 615
Harper, B. 525, 558
Harris, B. 244
Hartman, E. 318
Hastings, J. 316
Hatten, J. 318, 370, 442
Hatton, M. 354, 366, 369, 438, 522
Havelock, R. 318
Hawthorne, P. 318
Hayes, A. 318
Healey, W. 9, 36, 106, 174, 178, 245, 254, 264, 318, 319, 322, 355, 442, 450, 451, 471, 507, 508, 560, 620
Hedrick, D. 605
Heifetz, B. 559
Heise, G. 583, 620
Helbert, C. 15, 36
Herbert, E. 442
Herbold, D. 243
Hirsh, I. 620
Hoffman, L. 91, 109
Hoffman, M. 91, 109
Holderman, J. 319, 457, 508
Holliday, A. 546, 560

Hostrop, R. 281, 285, 319
Hubbard, C. 319
Hufstedler, S. 77
Hull, R. 263, 320
Hunt, J. 76
Hutchinson, E. 322, 512, 559, 560
Hyman, M. 370, 443

I

Illmer, R. 578, 620
Irwin, J. 15, 37, 370
Irwin, R. 319, 360, 443, 450, 459, 508

J

Jahoda, G. 319
James, H. 370, 443
James, T. 109
Jeffers, J. 319
Jeffrey, R. 243
Jelinek, J. 15, 36, 554, 558, 559
Jenkinson, P. 244
Jenson, T. 109
Jerger, J. 52, 71, 600, 606, 620
Jerger, S. 600, 606, 620
Jex, L. 606
Johns, R. 110
Johnson, L. 281
Johnson, T. 319
Johnson, W. 378, 443
Johnston, H. 109
Jones, J. 606
Jones, R. 319
Jones, S. 254, 471, 508
Journot, V. 319

K

Kagan, N. 228, 244
Kakalik, J. 319
Kalikow, D. 602, 620
Kane, A. 428, 444
Karp-Nortman, D. 318
Katz, J. 578, 606, 620, 621
Kavanaugh, J. 148, 174
Keith, R. 620, 621
Kent, L. 319
Kerr, C. 274, 319

Kimmel, G. 606
King, R. 364, 443
Kirk, S. 443, 605, 620
Kirk, W. 443, 605, 620
Kirtley, D. 221, 244
Klevens, D. 319
Knight, H. 148, 174, 467, 479, 481, 508
Konon, M. 319
Koppitz, E. 607
Kroth, J. 581, 620
Krouse, W. 110
Kunze, L. 604
Kvaraceus, W. 320

L

Landry, L. 319
Lauder, C. 491, 508
Lawrence, P. 320
Lazarus, C. 316
Lee, L. 361, 366, 443
Leland, B. 605, 619
Levy, K. 513, 559
Lewis, N. 620
Lichtenberger, A. 321
Lichtin, W. 581, 583, 620
Lieberman, I. 512, 559
Lindamood, C. 606
Lindamood, P. 606
Livingston, S. 320
Lorentz, J. 320
Lorsch, J. 320
Lukens, J. 167
Lynch, L. 525, 559
Lyness, S. 606
Lyons, J. 320

M

Mackenzie, R. 320
Mackie, R. 320
MacLearie, E. 457, 463, 508
Madaus, G. 316
Mager, R. 201, 244, 532, 535, 559
Male, M. 113
Mange, C. 54, 71
Manning, C. 605
Marge, M. 521, 559

Marland, S. 320
Martin, E. 119
Maruca, F. 623
Mason, R. 373, 374, 443
McBride, J. 513, 559
McCarthy, D. 366, 443
McCarthy, J. 443
McClain, B. 442
McClean, J. 15, 36
McCoy, P. 443
McDaniels, G. 116
McDonald, E. 368, 443, 461, 499, 508, 559
McDonald, J. 368, 443
McGregor, D. 320
McKee, B. 15, 36
Mead, M. 357, 444
Mecham, M. 606
Mencher, G. 581, 587, 620
Menyuk, P. 366, 443
Meyen, E. 320
Milisen, R. 109, 110, 360, 444
Miller, G. 583, 620
Millichap, J. 565, 566, 568, 621
Molly, J. 525, 558
Morely, R. 381
Morency, A. 604
Morphet, E. 110
Mowrer, D. 15, 36, 320, 465, 490, 491, 493, 498, 508
Mullen, P. 367, 443
Muma, J. 532, 559

N

Nash, H. 76
Nation, J. 348
Neagley, R. 109
Neal, W. 369, 411, 436, 437, 438, 443, 477, 485, 508
Neidermeyer, R. 15, 36
Nelson, C. 321
Nelson, G. 320
Newman, I. 115
Nikoloff, O. 38, 46, 53, 71
Nober, H. 468, 474, 481, 482, 507
Norman, M. 112
Norris, D. 467, 508
Northcott, W. 559

O

Odiorne, G. 320
Ogden, J. 356, 442
Ogilvie, M. 109
Omans, M. 214, 244
O'Neill, J. 520, 559
O'Toole, T. 244, 320, 412, 438, 508

P

Page, J. 15, 37
Paul, R. 585, 621
Pendergast, K. 174, 443
Perkins, W. 320
Peters, L. 320
Pfeifer, R. 498, 508
Piazza, R. 115
Pickering, M. 357, 443
Pinheiro, M. 621
Powers, M. 110, 153, 175, 373, 374, 443
Prather, E. 320
Prescott, T. 316
Proffit, W. 373, 374, 443
Pronovost, W. 376, 444, 605
Putnam, J. 321

Q

Quay, H. 320

R

Reagan, C. 605
Rees, N. 169, 175, 512, 559
Reller, T. 110
Reynolds, M. 264, 321
Rice, V. 444
Richardson, S. 587, 621
Rieke, J. 525, 559
Riley, D. 76
Rintleman, W. 619
Roberts, C. 321
Robertson, J. 321
Robertson, M. 149, 175
Roe, V. 360, 444
Rogers, C. 59, 71
Rogin, C. 318
Rosenshine, B. 321

Ross, D. 604
Rossmiller, R. 270, 321
Rupp, R. 582, 584, 621
Ruth, B. 321
Ruebhausen, O. 321
Rutenberg, W. 559

S

Sanders, D. 512, 559, 585, 621
Scalero, A. 15, 36, 554, 559
Schalk, M. 321
Schrag, J. 113
Schubert, G. 321
Schutz, R. 15, 36
Schwimmer, S. 619
Seaton, J. 554, 559
Seider, R. 443
Selmar, J. 443
Seltzer, H. 244
Shankweiler, D. 559
Shelton, R. 320
Sheretz, D. 316
Shores, R. 321
Shriberg, L. 321
Siegel, M. 381
Simon, C. 514, 559
Slingerland, B. 606
Smith, C. 615
Smith, E. 110
Soder, A. 443
Sokolof, M. 498, 509
Soltman, S. 525, 559
Sommers, R. 354, 357, 366, 368, 369, 374, 375, 380, 428, 444, 461, 498, 509, 522, 527, 529, 533, 546, 549, 559, 560
Stark, J. 169, 175, 604
Steck, E. 321
Stem, M. 113
Stevens, E. 560
Stick, S. 620
Stinnet, L. 357, 442
Stinnet, W. 559
Stinson, J. 321
Stormer, J. 318
Strickland, R. 515, 560
Strominger, A. 516, 560
Strong, B. 554, 560
Studebaker, G. 320

Sudderth, J. 442
Surles, R. 318

T

Templin, M. 367, 444
Thomas, H. 585, 621
Thompson, R. 321
Toffler, A. 322
Tolk, J. 585, 621
Tomblin, J. 516, 558
Torres, S. 115
Torter, R. 319
Townsend, R. 322
Trent, R. 244
Trudeau, E. 322
Tufts, L. 546, 560

V

Van Dusseldorp, R. 322
Van Hattum, R. 3, 4, 8, 12, 14, 15, 31, 36, 37, 38, 110, 348, 358, 365, 444, 448, 455, 456, 508, 530, 554, 559, 560, 619
Van Riper, C. 322, 361, 368, 370, 444
Vegley, A. 318
Venezky, R. 148, 175
Volkmer, C. 113
Volz, H. 319

W

Wahl, J. 606
Ward, L. 322
Weaver, J. 464, 509
Webster, E. 322, 542, 560

Werfelman, J. 559
Wechsler, D. 602, 621
Weiner, G. 621
Wepman, J. 578, 602, 604, 621
Wertz, R. 357, 444
Weston, A. 15, 37, 459, 508
Wheeler, G. 243
Whelan, R. 316
White, O. 322
White, R. 322
Whitehead, R. 367, 443
Wiedner, W. 457, 508
Wiggins, E. 317
Wiggins, J. 356, 442
Willey, N. 110
Williams, H. 320
Williams, S. 110
Willeford, J. 590, 599, 604, 605, 621, 622
Wilson, F. 370, 371, 444, 460, 509
Wilson, K. 244, 524, 560
Wing, D. 322
Witkin, B. 575, 605, 622
Witt, B. 525, 558
Wollersheim, J. 464, 509
Wood, K. 71
Woodcock, R. 590, 602, 605, 620
Work, R. 269, 322, 462, 476, 509, 510, 535, 559, 560

Z

Zani, W. 322
Zaslow, E. 412, 438, 508
Zemmol, S. 376, 444
Zettel, J. 110, 111
Zinkus, P. 577, 622
2600

SUBJECT INDEX

A

Activities
    for auditory learning skills 614
    for developing auditory perception 613
Accountability 197–202, 214, 241, 247, 291, 297, 313, 323, 334, 337, 469, 510
Administration 64, 75, 177, 182, 323, 325, 339
    consultation 148, 151–155, 378, 471, 542
    contracts 213
    cooperation 93, 179, 553
    establishing relationships 11, 14, 42
    informing 337, 494–495
    planning 12, 184, 250
    role 85–89, 181
    scheduling 456, 466, 473–489
Agencies 12, 30–31, 40, 102, 171, 172, 555–556
Aides (*see* Supportive personnel)
Alternating Speech Test 604
American Association for Children with Learning Disabilities 561
American Speech-Language-Hearing Association 7, 10, 29, 32, 39, 44, 96, 97, 107, 129–131, 147–148, 153, 161, 177, 190, 220, 225, 246–247, 254, 265, 270, 289, 298, 299, 302, 308, 338, 345, 355, 357, 360, 364, 373, 374, 411, 412, 413, 461, 486–487, 536, 542, 569–570
    Certificate of Clinical Competence 33, 44, 178, 235
    Code of Ethics 39–45
    conventions 33, 536
    membership 34–35
    national study 411–412, 436
    publications 33
    planning 246, 254, 289, 299
    Standards for Effective Oral Communication Programs 129–131
Articulation 14, 47, 48, 218, 366–369, 374, 376–377, 383–384, 390–392, 394–395, 408, 418–426, 458, 459, 489, 515, 526, 546, 549, 551, 583
Assessment of Children's Language Comprehension 604
Audiology 3, 8, 10, 39, 43, 75, 98, 176, 177, 178, 181, 182, 198, 216, 217, 220, 221, 229, 230, 231, 232–237, 265, 287, 326, 331, 417, 513, 561, 574, 575, 598–599
Auditory Discrimination in Depth 614
Auditory Discrimination Test 578, 604
Auditory Memory Span Test 604
Auditory Memory Training Exercises and More Auditory Memory Exercises 615
Auditory Perception Training Program 614
Auditory Perceptual Enhancement Program 615
Auditory Pointing Test 604
Auditory processes 613
Auditory processing 561
    disorders 4, 574–613
Auditory Processing Curriculum 615
Auditory Sequential Memory Test 604
Auditory Skills Curriculum 615
Auditory Training Manual 613

B

Basic Practice in Listening-Games and Activities 615
Behaviorally different 4, 14, 99, 271, 426, 427, 451
BiCycle Evaluation System 308–313
Bilingual population 518–520
Bill of Rights for Children and Their Communication Skills 5
Binaural Fusion Test 604
Binaural Separation Test 604
Block system 431, 454–465
Boards of Education 9, 75, 76, 83, 181, 182, 206, 208, 210, 294, 339
    consultation 151, 337, 542

function 75
Booklets, informational 67, 68
Boston University Speech Sound Discrimination Test 605
Broward County Schools 381, 390–411, 462
Budget 13, 185, 211–215, 220, 256, 269, 281, 283, 339

C

Carry-over 162–164, 166, 471, 549–550
Carter-Buck Articulation Test 461
Case finding 156–157, 354–365
Case history 55, 157, 168, 326, 327–330, 349–351, 523, 573
Case load 7, 11, 64, 149, 155, 268, 324, 367, 411–440, 450, 474, 477, 510
 composition 418–429
 determinants 11
 national study 418–429
Case selection 218, 365–411
Central tendency 47–48
Cerebral palsy 43, 58, 99, 269, 380, 521, 535
Certification 436
 Certificate of Clinical Competence 33, 178
 State 11, 33
Character 20–27
Child 23, 154, 159, 176, 229, 378
 ethical relationships 42
Child Services Review System 298–308
Classroom teacher 6, 14, 39, 66, 75, 88, 216, 340
 as supportive personnel 93, 165, 357–358, 554
 carry over 163–164
 consultation 148, 150, 155–160, 177, 358, 500, 519
 cooperation 98
 influence in case selection 365
 establishing relationships 11, 21, 43
 prevention 161–162
 referral 156, 358, 361, 370
 role 12, 89–91, 364, 365, 375, 492, 553, 554
 scheduling 90, 456, 457, 464, 466
 special education 166–167
 training 357–358
 understanding the program 165–166

Cleft palate 43, 58, 203, 380, 426, 521, 555
Clinician (*see* Speech-language pathologist)
College (*see* University)
Combined scheduling 462–465
Committee on the Handicapped 10
Communication
 development 160–162, 264
 deviations 162–164, 264, 364
 disorders 19, 164–165, 376–377, 418–426
 importance 3, 15
 in schools 338–346
Community
 agencies 30–31. 171, 172
 clubs 30, 171, 172
Composite Auditory Perceptual Test 605
Compressed Speech Test 605
Comprehensive Assessment and Service Evaluation System for Language, Speech and Hearing Programs 96–97, 107, 120–128, 270
Computers 296–297
Confidentiality 29, 231, 335, 355
Consultation 144–173, 378
 in the schools 144, 149–171, 267, 469–470
 nature of 144–146
 requisites 146
 to the community 171–173
 with teachers 500, 516, 517
Contracts 206–210, 494
Continuing education 28, 205
Coordination activities (*see* Office time)
Correlation 49–50
Council for Exceptional Children 32, 97
Counseling 38, 39, 53–70, 165, 169
 avoidance 57
 child 57–58
 emotional adjustment 54
 information sharing 67–68
 parents 63–70, 542
 public school setting 55–56
 secondary symptoms 57–58
 speech-language pathologist 56
 withdrawal and hostility 58–59
Counseling techniques
 catharsis 60–61, 67
 discussion 61
 non-directive 59–60
 role playing 61–63, 68
County schools (*see* Intermediate unit)

Subject Index

Cumulative record 333, 334-335, 352-353

D

Delphi Technique 277-280
Dental specialists 21, 44, 173, 373, 374, 555
Detroit Test of Learning Aptitudes 602, 605
Development 146, 160-162, 171, 177, 264, 329, 375, 376, 395, 516, 525
Developmental Sentence Analysis 366
Diagnosis 12, 14, 148, 255, 267, 288, 325, 326, 327, 330, 365-374, 469-470
Dialectally different 520
Differentiation of Auditory Perception Skills 605
Directors of Special Education 84, 179, 294
    consultation 151-152, 216
    planning 248, 542
    supervision 181
Dismissal 24, 326, 331-332, 549, 551-552
Dispersion, measures of 48-49

E

Education
    and communication disorders 147-148
    and public schools 74
    and the speech-language pathologist 152-155, 512, 513
    commitment to 73-74
    the local district 74-76
Educational team (*see* Team approach)
Educational Amendment of 1974 (Public Law 93-380) 355
Education of All Handicapped Children Act (Public Law 94-142) 4, 72, 77, 78, 80, 81, 90, 92, 95, 107, 110-111, 180, 188, 212, 215, 216, 245, 246, 249, 289, 324, 333-334, 343, 355, 364, 365, 374, 438, 449-453, 455, 460, 466, 467-470, 472, 473, 481, 482, 497, 512, 514, 531, 532, 542, 562
Emotionally disturbed (*see* Behaviorally different)
Equipment and materials 12, 13, 535-547
    budget 538
Ethical practice 8, 38, 39-45
    confidentiality 39-40
    coworkers 42-43
    guarantees 41
    outside employment 45

    parental permission 40
    parents 41-42
    private practice 44
    treatment by correspondence or telephone 41
Evaluation 157-158, 247, 251, 522-524
    auditory processing 597-607
    learning disabilities 572-574
    personnel 176, 224, 230-232
    program 176, 245-248, 287, 297-314
Exceptional children 6, 34, 83, 96, 145, 166-167, 216, 270, 380, 450, 510

F

Facilities 12, 540-542
    ASHA report 543-544
    availability 482-484
    importance for therapy 12
Federal government 185, 215, 284, 288, 312, 473-475
    and education 76-78, 79, 116-119
Filtered Speech Test-Frequency Distorted Speech 605
Fisher's Auditory Problems Checklist 591-597
Florida Language Screening System 512
Flowers Auditory Test of Selective Attention 605
Flowers-Costello Test of Central Auditory Abilities 605
Fluency 384-385, 392, 395, 408-409, 515, 526-527, 551-552 (*see also* Stuttering)

G

Games 27, 536-537
Goals 182, 199-201, 248, 257-259, 276
Goldman-Fristoe Test of Articulation 367
Goldman-Fristoe-Woodcock Auditory Memory Tests 605
Goldman-Fristoe-Woodcock Sounds-Symbols Tests 605
Goldman-Fristoe-Woodcock Test of Auditory Discrimination 605
Group sessions 26, 219, 529
Group therapy 150, 474
    scheduling 429, 431, 432, 435, 438, 439, 497-499, 512, 528-529

H

Hearing 17, 198, 214, 377, 380, 426, 427, 520–521, 578
Historical perspectives
  forward 13–18
  past 6–8
  present 8–13

I

Identification (*see* Case finding)
Illinois Test of Psycholinguistic Abilities 366
Individualized Education Plan (IEP) 87, 89, 91, 98–107, 111–115, 132–143, 145, 218, 246, 326, 327, 330–331, 333–334, 451, 452–453, 467, 471, 477, 488, 531–533
Individual sessions 26, 219, 429–430, 432, 435, 438, 515, 520–531
In-service training 165, 180, 183, 217, 218, 339, 340, 342–344, 357, 472, 476
  time for 217, 378, 472
Intensive system 455–467, 502–504
Intermediate units 83, 84–85, 181, 221
Intermittant system 431, 455–467, 501–504
Interpretation 158–160, 165–166
Ipsilateral-Contralateral Competing Message Test 605

J

Job descriptions 207, 230, 241
  speech-language pathologist 190–193
  supervisor, educational audiology 193–197
  supervisor, speech and hearing 186–190

K

Kindergarten Auditory Screening Test 606

L

Language 8, 9, 218, 510, 518, 572
  and case load 418–426
  and case selection 365–366, 376, 387–390, 410, 526–527
  dismissal 551
  disorders 8, 43, 169, 387, 399–403, 515
Leadership 34, 72, 176, 202–205, 221–222, 223
Learning disabilities 4, 8, 265, 521, 561–574
  and speech-language disorders 17, 571–572
Legal matters 251
Legislation 9, 145, 251, 562
Library 540
Licensure 33, 44
Lindamood Auditory Conceptualization Test 606
Local Education Agency (LEA) 83–84, 178, 180, 181, 206, 215, 246, 249
Local school district (*see* Local Education Agency)
Lyness Auditory Perception Test 606

M

MacDonald Deep Test
  screening 461
Management
  of program 245–248, 275–297, 313, 314
Management-by-Objectives 276–277
Management Information System 287–292, 293
Materials
  for screening 360–361
Maturation 14, 15
Mean Length of Utterance 366
Media 40, 50, 344–345
Medical specialists 7, 9, 19, 21, 39, 98, 148, 173, 284, 330, 365, 371, 524, 555–556, 574
Membership 34
Mentally retarded 4, 14, 99, 147, 171, 271, 428, 451, 460, 461, 521
Menyuk Sentence Repetition Task 366
Metropolitan Readiness Test 512
Modification of the Frontal Lisp 15
Montgomery County Intermediate Unit 381–390, 407–411
Multiply handicapped 22, 25

N

Negotiations 208–210, 241
National Education Association 73, 77
N.D.E.A. Act of 1958 76
New York State Education Department 10

Subject Index

Nonverbal communication (see Nonvocal communication)
Nonvocal communication 21, 403-408, 518
Northwestern Syntax Test 366
Number of schools served 476-477
Nurse 11, 43, 93, 148, 216

O

Objectives 201, 259-262
Occupational therapist 173, 216
Office time 473, 481-482
One person research 52
Operant therapy 432, 434, 435, 447, 459-460
Organizations 31-32, 34
Other school personnel
    consultation 167-168
    interaction 215-216

P

Paired Associates 15, 459-460
Parents 11, 23, 24, 41-42, 147, 171, 313, 329, 337, 340, 380, 485
    counseling 12, 29, 54, 63-69, 157, 378, 429, 439, 542, 544-547
    IEP 103-104, 132-134
    member of team 91-93
    parent groups 53, 65, 171, 343-344
    permissions 40, 365
    personal contacts 63, 472
    questionnaire 349-351
    role 69-70, 370, 546
Peabody Picture Vocabulary Test 366
Perceive and Respond Auditory Discrimination Program 614
Personnel policies 75
Personality and character 20-30, 205
Photo Articulation Test 367
Phonemic Approximation 15
Physically disabled 4, 147, 271, 451
Physical therapists 148, 173, 216
Physicians (see Medical specialists)
Planning
    program 10, 12, 27, 183, 184-185, 197-202, 204, 223, 245-275, 313-314
    staff involvement 184-185
Planning-Programming-Budgeting System 281-283

Political action 208, 210-211, 251
Predictive Screening Test of Articulation 369
Preschool 405-407, 515-516
Prevention 9, 12, 14, 160-162, 177
Principal 24, 75, 335, 343, 363
    consultation 152-155, 216, 337, 358, 362
    role 87-88, 553
Private practice 44
Profession 6-8, 21, 146-147
Professional, the (see Speech-language pathologist)
Professional relationships 19-20, 41-44
Profoundly handicapped 517-518
Program manual 13, 182, 183
Program philosophy 13, 511, 513-514
Program Planning-Evaluation 199-200
Prognostic testing 368-369
Psychologists 7, 11, 39, 43, 54, 55, 75, 93, 98, 148, 216, 284, 330, 365, 490, 553, 554-555, 574
    consultation 167-168
    cooperation 513
    mutual understanding 43
Publications
    American Speech-Language-Hearing Association 33
Public Law 94-142 (see Education of All Handicapped Children Act)
Public relations 11, 12, 64, 218
    and scheduling 473, 488-489
Pupil personnel files (see Cumulative record)

R

Reading 73, 148, 166, 361, 512, 516, 517
    specialists 17, 167, 169-170, 553
Recordings 326, 332-333
Records and reports 12, 14, 323-340
    content 326-333
    coordination with cumulative records 334-335
    cumulative speech-language-hearing record 333, 352-353
    documentation 324-326, 336-337
    purpose 337-338
    storage 287, 336-337
Recruitment 205
Referrals 12, 31, 63, 284

form 328.
principal 154
responsibility of SLP 30–31, 63, 524
source 326, 327
Release form 326, 333
Reliability 50–51
Remedial program (see Therapy)
Research 8, 12, 46, 52–53, 214, 325, 546
  relating to scheduling 453–454, 497–498
  statistical methods 46–53
Rules and regulations 11, 12, 13, 21, 256, 473–475

S

Sample schedules 500–505
Scheduling 12, 147, 153, 154, 218, 375
  clinical factors 489–494
  for the day 494–500, 501–505
  for the week 467–494, 501–505
  for the year 448, 449–467, 501–505
  research 431
Scientific method 38, 45–53, 310
Screening 12, 267, 294, 355–365, 522–524
Screening Test for Auditory Perception 606
Secondary schools
  scheduling 485–487
  screening 361–365
Self rating 28–30
Sequential therapy 524–525
Severely handicapped 77, 376, 474, 516–518, 530
Severity ratings 217–220
Short Term Auditory Retrieval and Storage Test 606
"s" Indicator 17
Slingerland Screening Tests for Identifying Children with Specific Learning Disabilities 606
Social workers 43, 75, 98, 148, 365, 513, 574
  consultation 167, 168–169, 216
  mutual understanding 43
Sound, Order, Sense, Level 1 614
Special Education (see Exceptional children)
Specific Learning Disability Test 606
Specific learning disabilities (see Learning disabilities)
Speech clinician (see Speech-language pathologist)

Speech disorders 8, 43, 77, 371, 515
Speech improvement 6, 7, 161, 432
Speech Improvement System 15
Speech-language pathologists 8, 9, 10, 146–147, 170–171, 287, 413–414
  and learning disabilities 569
  as an individual 18–30
  IEP 98–103
  job description 190–193
  role 93–98, 155, 467–468
  students 232–237
Speech-language specialist (SLS) (see Speech-language pathologist)
Speech notebooks 464, 537
Speech Perception in Noise Test 602, 606
Speech scientists 3, 45
Speech therapist 9–10, 11 (see also Speech-language pathologist)
Staff meetings 12, 171, 184, 216–217
Staggered Spondaic Word Test 578, 606
Standardization 50
State
  associations 29, 32
  certification 178, 232
  commitment to education 78
  conventions 32
  laws 146, 185, 209, 256, 268, 473–475
  licensure 44
  responsibility for education 78–83
State consultant 82–83, 294
Statistical methods 46–53
  central tendency 47–48
  correlation 49–50
  measures of dispersion 48–49
  sampling 51–52
  validity, reliability, standardization 50–51
Stimulus Shift Articulation Program 5
Stuttering 203, 218, 371–372, 377, 418–426, 455
Success in therapy 547–549
Superintendent
  consultation 151
  relationships 43, 216
  role 75, 76, 85–89
Supervision 12, 176–242, 432
  personnel 220–232
  practica 232–237
  program 181–219

Subject Index

Supervisors of speech-language-hearing 75, 84–85, 88–89, 179–181, 534
    critical work activities 186–187
    job description, educational audiology 193–197
    job description, speech-language 188–190
    leadership 202–205, 223, 248
Supportive personnel 12, 14–18, 356–357, 517, 553–554
    parents 69–70
    teachers 162
SWRL Program 15–17
Synthetic-Sentence-Identification Test with Ipsilateral Competing Message 600

T

Taped Articulation Therapy 15–17
Teacher of the Speech and Hearing Handicapped 10, 11
Teachers (*see* Classroom teachers)
Team approach 72–108, 146, 148–149, 154, 162, 164, 215, 361, 365–366, 375, 470, 513, 553, 573
Templin-Darley Articulation Test 367
Testing 158, 168, 358–360, 375, 469
    validity 366
Test of Auditory Comprehension 606
Test of Auditory Comprehension of Language 366
Testing of Listening Accuracy in Children 606
Test of Nonverbal Auditory Discrimination 606
Test of Compressed Speech 600
Therapy 12, 160–165, 354, 510–557
    auditory processing disorders 607–615
    games 536–537
    length of sessions 499–500
    parameters 527–528

    parents' role 542–547
    techniques and methods 533–535
    the session 528–531
Time 14, 27, 448
    consulting 469–470, 471, 500
    counseling 471
    habilitation 471
    testing 360, 469
    travel 478–482
Tongue thrust 373
Tradition
    and scheduling 473, 475–476
Traditional therapy (*see* Van Riper therapy method)
Travel time 479–481

U

United States Department of Education 76, 78, 79, 116–119, 411, 563
United States Office of Education-Purdue University Study 411, 436–440

V

Validity 50–51
Van Riper therapy method 432, 434, 435, 447, 460
Visual Aural Digit Span Test 607
Visually impaired 4, 77, 147, 521
Voice disorders 43, 218, 369–371, 377, 385–387, 392, 395, 409, 418–426, 515, 524, 526–527, 552

W

White House Conference on Education 73–74
Workshops 340, 342–344